Functional Neuroanatomy
Organized with Reference to Networks, Lobes of the Brain, 10-20 Sites, and Brodmann Areas

Michael Thompson, M.D., & Lynda Thompson, Ph.D.

Consultants: James Thompson, Ph.D., David Hagedorn, Ph.D., Andrea Reid-Chung, M.A., C.Psych.Assoc., Tammy Binder, M.D.

This Monograph comprises one section of
The Neurofeedback Book: 2nd Edition

Table of Contents

Part 1 Introduction/Orientation 1

Illustrations:

Lateral and Midsagittal Sections: Brodmann Areas, Lobes, 10-20 sites
Lateral and Midsagittal Sections: Networks Overview
Lateral and Midsagittal Sections: Gray's Anatomy for Gyrus and Sulci Locations
Lateral and Midsagittal Sections: Brodmann's Original Drawings
Electrode Positions: Expanded 75 sites including 10 – 20 sites

General Notes:

Korbinian Brodmann: Historical Note
Preliminary Comments about the Organization of this Section
Neurofeedback Training is Guided by Brodmann Areas and Networks
Brodmann Areas Overlap
Why Use Single-Channel Training?
Why Use LORETA Z-Score NFB?
Importance of Networks
Cortex-Basal Ganglia-Thalamus: How to Activate One Network – Inhibit Others

Functional Networks and Behavior

Frontal-Subcortical Circuits 15
Go vs No-Go: Direct, Indirect, and Hyperdirect Pathways 18
Relevance of these Pathways to SMR Production 20
Central Midline Structures (CMS): An Anatomical and Functional Unit 23
Default and Salience Networks.. 24
Why Training at Central Sites Affects Networks 26
Importance of Heart Rate Variability (HRV) Training: Heart – Brain Connections 27
Cortical Connectivity - Modules, Hubs and Nodes Maximize Efficiency 29

Part 2 Functions Related to Lobes of the Brain, International 10-20 Sites, and Brodmann Areas 32

Introduction
Table: Summary of Locations of Brodmann Areas 33
Figures: Lobes, Brodmann Areas, Functions (Networks) 34
Table: Order of Description of Functions 36
Notes on Doing Neurofeedback and Heart Rate Variability Training 37

Frontal Lobe 38

Introduction - Functions Related to the Frontal Lobes
Reasoning: Deductive & Inductive
Orbital Frontal Cortex and Links to the Temporal Lobe
Fz, F3, F4; BAs 8, 9: Prefrontal Lateral and Medial Aspect – Executive Network 44
FP1, FP2; BAs 10, 11, 46 Prefrontal Lateral and Medial Aspect – Executive Network
F3 (-F7), F4 (-F8); BAs 44, 45: Prefrontal, Lateral and Medial Aspect – Executive & Affect Networks
F7, F8; BAs (38), 44, 45, 46, (47): Temporal Pole & Inferior Frontal Cortex – Executive & Affect – Social Networks 50
Paul Broca: Historical Note 51
F9, F10; BAs 11, 47, 38: Temporal Pole & Inferior Frontal Cortex – Executive & Affect – Social Networks
F9, F10; BAs 47,12, Inferior Frontal Dominant; Inferior Frontal Non-Dominant
Memory (Semantic, Working, Episodic & Hippocampal Theta)

Orbital Frontal/Inferior Frontal Cortex **56**
F9, F10, BAs 11, 12: Orbital / Inferior Frontal Cortex, - Affect Network - Emotional/Social
Phineas Gage: Historical Note
Posterior Basal Forebrain: Nucleus Basalis of Meynert (Acetylcholine; Alzheirmer's)
Orbital Frontal – Ventral Medial Prefrontal Cortex

Central Regions 60
Cz, C3, C4; BAs 4, 6, and 1, 2, 3, 5: - The sensorimotor strip

Cerebellum 62
Cz, C3, C4; BA 6 Premotor Cortex 63
Cz, C3, C4; BAs 5 (& 7 Parietal Lobe) Somatosensory Association Cortex 64

Temporal Lobes 66
Introduction
Influencing Central and Midline Structures with Neurofeedback
Overview of Verbal and Pattern Encoding; Memory; Seizures
Overview of Left Dominant and Right Nondominant Hemisphere Functions
T7, T8; T9, T10; BAs 41, 42, 22; 21,43; 52; 20: Temporal Lobes - Lateral Aspect
then Inferior Aspects
Amygdala 74
T9, T10; BAs 28, 34, 36, 37, 27, 35, 36: Inferior Temporal Lobe - Medial Aspect:
Parahippocampal Gyrus, Fusiform Gyrus, - Memory and Affect Networks
Notes on: Memory, Papez Circuit, Cingulum, Symptoms Observed with Temporal Lobe Seizures
Figure: Hippocampal Commissure
F7, F9-T7; F8, FlO-T8; BA 38: **Temporal Pole:** A Junction of Inferior Frontal and Temporal Regions
through the Uncinate Fasciculus **78**

Insula 86
C3- T7; C4- T8; BA 13: Insula 86

Cingulate Gyrus 89
Introduction: Affect & Executive Functions (E.g., Depression)
Figure: Midsagittal Section Cerebral Hemispheres
Fz - Cz, BAs 32, 24, 25, 33: Anterior Cingulate (Rostral Portion)
Executive BA 32; Affect & Default BAs 24, 25, 33.
Cz; BA 24: Central ACC - Affect & Executive Monitoring
Pz; BAs 23, 31; 29, 30, 26: Caudal Division: Posterior Cingulate Cortex - Default, Sensory Integration,
Executive Memory Networks 95

Parietal Lobes 100
Introduction .
Anatomical Boundaries; Overview of Functions
Pz; BA 7: Parietal Lobes, Dorsal Lateral Aspect - Somatosensory Association Cortex 101
Gerstmann and Bálint Syndromes
Pz: BA 7: Parietal Lobes, Medial Dorsal Aspect – Cuneus, Precuneus 104

Temporal-Parietal Junction, Lateral Aspect **105**
Introduction: Effects of Lesions in Dominant and Nondominant Hemispheres
T7-P3 x C3-P7; BAs 39, 40: Dominant Hemisphere (Wernicke's); Nondominant (Sensory Aprosodia)
Introduction to Parietal Lobes - Lateral and Inferior
Historical Note: Carl Wernicke 106
P3 and P4; P7 and P8; BAs 40, 39, (37): Lateral Inferior Parietal lobes Supramarginal &
Angular Gyrus (note: only superior posterior corner of BA 37) 110
Vestibular Connections to Inferior Parietal – Temporal – Frontal Operculum region

Occipital Regions 114
O1, O2: BAs 17, 18, 19: Occipital Lobes – Visual Network

Appendices. 118
Table of Networks and Brodmann Areas
Table of Regions of Interest, Lobules, Brodmann Areas
Order of Description of Functions: Lobes, Networks, Brodmann Areas, 10-20 Sites
Summary of Locations of Brodmann Areas

Multiple Choice Questions 122
Answers 127

References 128

Part 1
Introduction/Orientation

For detail on 10-20 Sites, Brodmann areas and functions, go directly to Part 2 beginning on Page 32

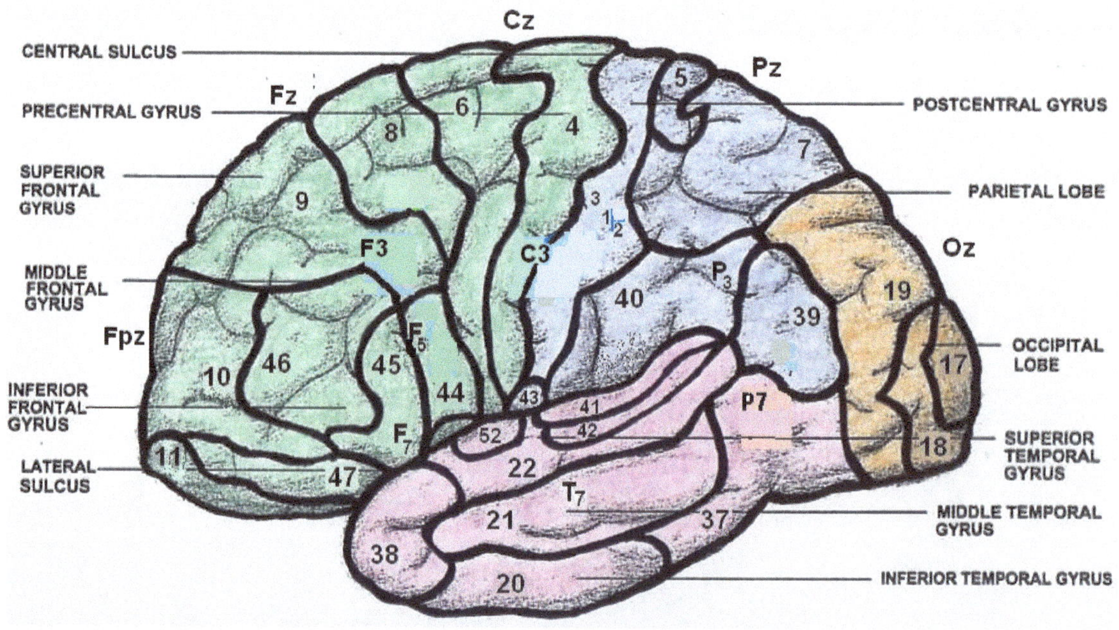

Lateral view to show lobes of the brain, Brodmann areas, and 10-20 electrode sites

(Drawing by Amanda Reeves and Bojana Knezevic)

On the diagrams the numbers go from 1 to 52, but do not frustrate yourself looking for every Brodmann area from 1 to 52 because there are some you will not find since the numbers jump from 12 to 17 and also from 47 to 52. This is because BAs 14, 15, and 16 are cell types found in the insular cortex of nonhuman primates and they are not found in the human cortex. The diagrams thus omit BAs 14, 15, &16. With respect to BA 13, it was identified by Brodmann in monkeys but neuroanatomists today feel it is also found in the human cortex where it acts as a bridge between the lateral and medial areas in the insula. Since the insula is an infolding of cortex, it would not, in any case, be visible in either the lateral (external side view) or the midsagittal view shown in these diagrams. BA 13 is included in the discussion because it is identified as a source using LORETA, and thus is relevant for people doing neurofeedback. With respect to BAs 48 through 51, BA 48 is in the retrosubicular area, a small part of the medial surface of the temporal lobe that is part of the hippocampal region, so it is not visible on the diagrams. BA 49 is found in rodents, and BAs 50 and 51 are found in monkeys. The last number, BA 52, is found in humans. You will find it in the diagrams, in the superior temporal lobe near the junction of the frontal, temporal, and parietal lobes.

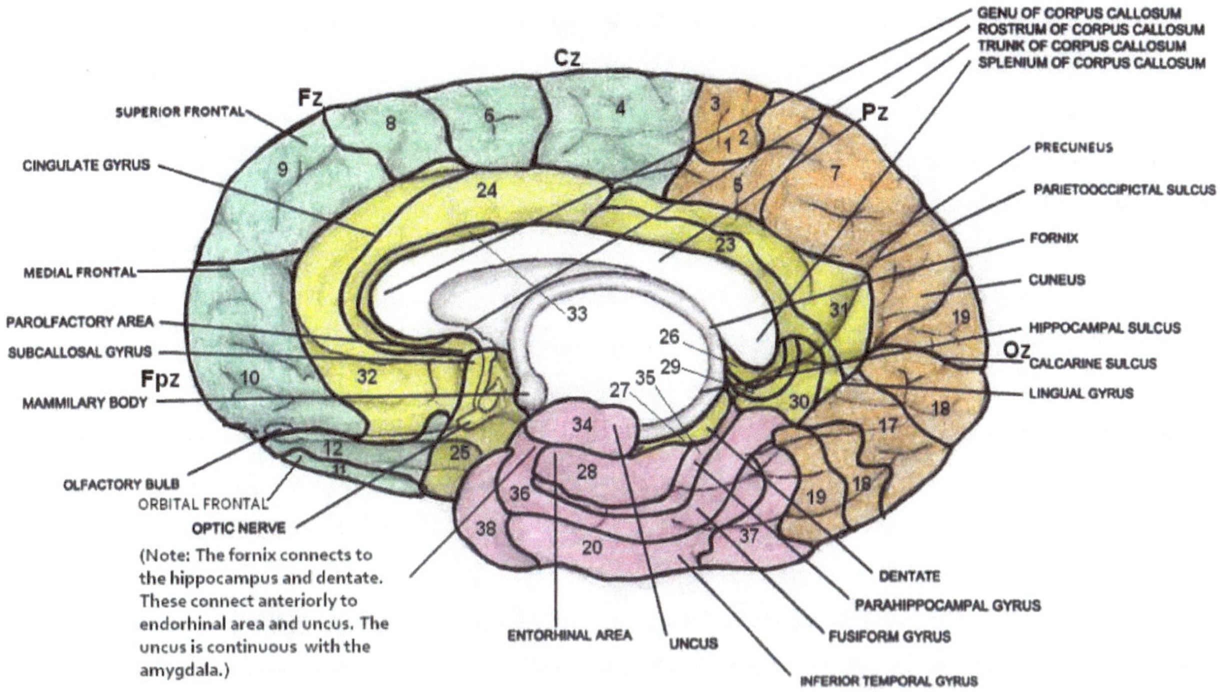

Midsagittal Section to show Lobes of the Brain, Brodmann areas, and 10-20 Electrode Sites

(Drawing by Amanda Reeves, Bojana Knezevic)

NOTE: These first two diagrams, along with brief notes on the main functions associated with each of the Brodmann areas, were first published as a four-page booklet through the International Society for Neurofeedback and Research (see www.isnr.org) in 2007. For quick reference, those booklets are still available on the ISNR website, and proceeds from the sales go to the ISNR Research Foundation.

The collaborative work on the original four-page document that was donated to the ISNR was done by Michael Thompson, M.D. (ADD Centre & Biofeedback Institute of Toronto, Canada), Dr. Wu Wenqing (Friendship Hospital & Capital Medical University of Beijing, China), and James Thompson, Ph.D. (Evoke Neuroscience, New York, N.Y.). These authors developed that document in an attempt to simplify and put in summary form work done by Korbinian Brodmann in the first decade of the twentieth century, combining his original maps of the human cortex with insights concerning functional correlates of the so-called Brodmann areas developed by many others who subsequently studied and added to this knowledge. The work was begun as part of the training of staff at the ADD Centre and was expanded during the time when James Thompson was doing his doctoral work at Pennsylvania State University concerning assessment of concussion in athletes. It was developed further during the six months that neurologist and epileptologist Dr. Wu spent at our ADD Centre while on sabbatical from his positions in Beijing. We hoped the information would be helpful to people who do neurofeedback in a thoughtful way that reflects its neuroanatomical underpinnings. There was a perceived demand for an expanded version of that short booklet and this book has been written to meet that need. We invite you to use the information and give us feedback regarding its utility.

In the Second Edition of *The Neurofeedback Book,* we expand on the discussion of each area and also link the primary functions of each Brodmann area with mention of the networks that involve those functions.

However, it must be kept in mind that each region/lobe of the brain functions in a number of networks that link modules and many Brodmann areas. The individual Brodmann areas do not have unique functions but rather have functions that overlap with adjacent BAs and they may also share functions with other Brodmann areas that are often in distant areas of the brain. In this manner, Brodmann areas are, for the most part, just component parts of complex networks.

Behavioral Interpretations of Intrinsic Connectivity Networks have been investigated in some detail and published by Laird et al. in 2011. Their publication is quite detailed and is based on about 30,000 MRI and PET scans. The reader is encouraged to read Dr. Thatcher's summary of the work by Laird et al. (Thatcher, Biver, & North, 2015). Laird's work defines 18 specific groupings of sites and functions. Their findings do not appear to differ from the functions and networks described in this text but it is a useful addition, providing an additional perspective, for practitioners who are doing LORETA z-score neurofeedback.

Primary Functions Related to General Areas of the Cortex

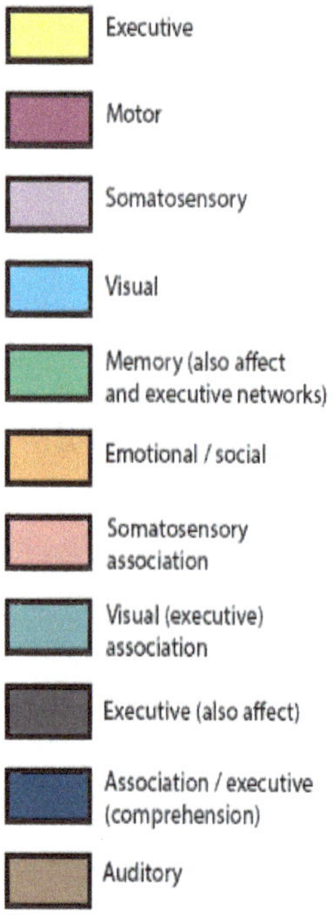

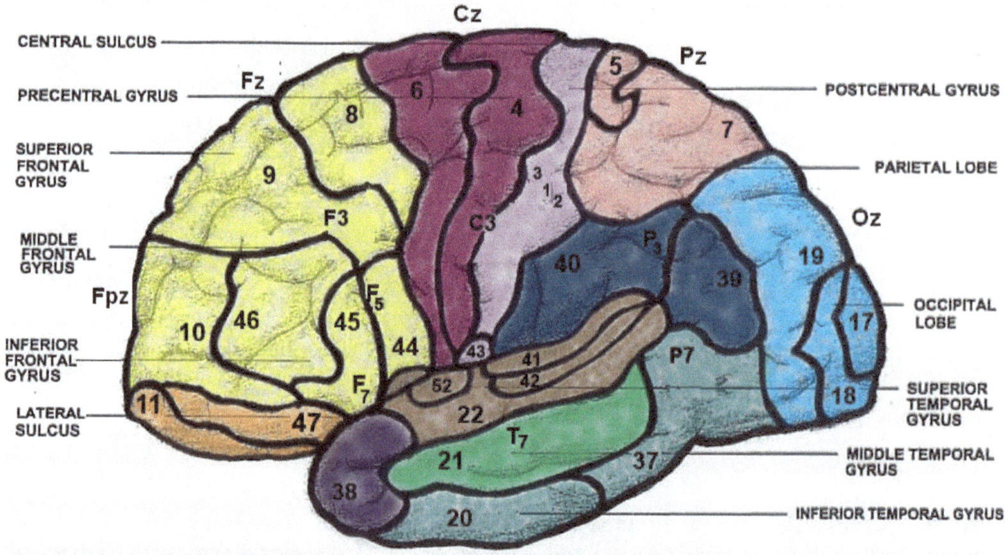

Drawing by Amanda Reeves, Bojana Knezevic, Maya Berenkey; Functional Areas by Michael Thompson

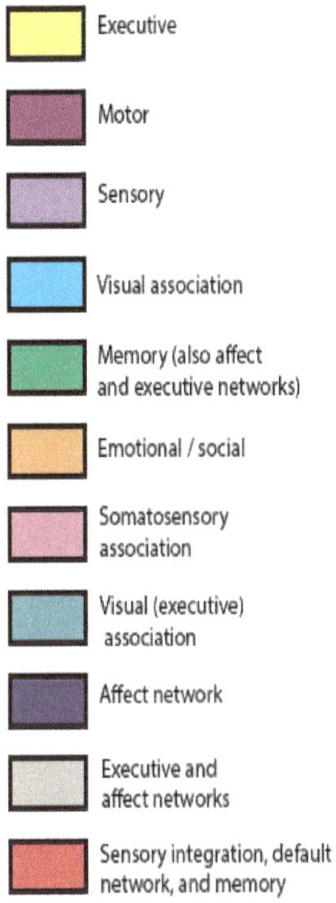

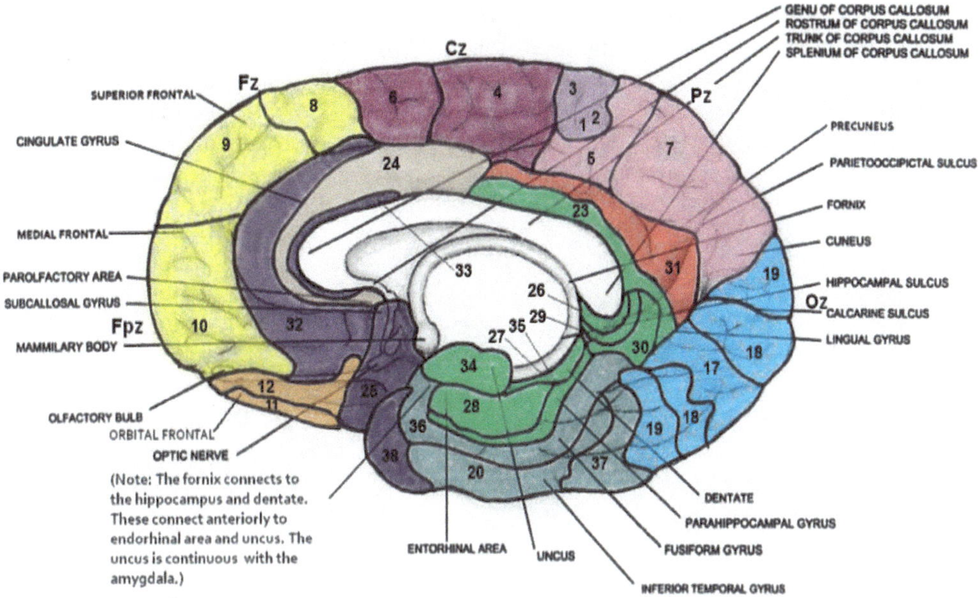

Drawing by Amanda Reeves, Bojana Knezevic, Maya Berenkey;
Functional Areas by Michael Thompson

Notes Concerning Illustrations:

1. *Attention, Salience, Default, and Memory Networks are too widespread to be usefully illustrated in this diagram.*
2. *Brodmann Area 32 is more executive than affect but is purple for color-contrast in diagram.*

These two diagrams provide very **broad overviews regarding how Brodmann areas relate to some of the functional networks in the cortex.** It is much too broad an overview and therefore, of course, basically incorrect. For example, memory and emotional regulation clearly must involve many more areas than indicated here. We have not labelled any area as 'attention' because that would include most of the areas that are already labelled! We also made the decision NOT to have four diagrams to show both left and right hemispheres, though there are some differences in functions of the dominant and non-dominant hemispheres that will be mentioned in the text. That kind of detail seemed inappropriate in an overview diagram. We attempted to use general but appropriate terms for areas. For example, the word 'comprehension' for BAs 39 and 40 can be understood, after reading the text, as being primarily language comprehension (Wernicke's area) and other aspects of learning in the dominant hemisphere, while covering nuance, innuendo, emotional, and nonverbal, even spatial reasoning, in the nondominant hemisphere. The finer points will be apparent as you read further: these are just overview diagrams to help the reader get oriented before we move on to more detail.

Thanks Are Extended

Special thanks are extended to Mark Dubin, Dan Lloyd, Richard Soutar, Bob Thatcher, David Kaiser, and Jonathan Walker, who either gave us their direct input concerning Brodmann areas and their functional correlates or whose work on Brodmann areas is available on the Internet. These people were consulted or used as primary references because all have spent considerable time compiling data on this subject. With respect to understanding basic features of neural networks, special thanks are given to Juri Kropotov and his work on event-related potentials, which has helped to delineate networks in the brain. Thanks are given to Jay Gunkelman, Barry Sterman, and David Hagedorn for assistance in the interpretation of EEGs.

Caution

When you read this text, please keep in mind that a Brodmann area (BA) does not (necessarily) correspond precisely to a named gyrus on the cortex. In the following we have tried to give as close a correspondence as possible regarding how specific International 10-20 sites relate to the Brodmann areas on the surface of the cortex. Always keep in mind that there are individual differences and thus variations in the brain's topography across individuals. There are also developmental changes in brain structure, particularly with respect to frontal lobe maturation, which is not complete until about age 25. As more fibers become myelinated and the frontal lobes become larger, there is a slight forward shift in locations. Thus, what is seen at CZ in a child may be better measured at FCZ (half-way between CZ and FZ) in an adult.

Brodmann dissected adult brains, so this section is based on findings in adult brains, though the information can certainly be extrapolated to work with children. Also note that Brodmann himself cautioned about the limitations of his maps due to the fact that labelling the surface gyri does not show the large areas of the cortical surface that are hidden in the infolding of the cortex at each sulcus and fissure.

Lateral view of the Left Cerebral Hemisphere.

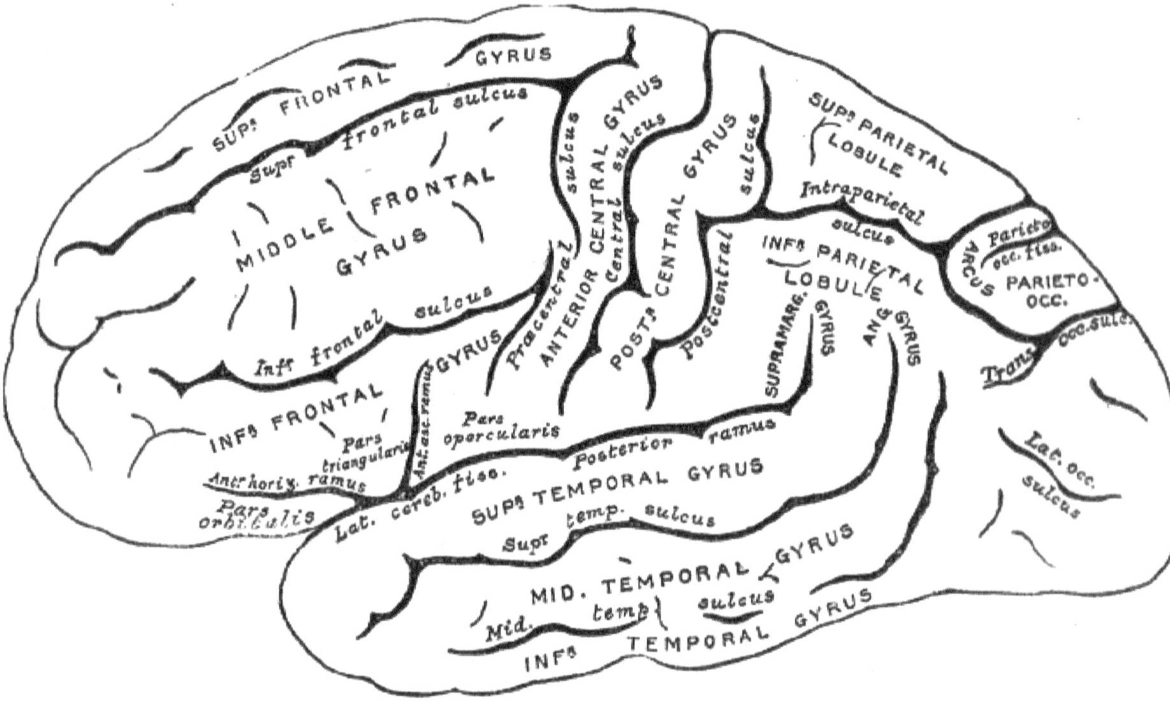

This figure is a Lateral view of the Left Cerebral Hemisphere from Henry Gray, Gray's Anatomy of the Human Body, *1918. This lateral view and the medial view below are shown here to illustrate sulci and gyri that are not labelled in our other diagrams.*

"Gray726." Licensed under Public Domain via Wikimedia Commons - http://commons.wikimedia.org/wiki/File:Gray726.png#mediaviewer/File:Gray726.png

Midsagittal View of the Left Cerebral Hemisphere

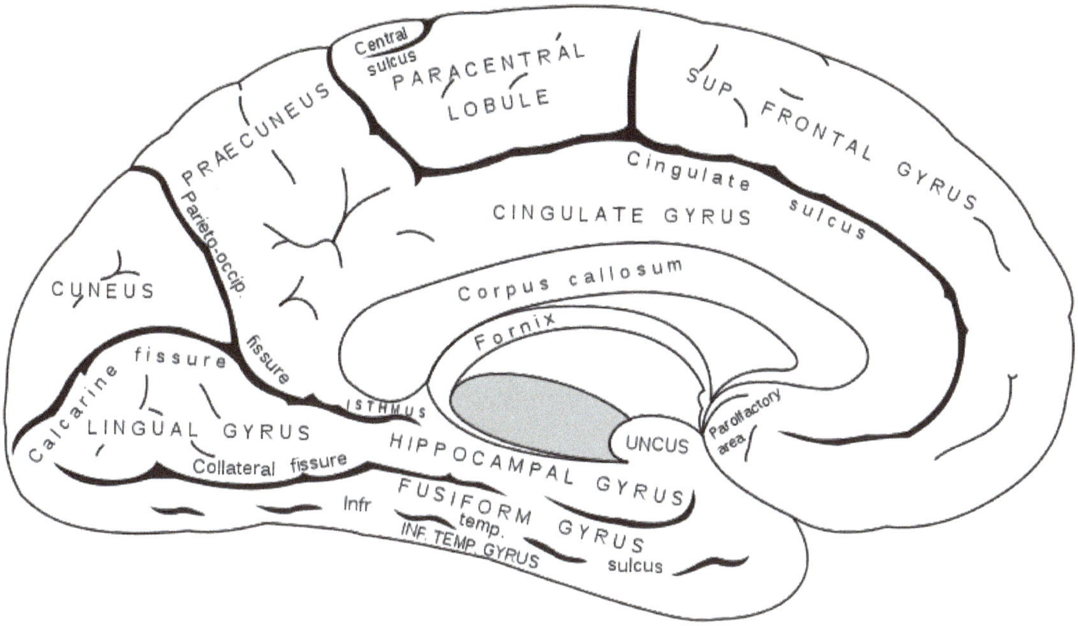

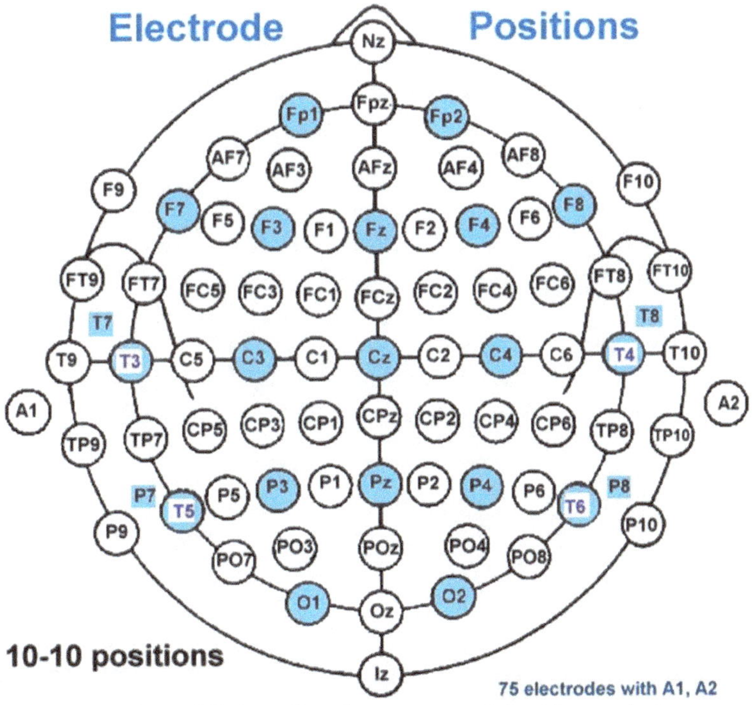

From David Kaiser (Brodmannarea.info) with permission.
The 19 sites that we will refer to in the following discussion are shaded.

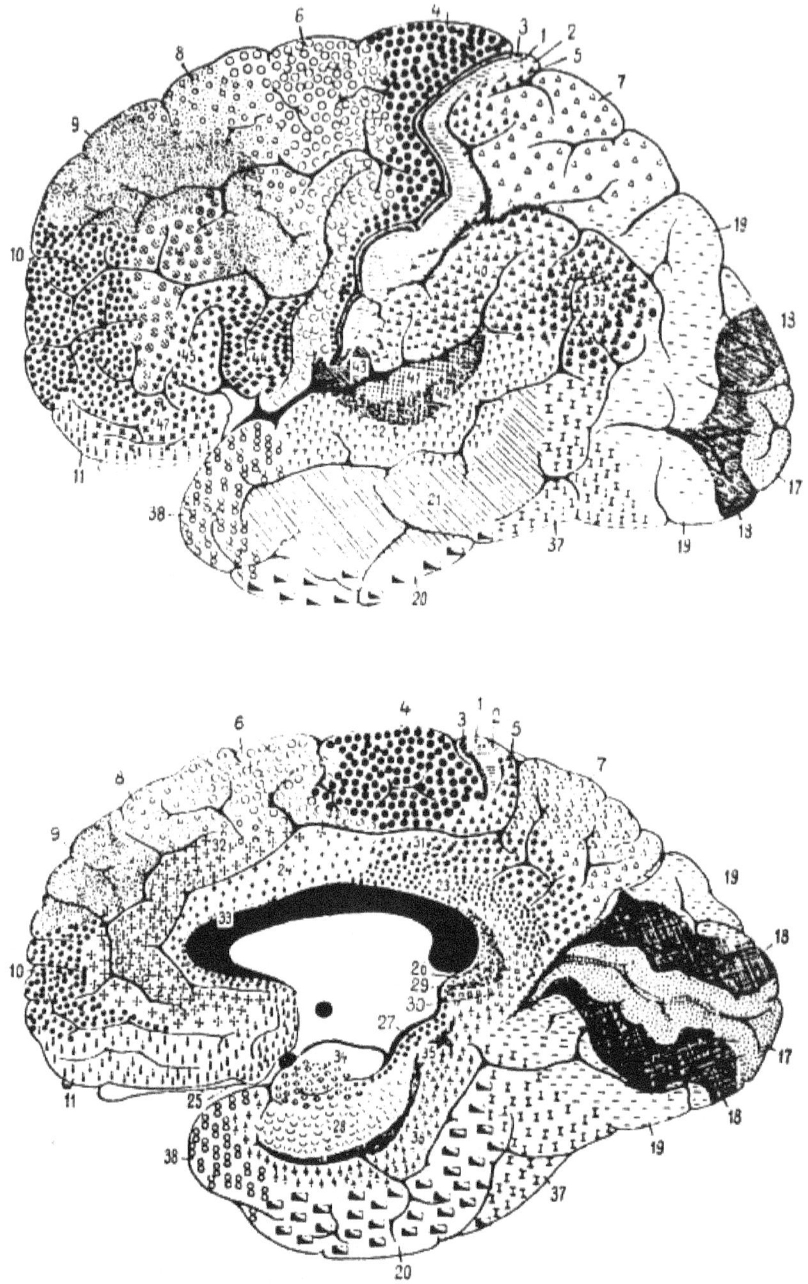

Cytoarchitectonics of human brain according to Brodmann (1909), (public domain)

Korbinian Brodmann said, "One thing must be stressed quite firmly: henceforth functional localization of the cerebral cortex without the lead of anatomy is utterly impossible in man as in animals. In all domains, physiology has its firmest foundations in anatomy."

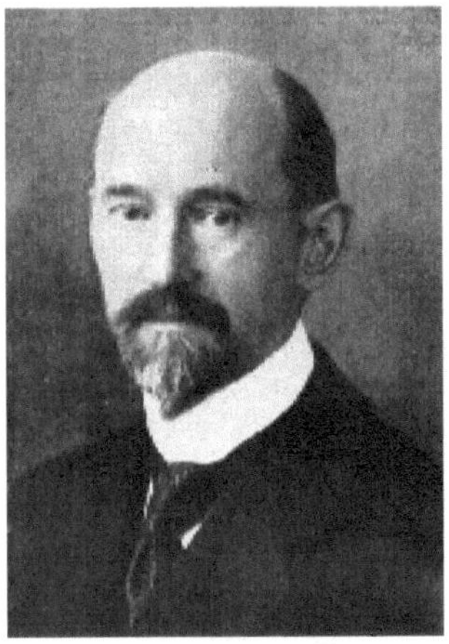

Dr Korbinian Brodmann, German Neurologist
(November 17, 1868 – August 22, 1918)

Historical Note Concerning Korbinian Brodmann

His work: It is now more than 100 years since Korbinian Brodmann published his work on mapping the mammalian cortex according to different cell types, their spacing and organization. It was while working from 1901-1910 at the Neurobiologishes Laboratorium in Berlin, part of an Institute for Brain Research founded by Oskar and Cecelia Vogt, that he conducted these studies. At that time he also became editor of the *Journal fuer Psychologie und Neurologie,* which survives today as the *Journal of Brain Research.* Between 1903 and 1908 he published his findings delineating areas of the brain according to cell morphology, or cytoarchitecture, in that journal. His best known work from that series is the article about the human cortex published in 1908. In all, he studied 64 different species of mammals.Doubtless inspired by the interest at the time in evolution, he focused on comparative anatomy, developing the idea that there was an old cortex shared across various mammalian species and a more recently evolved neocortex that had developed to a high degree in primates, particularly in humans. In 1909 an expanded version of his work, *Vergleichendes Lokalisationslehre der Grossgehirn-rinde*, was published by J.A. Barth in Leipzig. The goal mentioned in the book's preface was to produce a comparative, organic theory of the cerebral cortex based on anatomical features. In 1994 this work was finally translated into English by Laurence Garey with the title *Localisation in the Cerebral Cortex,* but Brodmann maps were being widely used long before the monograph was translated. Brodmann's observations remain relevant today.

His maps were created by doing meticulous dissections and then, using a microscope and a method of staining cells that he learned from Franz Nissl, to examine a slice of cortex. He began with cells in the middle of the lateral side of the brain in the post-central gyrus, calling that area 1, and then proceeded to give a number to each subsequent group of cells that had a different and distinct cytoarchitecture; thus, the morphology, or shape, and organization of the cells differs from one Brodmann area to another. He had become interested in neuroanatomy and its relationship to psychiatric disorders when working for a year (summer 1900 until August 1901) at the Municipal Mental Asylum in Frankfurt, where he met and was greatly inspired by Alois Alzheimer. This mentoring ignited the passion for neuroanatomy that he was to pursue intensively while working as a researcher in Berlin for the next ten years of his life.

His Life: His famous work, which was actually not as well appreciated when he was alive as it came to be later, built upon a steady academic trajectory that began in the local elementary school in Hohenfels, a village north of Lake Constance in southern Germany where he was born. (There is now a Brodmann Museum in the town hall, open the first Monday afternoon each month.) He finished high school at a Gymnasium in Konstanz in 1889 and then pursued medical studies, graduating as a doctor in 1895. He took a position in a clinic in Munich for his final training but, due to coming down with diphtheria and having to convalesce, he did not proceed with his original plan of starting his own medical practice in the Black Forest area. Instead he embarked in 1896 on further studies in Psychiatry, Neurology and Psychology in Berlin and other cities. Final training in Frankfurt that included working with Alzheimer was followed by taking the position in Berlin at the Vogt's brain institute from 1901 – 1910. When the University of Berlin failed to grant him his doctorate in 1910, which was required to become a professor and have a steady income, he left for the University of Tuebingen where he worked from 1910 – 1916 in the anatomical laboratory of the University Clinic. The war disrupted his research and curtailed further publications concerning his work as he began working with neurological patients at the military field hospital in Tuebingen. He was recognized for his services and then, finally, was given a paid position in Halle, where he met and married a much younger woman, Margarite Franz, in April 1917. In 1918, the year their daughter Else was born, he was appointed as the Director of Anatomical Topography at the German Research Institute in Munich. Just as his life was looking happier and more secure, he developed a blood infection, likely from a small cut incurred while doing an autopsy, and he died of sepsis on August 2, 1918. One is left to speculate on what further knowledge he might have added to the field of functional neuroanatomy had he lived into his late eighties like his colleagues Oskar and Cecelia Vogt who died in 1959 and 1962 respectively. Oskar Vogt, in his retirement, wrote a biography of his colleague.

Preliminary Comments about the Organization of this Section

The Brodmann areas (BAs) are discussed in this text by working through **each anatomical area according to the lobes** in which they are located and the related 10-20 electrode placement sites, rather than by listing the Brodmann areas in numerical order. This is because the individual Brodmann areas do not have unique functions but instead have functions that overlap with adjacent BAs and share functions with other Brodmann areas that are often in distant areas of the brain. Each Brodmann area is, for the most part, just one part of one or more complex networks.

Thus, though neuroanatomy is involved, this section is written with the sole goal being to summarize some of the functions within networks that may be expected to respond to neurofeedback (NFB) + biofeedback (BFB) operant conditioning techniques. We decided NOT to merely 'list' functions under each Brodmann area (BA), though there is a summary table at the end. In addition to our previous comments regarding lack of specificity, the lists can be long and there is so much overlap between areas that they lose their clinical usefulness and become overwhelming for anyone without an eidetic memory.

Since this is not an anatomy textbook, but rather a **text written to assist people doing clinical practice where neurofeedback and biofeedback** and, at times, transcranial direct current stimulation (tDCS) are the principle methods of intervention, the organization of the information starts not in the middle, as Brodmann did, but rather with the frontal lobes and electrode sites Fz, F3, and F4. We provide a general overview of the functional significance of cortical areas. Then each Brodmann area for that area of the brain is discussed. The areas are covered in the following order: Frontal Lobes, Central (Cz, Pz), Temporal Lobes, Cingulate Gyrus, Parietal Lobes, and Occipital Lobes.

Things to Keep in Mind

Please remember when reading this explication of functional neuroanatomy with an emphasis on Brodmann areas that each Brodmann area (BA) delineates cortical areas that are differentiated by discrete cell histology and the hypothesis is that each of these areas may have a primary function and also many different functions associated with it. This summary gives rudimentary information associating Brodmann areas with the standard sites of the International 10-20 System of electrode placement. The updated site names are used for the temporal and parietal areas; that is, rather than the old sequence of F7 – T3 – T5, we have used F7 – T7 – P7. In the right hemisphere, the longitudinal sequential placements F8 – T4 – T6 became F8 – T8 – P8. Since most of the databases used in the neurofeedback field were developed before the neurologists changed the nomenclature, you will find both the old and new designations for T3/T7, T4/T8, T5/P7, and T6/P8 used.

The description of Brodmann area functions leads into a discussion concerning neural networks that we posit can be affected using a combination of neurofeedback (NFB) plus biofeedback (BFB).

Neurofeedback Training is Guided by Brodmann Areas and Networks

Brodmann Area Functions Overlap

The primary functions for each Brodmann area (BA) are given in the next section of this monograph. The functions described in the text represent a best guess, based on our clinical observations and on the published and unpublished work of others. Please be advised at the outset that the detail of functions for each Brodmann area is necessarily FALSE. Why? Because all functions emerge from the interaction of many areas and they are not localized to a single area of the brain. This is not a twenty-first century version of phrenology. An expert in Brodmann areas, Dan Lloyd of Trinity College, Hartford, CT, writes, "The **typical BA is differentially engaged in 40% of behavioral (cognitive, perceptual, emotive) domains"** (Lloyd, 2007, personal communication). What lies behind this observation is the fact that **each Brodmann area represents just one area out of many that are involved in one or more neural networks** that involve cortical-subcortical connections; thus each BA becomes involved in a coordinated activity with many other functionally related cortical areas, **depending on what task the brain is doing**.

This may be one reason why practitioners have obtained good results when only doing neurofeedback (NFB) over a single site, such as Cz. That one site lies above BA 4 (primary motor cortex). BA 4 lies above BA 24, the anterior cingulate, which is involved in multiple networks.

Why Use Single-Channel Training?

Training Over Central Midline Structures

Approximately 50% of the EEG amplitude at any single site, such as Cz, arises from neurons directly beneath the electrode, and 95% arises from an area within a 6 cm distance around the site (Thatcher, 2012, quotes Nunez et al., 1981, 1995, 2006). Training at central midline sites such as Cz, Fz, and Pz is hypothesized to **influence key areas**, such as the cingulate gyrus, that are involved in many networks including, but not limited to, the **Executive, Affect, Salience, and Default networks. These** are discussed in more detail in the following section.

A network serves to synchronize the functions of groups of neurons in many different but related sections of the cerebral cortex. The **Attention network,** for example, which is one of the Executive networks, may be affected by training at Cz, and this network **synchronizes the functions of neurons** in the frontal and parietal lobes, anterior cingulate gyrus, hippocampus, the frontal eye fields, and the intraparietal sulcus (Coul and Nobre, 1998). In addition, there appear to be areas that act to switch the brain from one network to another. For example, when the **Attention network is on, the Default network is off** (Sridharan et al., 2008; Fox et al., 2005). The insula is postulated to operate as **a switch** that turns the Default network off and the Attention network on, and vice versa (Sridharan, 2008).

Both the Attention and the Default networks show markedly decreased activity during sleep. The posterior cingulate gyrus shows significant deactivation in both sleep and anesthesia. These examples show how complex the interactions are and how any single BA can be involved in multiple networks at different times.

Doing neurofeedback (NFB) using a referential placement with the active electrode at Cz and the reference electrode on one earlobe, we have seen many case examples where training has apparently had an effect on several networks. This is possibly due to NFB influencing a number of areas within the **anterior cingulate cortex (ACC)**. As noted above, the ACC is a central structure that is involved in a number of neural networks including the Executive (and Attention) network, the Affect (and distress) network, and the Salience network. We have chosen to use the singular for each network but in reality each network is a group of networks.

If the practitioner **combines NFB** for improved attention **with BFB** for relaxation and includes heart rate variability training, then symptoms that relate to anxiety usually decrease. If the practitioner combines the NFB with teaching **metacognitive strategies** ("learning to learn" techniques) and does some training on-task, then an increase in academic performance and in intelligence, as measured by IQ tests, has been found in conjunction with an increase in attention span and concentration (Lubar et al., 1995; Thompson & Thompson, 1998; Thompson & Thompson, 2010).

We hypothesize that we must be affecting complex networks that involve many different cortical and subcortical areas in order to achieve such wide-ranging changes in cognitive and affective functioning with relatively simple single-channel feedback procedures. Indeed, it may be possible that single-channel NFB training, in some patients, could have a **theoretical advantage over training that involves multiple sites**. By having an effect on a network from a single central site, and by only having a direct influence on one site, single-channel NFB may **allow the brain to balance** the degree to which other areas within a network are changed.

NFB at one site avoids making incorrect decisions about the degree to which multiple sites are being 'normalized' when we use z-score directed LORETA NFB. It could be argued that single-channel NFB might be a more 'balanced' approach to changing the brain, and it does not have the theoretical danger of adversely affecting a site that is outside database norms due to genius or due to compensatory mechanisms. This theoretical dilemma can only be resolved by years of data collection and research.

Why Use LORETA Z-Score NFB?

Nevertheless, with some complex cases, the practitioner may wish to be more precise and try to have an effect on a number of different areas with some of them being distant from surface electrode sites. One may also want to simultaneously train a number of different parameters, such as amplitude, phase and coherence. For these clients we use LORETA z-score neurofeedback (LNFB).

Importance of Networks

In our work using NFB we are practically always attempting to optimize the performance of neural networks. **Networks are** 'chains' of linked groups of neurons that function together to accomplish a goal. In this context it may be useful to recall what our grandmothers said and our coaches emphasized, "The chain (team, network) is **only as strong as its weakest link**." Thus with cortical dysfunction, our NFB training must either strengthen the performance of that 'link,' or help the network readjust in order to compensate for its dysfunction. The brain has a **plasticity** that should allow this to take place, as has been the case with other interventions, too. (For excellent examples of a range of neuroplastic changes, see Norman Doidge's 2010 book, *The Brain that Changes Itself*, and its 2015 sequel, *The Brain's Way of Healing*.

Cortex-Basal Ganglia-Thalamus: How to Activate One Network – Inhibit Others

In order to have such broad effects, the cortical area to which we are directing our NFB must have a way of connecting to many functionally related, though spatially distant, cortical areas. At the same time, other functionally nonrelevant areas of the cortex must be inhibited. In this manner, many functionally related cortical areas are synchronized and recruited to operate as a specific network to accomplish the task at hand.

The brain is constantly working to reduce uncertainty and make the environment both consistent and predictable. It is finding meaning in information, making patterns and associations. It is continuously analyzing and reanalyzing information in order to understand it in a personally relevant manner. Thus, when we do an assessment, whether it be eyes closed, eyes open, or on a specific task, the brain is always working. There is no true 'resting' state. The brain is continuously activating specific networks and the Default network comes into play when a person is awake but not focused on a particular task. With activation of relevant networks happening, how does inhibition of pyramidal cells and then of systems of whole nonrelevant networks come about?

Remarks Concerning Inhibition in the Cortex

Local inhibition of specific pyramidal cells is done immediately after a pyramidal cell fires by basket cells that are close to the pyramidal cell. Basket cell firing may have other important functions, and it has been noted that gamma synchronization of basket cell inhibition of pyramidal cells may be one key for understanding some aspects of cerebral dynamics. This, however, is not a subject for a basic textbook and it will not be discussed here. What, then, is one possible mechanism that could be responsible for activating a single network while inhibiting often widely distributed nonrelevant cortical areas in order to focus attention and action on a single function to accomplish the task-at-hand? An inhibitory mechanism that is available, which can affect widely distant cortical areas, involves links from the cortex to subcortical structures that are broadly labelled the 'basal ganglia.' These connections, from the cortex to the basal ganglia and then back to the cortex via the thalamus, can focus action while simultaneously inhibiting areas that are not necessary for a particular task.

The Basal Ganglia

The structures that comprise the basal ganglia include the dorsal striatum (putamen and caudate), subthalamic nucleus, the substantia nigra (pars compacta (SNc) that produces dopamine and pars reticulata (SNr) that has functions similar to the pallidum), and a limbic sector that includes the nucleus accumbens (ventral striatum), ventral pallidum, and ventral tegmental area (VTA). VTA efferents provide dopamine to the nucleus accumbens (ventral striatum) in the same way that the substantia nigra provides dopamine to the dorsal striatum and the globus pallidus. You will also hear another term 'lentiform nucleus,' which means shaped like a lens. The lentiform nucleus comprises the putamen laterally, globus pallidus medially and the innominate substance, which contains the anterior perforated area, inferiorly.

Figures to Help Visualize these Structures

Several figures are given below to remind the reader of the locations of some of these structures. Four of these figures have been taken from other parts of *The Neurofeedback Book* to help you see the relationship between the basal ganglia, the thalamus, and the cortex. Note when reading the text and looking at the figures that 'dorsal' is towards the top of the head, but in the brainstem and spine, it is at the back. 'Ventral' is towards the base of the skull but, in the spine, it would be towards the front of the body. Lateral means towards the side and medial is towards the middle of the head. Thus a medial or midsagittal section would slice down the vertical plane in the middle of the head from anterior (front/forehead) to posterior (back/occiput).

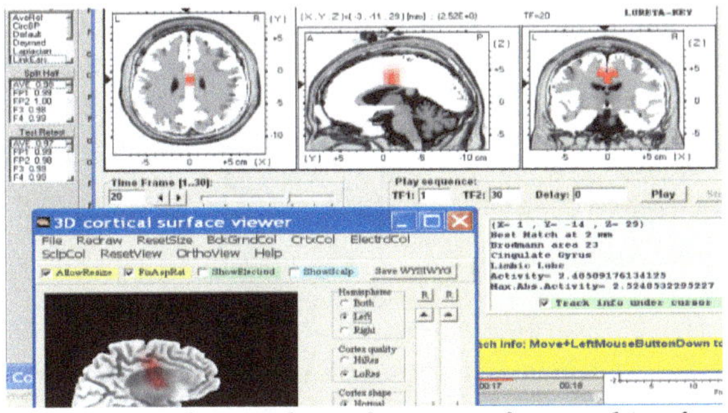

The 'slices' shown along the top in the graphic above are LORETA images: Horizontal, Sagittal and Coronal respectively. In the bottom left hand corner is placed the three dimensional sagittal slice from the LORETA program.

This figure, taken from an analysis done with Neuroguide, shows the 'slices' of the brain as they are seen using LORETA. It shows a LORETA source correlation in Brodmann area (BA) 23, cingulate gyrus. The activity was 2.5 standard deviations above the database mean using the Neuroguide program. This finding reflected excessive amplitude of 20 Hz activity in a 42-year-old woman who had anxiety symptoms (affect network).

Note that LORETA images, though they look like MRI scans, are mathematically derived from surface EEG data. For cortical sites, there is correspondence between LORETA source localization and MRI findings. LORETA however, does not reveal subcortical sites.

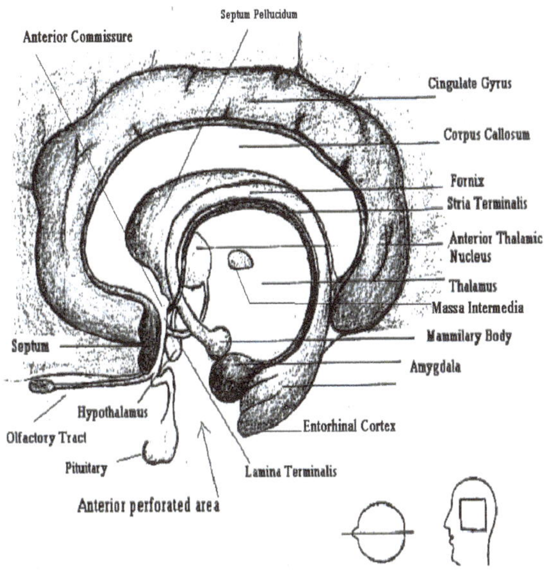

The above figure is a midsagittal section that shows the position of the thalamus below the cingulate gyrus and the corpus callosum.

The figure below is a coronal, also called transverse, section that shows the relationship between the putamen, the globus pallidus, and the thalamus as you move medially from the right lateral aspect of the cortex (an infolding of cortex called the insula) towards the centre of the brain where you see the third ventricle. The same structures are mirrored in the left hemisphere.

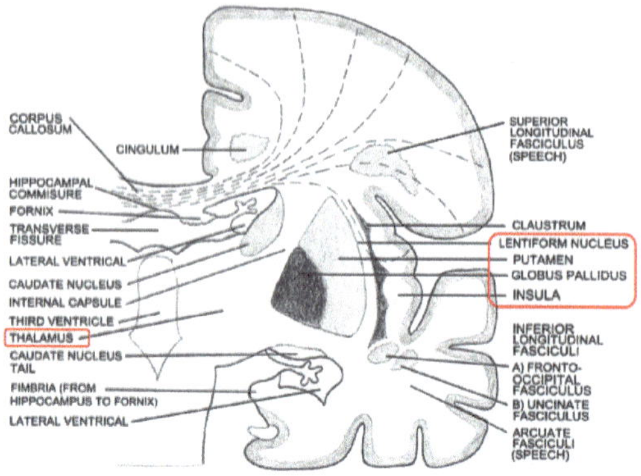

Schematic diagram of a transverse section through the right cerebral hemisphere (Amanda Reeves, after Smith 1962).

The figure below shows these same structures plus nuclei that influence them. The basal ganglia and the cortex are directly influenced by the substantia nigra, which produces dopamine. The following diagram includes the basal ganglia, the thalamus, and the substantia nigra.

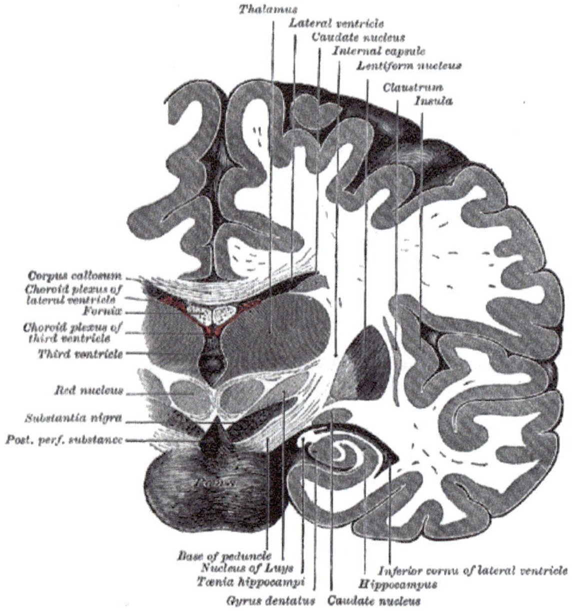

Gray's Anatomy *(public domain). Schematic Diagram of a Transverse Section Through the Right Cerebral Hemisphere and midline structures (after Smith 1962) to show the Red Nucleus and the Basal Ganglia and the Substantia Nigra (Nucleus of Luys is more often called the subthalamus).*

The following figure shows the thalamus and a broad general overview of its projections to different cortical areas. All sensory information except smell passes through the thalamus before going on to the cortex. The thalamus has two lobes (a left thalamus and a right thalamus) connected, in about 85% of people, by the *massa intermedia* (shown in a previous figure), which goes through the third ventricle. The nuclei within the thalamus project to specific areas of the cerebral cortex, as seen in the next diagram.

Note: The temporal lobe (at top of figure) has been 'folded up' to show the auditory area (red).

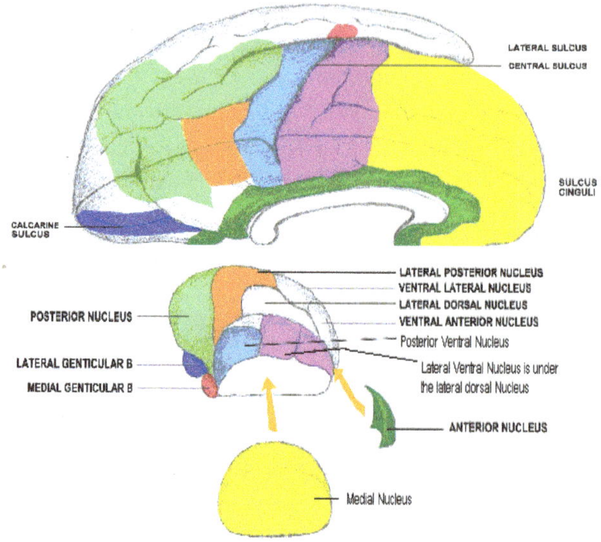

The thalamic nuclei and their functionally related cortical areas (adapted from Smith, 1962)

The above figures are **included to assist the reader, when we outline cortex-basal ganglia-thalamus-cortex loops,** to picture how influencing a single area of the cortex may have the effect of activating one neural network and simultaneously inhibiting others. For example, feedback at Cz might affect BA 24 within the anterior cingulate gyrus, and LORETA NFB might affect this area even more directly. As we will see in greater detail below, this area connects to the ventral striatum in the basal ganglia. Lateral inhibition within the striatum will select one specific network to become active while other networks, and therefore cortical areas that were less relevant to a specific function at that moment in time, are inhibited.

In basic overview terms, the putamen inhibits the globus pallidus (GP) (pallidum). The GP fires at a very high frequency inhibiting the thalamus. Each of these three structures can be thought of as being 'functional maps' of the cortex. Thus if, for example, a motor area of the cortex activates a specific functional area of the putamen then that area will inhibit a specific functionally related area of the GP. This inhibition stops the GP high rate inhibitory firing to a corresponding specific area of the thalamus. Since the thalamus is connected to all the areas of the cortex, this means that only that one functional gate is opened while the others remain inhibited. The result is that areas of the cortex that are functionally related areas to this open gate (a network) are activated while other networks within the cortex remain inhibited.

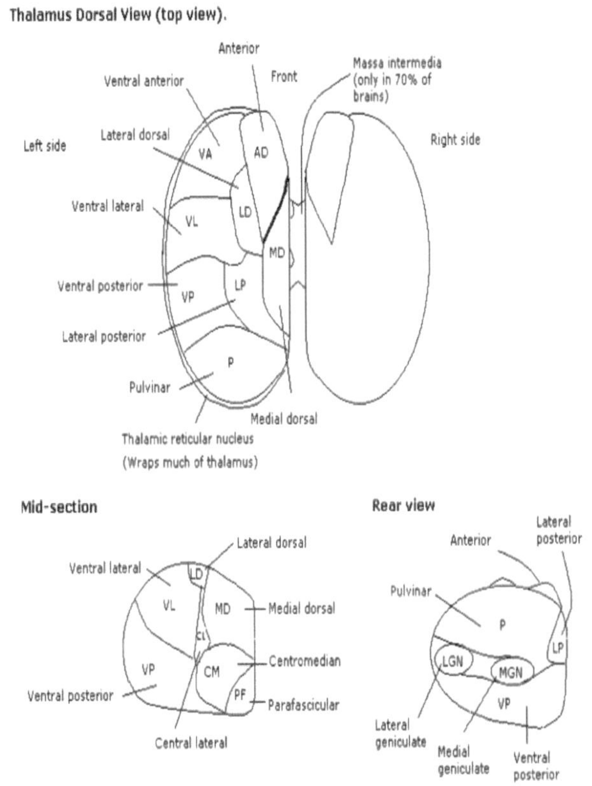

Nuclei of the Thalamus

Permission is granted to copy, distribute, and/or modify this document under the terms of the GNU Free Documentation License, Wikipedia.

Other diagrams can be found on the internet under *Human Neuroanatomy: An Introduction.* James R. Augustine. (2008) Elsevier.

Functional Networks and Behavior

Frontal-Subcortical Circuits

(Special thanks to Tammy Binder, M.D. for her complete revision of this section)

Five Examples of Cortical – Basal Ganglia Circuits

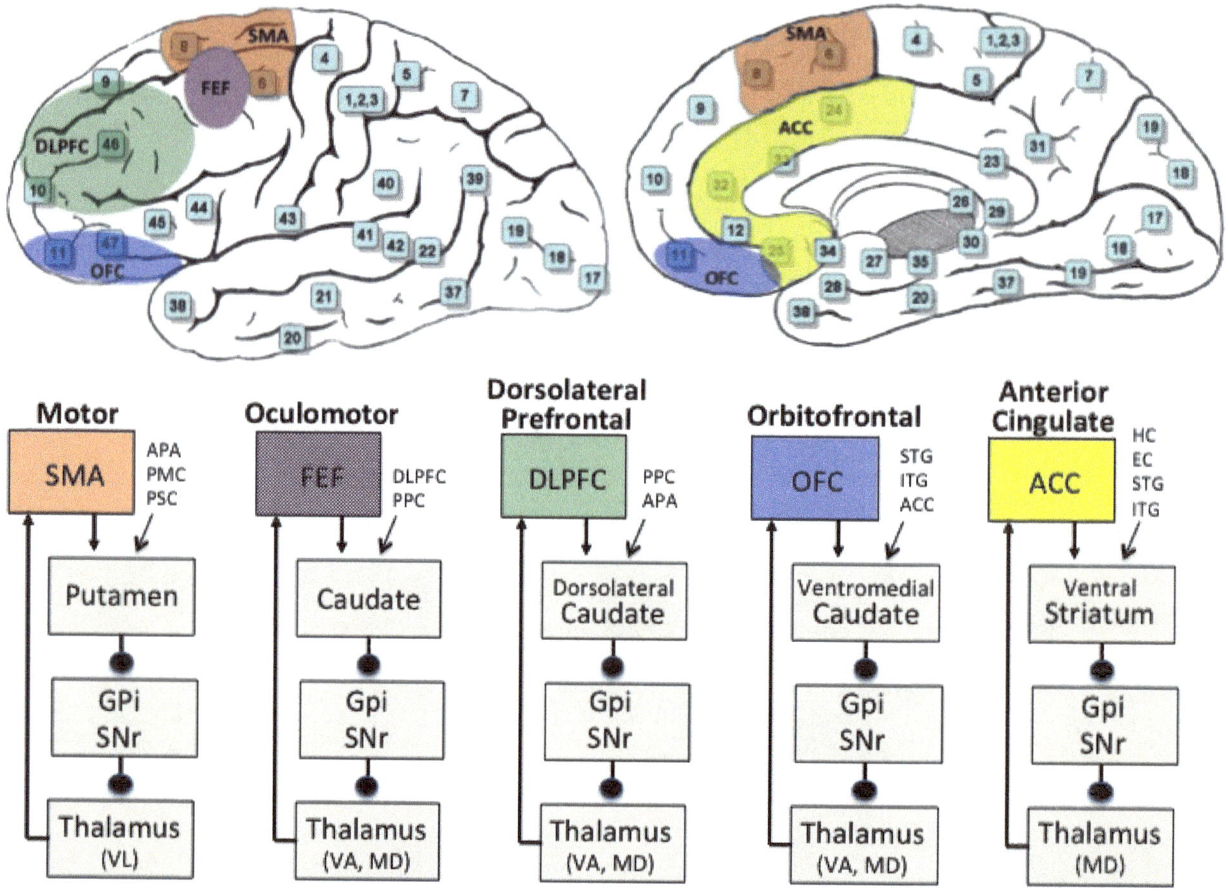

Circuits adapted from Alexander et. al. (1986). Colored boxes at the top of each circuit represent cortical areas from left to right: SMA (supplementary motor area); FEF (frontal eye field); DLPFC (dorsolateral prefrontal cortex); OFC (orbitofrontal cortex); ACC (anterior cingulate cortex). Uncolored boxes represent subcortical structures: GPi (internal segment of globus pallidus); MD (medial dorsal nucleus of thalamus); SNr (substantia nigra, pars reticulata); VA (ventral anterior nucleus of thalamus); VL (ventral lateral nucleus of thalamus). Abbreviations used outside of boxes represent 'open loop' contributions to the circuit and likely provide 'context' to the striatum: APA (arcuate premotor area), EC (entorhinal cortex), HC (hippocampal cortex), ITG (inferior temporal gyrus), PPC (posterior parietal cortex), PMC (primary motor cortex), PSC (primary somatosensory cortex), and STG (superior temporal gyrus). Diagram of Brodmann areas modified from the 20th U.S. edition of Gray's Anatomy *of the Human Body, available on Wikipedia.*

The striatum is a relatively quiet structure. By contrast, the internal segment of the globus pallidus (GPi) and the substantia nigra pars reticulata (SNr) have high baseline rates of activity that provide tonic inhibitory drives to specific nuclei of the thalamus.

The five circuits shown in the diagram remain remarkably anatomically segregated as they traverse the subcortical structures. They are named according to their cortical area or function.

The frontal lobes have long been considered the centre of 'executive function,' which Kropotov (2009) defines as "the coordination and control of motor and cognitive actions to attain specific goals." Other components of executive function include: voluntary control of attention, inhibition of inappropriate and/or unwanted behavior, planning, decision making, working memory, monitoring, and the use of feedback to improve performance.

As shown above, on the basis of neuroanatomy and function, Alexander et al. (1986) described five parallel frontal-subcortical circuits. Each circuit has the same general structure: a specific area of frontal cortex projects to specific areas of basal ganglia, then thalamus, before returning to the originating region in frontal cortex and to functionally related areas.

In his book *The Frontal Lobes and Voluntary Action,* Richard Passingham (p. 220) proposes that the frontal-basal ganglia system as a whole is involved in the process of deciding "what to do...what response is appropriate."

'Appropriate' behaviors often require that deliberative, planned actions occur rather than more reactive, automatic or over-learned actions that are usually faster to execute. Consider, for example, a quarterback who calls for a short pass play that he and his tight end have practiced many times. Now consider the possibility that just as he is about to make the pass he notices that his star wide receiver has just broken free of the defense and is wide open, halfway down the field. In the current context, the quarterback suddenly needs to inhibit the 'preloaded' motor program for the short pass in order to plan and execute the long pass. How does the quarterback do this?

Our brains often prepare competing plans of action in parallel. In the case described above, the motor plan for the long pass needs to compete with and win over the faster, preloaded and over-learned short pass motor plan. In order for this to occur, the brain must be able to inhibit all potential movement plans until the best plan can be chosen given the current goals and circumstances. The brain achieves this by creating programmable movement gates. These gates help prevent the fastest plan (in this case the short pass) from always 'winning.' Gating of movement until a single winning plan emerges is also important to prevent 'blended' movements in which two or more motor plans are performed at the same time. In the case of the quarterback, this would result in the ball being thrown somewhere in between the two receivers, which is clearly not a desirable outcome. The organization of multiple parallel circuits through the basal ganglia, together with basal ganglia inhibition of the thalamus, serves to create a large number of programmable gates. Note that baseline firing rates of GPi (the internal segment of the globus pallidus) and SNr (substantia nigra, pars reticulata) are high, resulting in tonic inhibition of thalamic neurons. In other words, at baseline, the gates are closed.

Now imagine cortical plans of action sending excitatory projections to the striatum. Each plan activates striatal neurons in its own segregated circuit. These excited striatal neurons inhibit striatal neurons in other circuits (activated by alternative plans of action) by lateral inhibition (either directly or mediated by inhibitory interneurons) and, in this way, different plans of action can compete. At the same time, the active 'winning' plan's striatal neurons also inhibit the tonically active GPi neurons within its own circuit, causing a pause in their activity. This pause in the activity of GPi neurons releases the thalamic cells in the same circuit from inhibition. The transient excitation (i.e. disinhibition) of the thalamic cells provides an excitatory signal back to the area of frontal cortex that generated the winning plan – a kind of 'go' signal – allowing the plan to execute.

Please note that the above discussion is a simplification. For example, neurons that receive 'go' signals from the thalamus to execute a particular plan are in the same cortical area but in a different cortical *layer* than the neurons that generated the plan. (Recall that the cortex of a mammal has six layers.) For more details, refer to Brown et al. (2004).

Let's now consider each circuit in turn:

Motor Circuit

The **motor circuit** is involved in the planning, execution and inhibition of voluntary movements of the body. Disruptions at any level in this circuit lead to disorders of motor control such as those seen in clinical conditions like Parkinson's disease, where basal ganglia dysfunction results in excessive inhibition of movement called bradykinesia (slowed movement), which can be thought of as difficulty in opening movement gates, as well as inappropriate opening of movement gates, which causes tremor.

Oculomotor Circuit

The **oculomotor circuit** is involved in the planning and execution of voluntary eye movements. Disruptions at any level in this circuit interferes with the ability to voluntarily choose to look at a particular object or location while resisting the natural tendency to make eye movements to look at compelling distracters or competing objects. This circuit is also necessary to make eye movements to remembered locations.

Dorsolateral Prefrontal Cortex (Executive) Circuit

The **dorsolateral prefrontal cortex** is involved in many aspects of executive function including the ability to solve complex problems, plan ahead, focus and sustain attention, regulate actions according to task demands, and shift gears when task demands change. It also plays an important role in working memory: the ability to keep things in mind long enough to direct action, such as remembering a new phone number long enough to dial it. Patients with a disruption at any level of the dorsolateral prefrontal circuitry exhibit a classic 'dysexecutive' syndrome characterized by being concrete, perseverative, inattentive and disorganized, with poor memory search strategies, impaired reasoning and reduced mental flexibility (Tekin and Cummings, 2002). They are particularly impaired on the Stroop task in which a person must override the more automatic skill of reading words in order to name the color of the ink that the word is printed in. This becomes challenging because there is a conflict between the word itself and the color it is printed in. For example, when a subject sees the word 'RED' printed in large block letters in blue ink, the correct response is to say 'blue.' This requires the ability to suppress – or gate – the strong tendency to simply read the word, that is, to say 'red.'

Orbitofrontal Cortex (Social) Circuit

The **orbitofrontal cortex** "is the neocortical representation of the limbic system" (Bonelli and Cummings, 2007). The **orbitofrontal circuit** mediates empathic and socially appropriate behavior (Chow and Cummings, 1999) and may select objects and actions based on their subjective value (Dranias, 2008). Damage to this circuit results in behavioral disinhibition, emotional lability, poor judgment, and irresponsibility toward family and social obligations (Bonelli and Cummings, 2007). For example, a patient with damage to this area may not be able to apply social norms to prevent helping themselves to food from someone else's plate if they are hungry and the food is appealing. That is, the value of socially appropriate behavior is no longer biasing behavior, so more reflexive responses reflecting more basic drives (in this case eating when hungry) drives behavior.

Anterior Cingulate Cortex (Affect) Circuit

The **anterior cingulate cortex (ACC)** has different functional zones (Nee et al., 2011) that can be seen on the diagram of Central Midline Structures that appears at the beginning of the next section.

i) **Pre-** and **subgenual ACC (PACC)** is thought to be linked to emotional networks that activate when an error in performance has occurred. Brodmann area 25 is a part of PACC that has received particular attention by virtue of its consistent overactivity in depression. Remarkable remissions of severe, treatment-resistant depression have occurred when this abnormally high activity is disrupted by deep brain stimulation (DBS) (Mayberg et al., 2005; Holtzheimer and Mayberg, 2011). It is as if DBS to BA 25 'closes the gate' to overwhelming negative mood states. (See Dobbs, 2006, for a very readable history behind this intervention.) Neurofeedback combined with psychotherapy has also been shown to influence BA 25, and also other areas linked to depression (Paquette, 2009).

ii) A more dorsal area of ACC called the rostral cingulate zone (RCZ) or **supragenual ACC (SACC)** has an anterior portion involved in monitoring cognition to predict errors that suggest increased cognitive control is required (Brown and Braver, 2005). Such requisite increased vigilance or arousal might then be achieved through ACC projections to the brainstem **locus coeruleus (LC)** (Aston-Jones and Cohen, 2005) that, in turn, sends noradrenaline (NE) back to many areas of cortex. The increased noradrenaline available to cortical neurons is believed to sharpen their responsiveness to input and the widespread simultaneous changes in cortical neuron activity modulates cognitive performance. There is an inverted U-shaped relationship between tonic LC activity and performance on tasks that require focused attention. This means that poor performance occurs at both low (underaroused) and high (anxious) levels of tonic LC activity. Optimal performance occurs at moderate tonic LC activity, which allows for the largest phasic LC activations in response to goal-relevant stimuli (Aston-Jones and Cohen, 2005; please also see Sara and Bouret, 2012, for a recent review of LC effects on cognition). It is tempting to speculate that ACC/LC interactions play an important role in learning to self-regulate arousal and attention to meet task demands.

Large bilateral lesions to the ACC lead to akinetic mutism, which is seen as an awake but underaroused state of "profound apathy" (Bonelli and Cummings, 2007). Such patients rarely move or talk spontaneously and have limited or no response, even to direct questions and requests. They are indifferent to pain, thirst, or hunger. Thus neurosurgical lesions have occasionally been deliberately placed in the ACC of patients with severe, intractable pain. People with damage to the ACC circuit have also been reported to experience "a diminished ability to conceive new thoughts or participate in creative thought processes" (Chow and Cummings, 1999).

iii) The **posterior part of SACC** is more connected to motor networks and may be involved when uncertainty or conflict make appropriate response selection challenging (Nee et al., 2011). For example, in the go/no-go task, subjects may be asked to push a button (a 'go' trial) when they see the letter 'A' but to inhibit their response (a 'no-go' trial) when they see the letter 'B.' Usually subjects are exposed to more 'go' trials and develop a predisposition to respond (i.e. push the button) that must be inhibited in order to perform correctly on subsequent 'no-go' trials. In addition to the apathy syndrome described above, patients with ACC lesions typically perform poorly on this task.

Go vs. No-Go: Direct, Indirect and Hyperdirect Pathways

Note that the circuit diagrams above and much of the discussion so far has focused on the 'direct' pathway through the basal ganglia and how this generates 'go' signals. There is also an 'indirect' or 'no-go' pathway whose neurons inhibit direct pathway neurons (within the striatum) and also inhibit tonically active neurons of the external segment of the globus pallidus (GPe). The GPe tonically inhibits several structures but only its output to the **subthalamic nucleus (STN)** is illustrated below. Activation of the indirect path can therefore lead to increased activity in the STN (via disinhibition) while the 'hyperdirect' pathway activates the STN directly.

Increased STN activity can generate 'no-go' signals by sending glutaminergic *excitatory* inputs to the neurons of the GPi/SNr, thereby **enhancing thalamic inhibition**. Recall that the 'direct' path has the opposite effect on GPi/SNr: cortical signals transmit through the striatum to transiently *inhibit* GPi/SNr cells, resulting in transient disinhibition of the thalamus. The opposing effects of direct 'go' and indirect and hyperdirect 'no-go' pathways on the GPi/SNr are shown below.

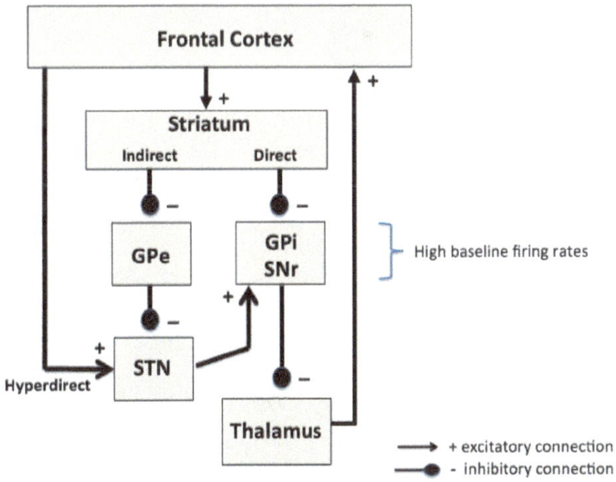

*Simplified frontal-subcortical circuits illustrating selected aspects of the direct, indirect, and hyperdirect paths. Activation of striatal neurons in the '**direct**' pathway leads to inhibition of neurons in the internal segment of the globus pallidus (GPi) and substantia nigra pars reticulata (SNr). Activation of striatal neurons in the '**indirect**' path leads to inhibition of tonic activity in the external segment of the globus pallidus (GPe). This inhibition of GPe disinhibits the subthalamic nucleus (STN), which then provides an excitatory drive to the GPi/SNr. The frontal cortex can also excite STN cells directly via the '**hyperdirect**' pathway.*

By adding extra excitatory drive to the GPi/SNr neurons, high STN activity opposes and sometimes even overcomes the direct pathway's inhibition of the GPi/SNr. In this way, STN activity can slow down, and may even prevent the direct pathway's disinhibition of the thalamus, thereby disrupting the transmission of a 'go' signal back to the cortex.

Indeed, abnormally high STN activity is seen in Parkinson's disease (PD) and contributes to the slowed movement that is seen in this disease. In fact, knowledge of this circuitry led to the development of neurosurgical techniques, including deep brain stimulation (DBS) of the STN, to specifically disrupt these pathologically strong 'no-go' signals in PD.

In normal functioning, 'no-go' signals are important to interrupt behavior when new information, such as a new goal or target, becomes available. Consider once again the example of the quarterback who has called for a short pass and is in the beginning stages of executing the motor program to make this pass. This means that the short pass motor program has already 'won' in the direct path of the striatum. However, if at the last moment he notices a wide receiver with excellent field position, 'no-go' mechanisms can intervene and interrupt the already selected motor program.

One 'no-go' mechanism that may be particularly relevant to behavioral interruption and task switching involves strong projections from the thalamus to the striatum. Neurons of the centromedian-parafascicular complex (CM/Pf) of the thalamus are activated by unexpected salient stimuli, and project to striatal cholinergic interneurons. Activation of these striatal cholinergic interneurons (known as tonically active neurons or TANs) transiently produces increased outflow of the indirect pathway and decreased outflow of direct pathway. This shift in processing to favor the indirect path's output results in the interruption of the current motor program and transient movement suppression (Minamimoto, 2008; Ding, 2010; Tan and Bullock, 2008, Smith, 2011). Following this, a new competition in the direct pathway of the striatum can be initiated. In this new striatal competition, the high reward possibility of the long pass can outcompete the short pass, 'win' and be executed.

In addition to (i) task switching and (ii) interruption of ongoing behavior, indirect and hyperdirect pathways are thought to play important roles in (iii) delaying voluntary action, (iv) locking out competing responses to allow a selected program to fully execute, (v) inhibiting motor programs once they have been executed in order to prevent perseveration, and (vi) shifting to the next motor program in a smooth sequence of action. These last two roles are explicitly incorporated in a computational model of speech production that, when 'lesioned' (by abnormally high levels of dopamine in the striatum or by specific and localized white matter abnormalities), reproduces many features of stuttering (Civier et. al, 2013).

Shifts in the relative activation of direct, indirect, and hyperdirect pathways are also thought to affect speed vs. accuracy trade-offs, a long-observed phenomenon in behavior whereby forcing quicker decisions can lead to a loss of accuracy, whereas emphasizing accuracy in decision-making can lead to slower responses (see Bogacz, 2010, for review).

Note that increased dopamine in the striatum increases activity in the direct path (via excitatory D1 receptors on striatal neurons in the direct path) and decreases activity in the indirect path (via inhibitory D2 receptors on striatal neurons in the indirect path). The net effect favors direct over indirect pathways. In this way, dopamine release into the striatum can speed performance. But too much dopamine can also produce aberrant performance. (See Civier, 2013, for an example.)

Mechanisms that favor the indirect and hyperdirect pathways over the direct pathway have the opposite effect and can slow performance. Consider the example of increased activation of GPi/SNr by the STN. The more active GPi/SNr neurons would then require stronger-than-typical outputs from the direct pathway to become inhibited (in order to disinhibit the thalamus and generate a 'go' signal back to cortex). The extra time it takes to generate this stronger–than-typical direct pathway output results in slower performance. At the same time, this delay gives selection mechanisms within the striatum more time to operate and allows later arriving or initially weaker inputs a better chance to compete and grow in activity than they otherwise would have, if quick responses were demanded.

Consider once again the Stroop task, where faster reading of words competes with the slower process of naming the color of the ink that the word is printed in, especially when there is a conflict between the word itself and the color of its ink. When we view the word 'RED' printed in large block letters in blue ink, two potential verbal responses are prepared in cortex and send competing bids to striatum. Because the pathway for reading words is overlearned, it is faster, and so the verbal plan for 'red' is generated more quickly, going on to quickly activate striatal output neurons in the direct path. If at this point these striatal neurons are active enough to inhibit GPi/SNr activity, then a 'go' signal will be sent back to cortex and an incorrect response to the task will have been made since the person will say 'red.'

On the other hand, if STN excitatory drive increases GPi/SNr activity, then a higher activity level is required of striatal neurons to generate a 'go' signal; the initial activity level of striatal neurons in the 'red' direct pathway won't be sufficient. In this way the higher GPi/SNr activity level has set a higher 'response threshold' that prevents the impulsive response 'red,' and gives the later-arriving striatal bid from the verbal plan for 'blue' a chance to compete.

Note that the task demand – in this case the instruction to report the color – is likely encoded in lateral prefrontal cortex. As long as this task demand is kept 'in mind' and active, it can provide contextual signals to bias cortical and striatal competitions towards the correct 'blue' verbal response. To summarize, correct performance on the Stroop task requires at least three elements: a high enough response threshold to prevent fast but incorrect responses, the ability to keep task demands in mind, and enough time to allow task demands to help grow the slow but correct response to a high enough activity level to win cortical and striatal competitions.

Recall from the previous description of the anterior cingulate cortex (ACC) that it is involved in performance monitoring and predicting when errors are likely to occur. These roles led Frank (2006) to propose that ACC inputs to STN could be a mechanism for increasing response thresholds when errors are more likely, resulting, as we have seen, in slower but more accurate responses. While this hyperdirect pathway hypothesis is currently an influential model, other 'no-go' mechanisms such as the previously described centromedian-parafascicular complex (CM/Pf) thalamostriatal pathway may prove to be even more relevant.

Relevance of These Pathways to SMR Production

At this point, it is interesting to consider the possibility that the sensorimotor rhythm (SMR) arises from a basal ganglia 'no-go' state and that SMR training enhances the ability to voluntarily shift into this 'no-go' state. This is consistent with findings (see Sterman and Thompson, 2014, for review) that SMR is associated with immobility and was originally observed when cats needed to inhibit a previously rewarded response. The finding by Boulay et al. (2011) that reaction time tracked SMR production in a go/no-go task (i.e. longer reaction times during high SMR production and shorter reaction times during low SMR production) are exactly what would be predicted by 'no-go' and 'go' modes of basal ganglia functioning respectively. The proposal that SMR is produced by a 'no-go' state is also consistent with the observation of increased fMRI activity in the striatum during SMR production (Birbaumer, unpublished results reported in Sterman and Thompson, 2014), and after successful SMR training, while performing a Stroop task (Levesque et al., 2005). Because the striatum is known as a 'silent structure' due to the low percentage of neurons active at any time, it is likely that these fMRI findings reflect 'no-go' inhibitory mechanisms, which are more likely to be synchronous and extend over larger areas (Bullock et al., 2009) compared to more focal 'go' pathways.

The view that SMR training might actually be striatal 'no-go' training is also consistent with what is already known about mechanisms underlying SMR generation. The rhythm itself arises from interactions between two populations of neurons within the thalamus: inhibitory neurons in the thalamic reticular nucleus (nRT) and excitatory thalamocortical neurons in the ventrobasal (VB) complex.

A crucial property of thalamic neurons that underlies their role in generating a wide variety of cortical rhythms is that, when they are inhibited strongly enough, they move from tonic activity to a bursting mode of firing. In the case of SMR, strong enough inhibition of neurons in VB causes them to become hyperpolarized. They recover from hyperpolarization with a burst of activity that excites nearby nRT neurons. The excited nRT neurons then reciprocate by inhibiting the VB neurons that excited them. This will once again hyperpolarize the VB neurons and the cycle will repeat. In this way, alternating bursts of activity continue between these two thalamic nuclei. Because VB also sends excitatory projections to primary somatosensory cortex (S1), the oscillatory activity in VB results in oscillatory activity in S1, detectable by EEG.

The thalamocortical oscillations that underlie SMR have been known for some time. What has been less clear is what might initiate the process during voluntary SMR production. Given that behavioral correlates of SMR are consistent with 'no-go' activity in the basal ganglia, it is interesting to note that GPe, the main output of the 'no go' indirect path, projects to nRT (Bullock, 2009). At baseline, GPe provides tonic inhibition to nRT. However, in the 'no-go' state, the indirect pathway's output would inhibit GPe neurons, thereby *disinhibiting* neurons in the nRT. The resulting increased activity in nRT could then initiate the oscillatory process described above (i.e., by inhibiting VB neurons enough to trigger their bursting.)

Same Frontal-Subcortical Circuits, Emphasis on Open-Loop Integration

Understanding how the brain learns to select and enact the most adaptive behavioral plan given the circumstances will certainly involve understanding the flow of activity through frontal-subcortical circuitry. Potential cognitive and other action plans are generated in frontal areas that are part of the closed loops that are emphasized in the original circuit diagrams shown previously. The loop is 'closed' when thalamic projections carry the 'go' signal back to the originating frontal area. The 'open loop' contributions to each circuit can be thought of as carrying contextual information. These circuits are sometimes drawn with equal emphasis on the closed and open loops to highlight how the basal ganglia can coordinate wide areas of cortex in the service of a particular task.

A Motor Network

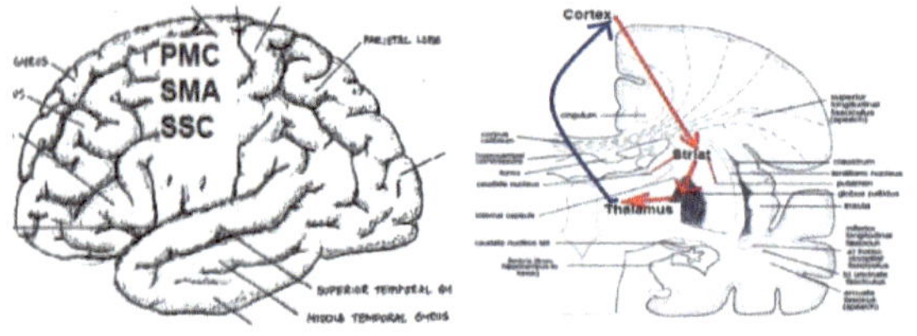

Motor plans from supplementary motor cortex join with motor state information from primary motor and somatosensory cortex in the putamen, then 'winner' outputs to internal GP/substantia nigra, pars reticulata, then to ventrolateral *and* ventroanterior *thalamus, then back to supplementary motor cortex.*

For example, in the motor network, note that supplementary motor cortical plans (BAs 6,8) join with information on the current state of the motor system provided by arcuate premotor (BA 8), primary motor (BA 4) and sensorimotor (BAs 3,1,2) cortices to select the best action, taking into account the current motor state. Neurons from all these functionally related cortical areas will project to partially overlapping populations of **striatal medium spiny neurons** (**MSNs**) in the putamen. Here it is important to recognize that there is a clear funneling of inputs from a large number of cortical neurons to a much smaller number of MSNs. In fact, each MSN is estimated to receive approximately 10,000 afferent inputs from different areas of cortex (Lawrence, 1998).

The forced intermingling of inputs from different cortical areas on the same MSN makes MSNs well suited to be pattern classifiers that can come to learn – through previous reinforcement learning – what plan, given the detailed information about the current context (from both closed- and open-loop areas) is most likely to be successful and rewarded in the present moment. The MSN that receives the best *combination* of plan, context, and goals will be the most active, resulting in the execution of the plan that activated it (by the flow in the circuit through GPi and thalamus as described previously). At the same time, its high activity will lead to the inhibition of other MSNs (through lateral inhibition), ensuring that competing plans that are not as well suited to the current situation are not performed.

A Spatial Network

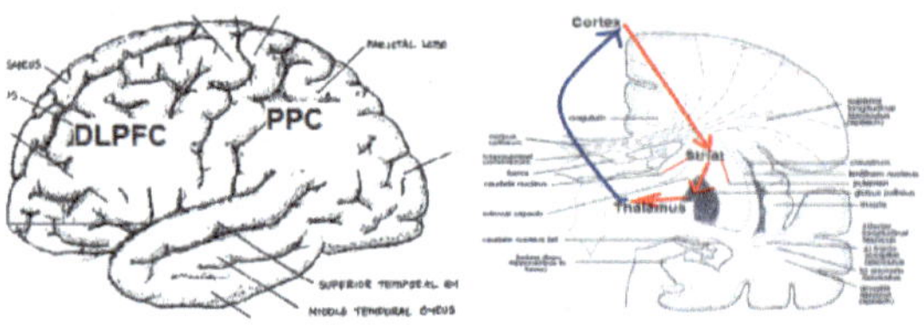

Spatial information goes from posterior parietal and dorsolateral prefrontal to head of caudate to internal GP/substantia nigra, pars reticulata, then to ventro-anterior and mediodorsal thalamus, back to cortex.

Lawrence et al. (1998) modified the original circuits in a way that highlights distinct parts of the lateral prefrontal cortex. The more dorsal part, referred to as **dorsolateral prefrontal cortex** (**DLPFC**) consists of BA 9, and the dorsal aspects of BAs 10 and 46. The DLPFC circuit receives spatial information from **posterior parietal cortex** (**PPC** BA 7) and is known to be involved in spatial working memory, such as the ability to hold a particular location in mind when the cue for that location disappears. Note that PPC is part of the 'where' visual stream. (The 'what' visual stream is more ventral and includes the ventro-lateral prestriate cortex (parts of BAs 18, 19) and the inferior temporal cortex.)

More ventral parts of BAs 10 and 46 are referred to as **ventrolateral prefrontal cortex** (**VLPFC**). This circuit receives object information from **inferior** and **superior temporal gyri** (**IT** BA 20 and **ST** BA 22), and is involved in working memory for objects. Note that this is part of the 'what' visual stream involved in object recognition.

A Visual Network

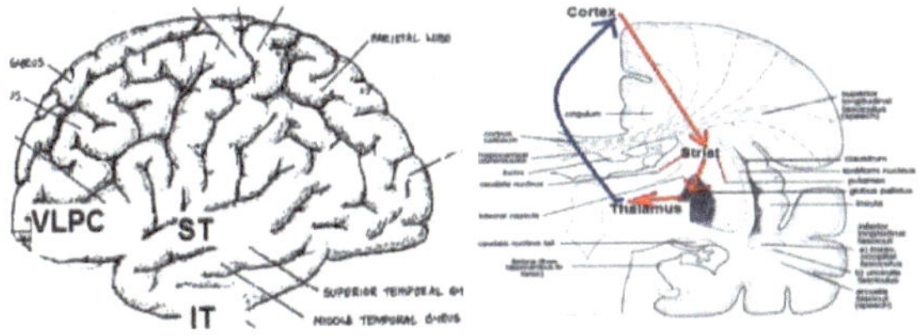

Visual information from inferior and superior temporal joins ventrolateral *prefrontal inputs in* tail *of caudate, then 'winner' outputs to internal GP/substantia nigra, pars reticulata, then to ventroanterior and mediodorsal thalamus, then back to VLPC.*

Lawrence et al. (1998) also modified the original circuits by separating the lateral prefrontal cortex into the VLPFC described above and the **orbitofrontal cortex (OFC)**. They then combined orbitofrontal and **anterior cingulate** cortices into one 'Affect Network' and added known, important contributions from the **amygdala** to the **hippocampal** and **entorhinal** inputs to this network.

Affect Network

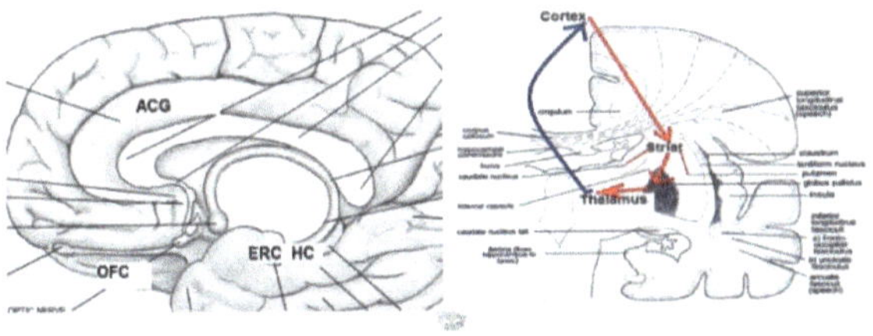

Affective information from orbitofrontal and anterior cingulate joins information from hippocampus, entorhinal and amygdala in nucleus accumbens, then 'winner' outputs to ventral pallidum to medial dorsal thalamus, then back to orbitofrontal and anterior cingulate to regulate mood and emotional reactions.

Drawings by Amanda Reeves, modified from Kropotov, 2009 and Lawrence et al., 1998.

Affect Network: Affect Information Flow

In simplest terms, information related to 'affect' or emotion may traverse from the orbital frontal cortex (OFC), medial frontal cortex, anterior cingulate gyrus (ACG), hippocampus (HC), amygdala, and entorhinal cortex (ERC)/uncus area to the basal ganglia, including the nucleus accumbens and ventral pallidum. From there, signals go to specific functionally related areas of the thalamus, such as the medial dorsal and anterior nuclei of the thalamus. The thalamus then connects back to areas of the cortex including the anterior cingulate, which has functions related to control of the Affect network. The result is regulation of mood and emotional reactions (after Kropotov, 2009).

The orbital and medial prefrontal cortices as well as the amygdala are key areas for understanding anxiety (Davidson, 2002; Thayer, 2012), as is the anterior cingulate cortex (Matthews et al., 2004). The anterior cingulate involvement in depression was described earlier.

Also described earlier in the separate sections on the orbitofrontal and anterior cingulate circuits, other functions of this network include: 1) the selection of goals (objects and actions) on the basis of their subjective value, and 2) the monitoring of error likelihood in order to increase arousal and vigilance to better match challenging task demands.

Concluding Remarks

In summary, when cortical-basal ganglia-thalamocortical circuits are functioning properly, the best cognitive or behavioral plan, given the current context, previous learning, and current goals, will be selected with the aid of the basal ganglia. As we have seen, the basal ganglia coordinate wide areas of cortex into functional networks. When not operating properly, the current context and goals have less influence, and overlearned, reactive responses may dominate. 'Gating' mechanisms slow down prepotent responses to allow potentially better plans a chance to be selected. Complex interactions within the basal ganglia together with the structure of 'go' and 'no-go' pathways create many opportunities to select, interrupt, and otherwise control behavior in real time.

Central Midline Structures (CMS): An Anatomical and Functional Unit

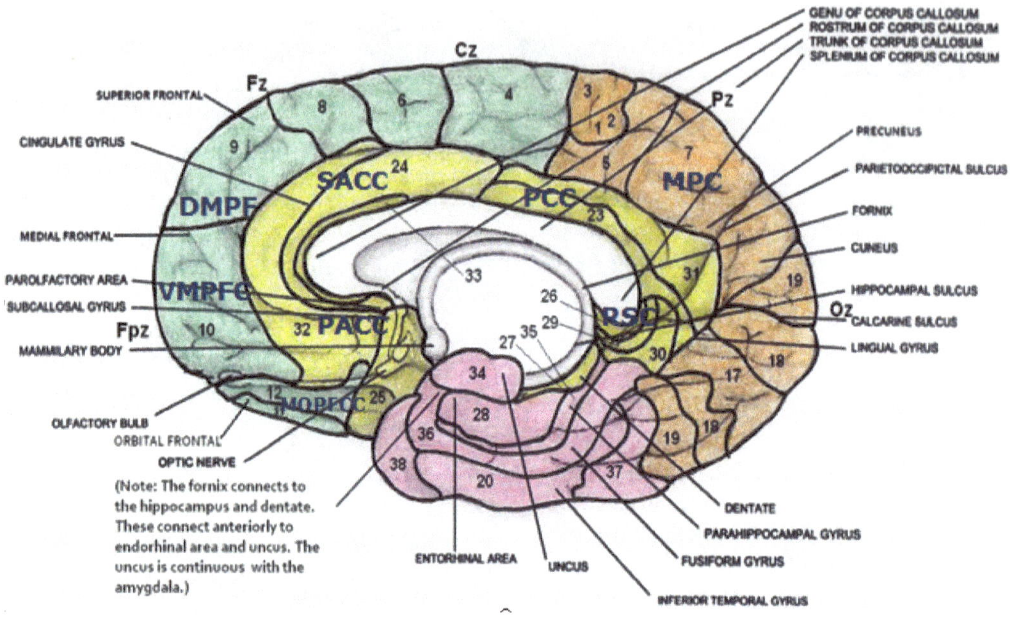

Central midline structures in BOLD (after Northoff, 2006). We superimposed bold letter abbreviations in the above figure to indicate areas that are considered to be important central midline structures. We suggest that one should also include in discussions of CMS, in both hemispheres, the hippocampus, the entorhinal-uncus area, and the insula.

***SACC** = supragenual anterior cingulate cortex (BAs 24, 32)* ***DMPFC** = dorsomedial prefrontal cortex (BA 9)*
***MPC** = medial parietal cortex (BAs 7, 31)* ***PCC** = posterior cingulate cortex (BAs 23, 31)*
***RSC** = retrosplenial cortex (BAs 26, 29, 30)*
***MOPFC** = medial orbital prefrontal cortex (BAs 11, 12);*
***VMPFC** = ventromedial prefrontal cortex (BAs 10, 11);*
***PACC** = pre- and subgenual anterior cingulate cortex (BAs 24, 25, 32);*

CMS areas are involved to different degrees in all the major neural network systems: **Affect, Executive, Salience, and Default**. They are vital structures in our understanding of most human behavior.

Neural Foundation of a Sense of 'Self'

Central midline structures are involved in our sensing of who and where we are, both with respect to how we relate to others and with respect to how our body relates to the space around it. It has been stated that patients with lesions in ventral CMS are unable to develop a coherent model of their own self (Damasio, 1999). Damasio noted that lesions that compromise the ability to **experience emotional feelings** and to sense the body are often located on the right side of the somatosensory complex and involve, in particular, the **right insula**. These patients have a compromised **sense of self**. He notes that activity at the level of the parabrachial nucleus (PBN), the **nucleus tractus solitarius (NTS)** and the hypothalamus may be important in establishing a sense of self. (The PBN and NTS structures are discussed later in detail under Heart Rate Variability training.) The NTS and the PBN convey information to the right insula via the ventral-medial nucleus of the thalamus, and some sense of self may emerge at this level. The insula connects to the anterior cingulate cortex and the medial frontal cortex. These areas are also all key structures in the Affect network. Damasio concludes that all of these structures and connections are the **neural foundation for the self,** the grounding of the material 'me' (Damasio, 2003).

Default and Salience Networks

The Executive, Attention, and Affect (Emotional) networks are quite well known, and functions related to these networks will be described when Brodmann areas that relate to their functions are discussed in Part II. Two more recently delineated networks, the Default and the Salience networks, deserve some additional comment here.

Default Network

When nothing is consciously going on, your brain is still active. Your thoughts may include: **insight, imagination, judgment, thoughts about self and self in relation to others**, as well as autobiographical memory. The Default network plays a vital role in forming a sense of identity, self-concept, self-perception, and, more broadly, one's concepts of social and family systems. This **self-reflection** activity is one important aspect of homeostasis within the brain – the set-point to which brain function returns after being engaged in other mental activity.

Aspects of the Default network are laid down in infancy and thus can be significantly **damaged by negative emotional experiences in early childhood.** Its connections with all the key areas involved in the Affect network mean that early negative experiences can be expected to have major effects on self-concept and emotions in later life. This is particularly true due to the fact that, to the infant, the mother (or the mothering-figure) is the universe (Thompson & Patterson, 1986). Any disruption in this relationship will alter the psychosocial development of the child (McCrone, 2002).

Anatomy of the Default Network

The **Default network** comprises a number of central midline structures including the ventral-medial prefrontal cortex, anterior cingulate cortex and, for spatial self-reference, lateral parietal cortex, cuneus and precuneus, and the posterior cingulate. All of these areas are concerned with understanding and constant monitoring of *self and self in relation to others (*Supekar et al., 2010*)*. Thus the Default network is involved in self-referential processing and understanding others' intentions. These functions are important in our work with autism spectrum disorders (ASD). Remember that the Default network becomes active when the brain is not engaged in specific cognitive or motor tasks.

The **Default-mode network** (DMN) includes the dorsal and ventral medial prefrontal cortex (dMPFC and vMPFC; Brodmann areas (BAs) 10, 9, 32, and 24), the posterior cingulate cortex (PCC, BAs 23/31), retrosplenial cortex (RSC, BAs 29/30), and the lateral posterior cortex (LP, BAs 39/40) (Buckner et al., 2008; Fox et al., 2005; Greicius et al., 2003; Gusnard and Raichle, 2001; Raichle et al., 2001).

The Default network also has **connections to Mirror Neuron areas** and these are critical in forming a concept of self and self-in-the-world. Using fMRI, regions can be observed to become active (light up) in the medial orbital and medial prefrontal areas and in medial parietal areas when activities related to the Default network are involved. Thus these areas and functions are subsumed under the term 'Default Network' (Raichle, 2010). The posterior cingulate and subgenual cingulate areas may be involved in depressive ruminating (Berman et al., 2011).

The Default network has been divided into dorsal and ventral areas, but here we are treating it as a single functional unit. In very general terms, one can say that when executive and/or motor networks are active, the Default network is turned off. The opposite is true when executive cognitive functions or motor functions are turned off. In that situation, the Default network is active.

It is thought that the Default network may not be functioning normally in people with autism spectrum disorders.

The Salience Network

The frontal lobes are also important in determining the 'salience' of information; that is, deciding what incoming information is relevant or important. The Salience network (Seeley, 2007) includes the dorsal and anterior cingulate gyrus (BAs 24 and 25), insula, middle superior frontal area, and the para-central area (BAs 4, 5, 6), subcallosal gyrus, entorhinal area (BA 28) and uncus (BA 34), parahippocampal gyrus (BA 27), hippocampus (BA 35) and fusiform gyrus (BA 36). As with other networks, it is apparent that we cannot isolate a function to a single area or lobe of the brain. We must think more in terms of how areas function together in a network that subsumes a particular function. Clearly one would expect overlap with memory areas as well as areas involved in emotions and sense of self when determining relevance.

The right dorsal anterior cingulate cortex (dACC) and the right insula **may together act as a switch** between the frontal-parietal Executive network and the Default network when determining salience (Sridharan et al., 2008). It is also apparent that the ACC will switch between the Affect network and the Executive network when executive tasks are activated, such as when there is a task demanding divided attention (Devinsky et al., 1995).

However, there are always **other networks that subsume similar functions** but in a different context. This is clearly true for determining 'salience.' An example is a salience map (or network) to rank items in the visual field for locus of attention (Bisley, 2006). In this Salience network, the lateral intra-parietal area (LIP) connects to the frontal eye field (FEF) (as does the upper auditory cortex), superior colliculus, pulvinar nucleus, and inferior temporal area (BA 20) (visual pattern recognition). This network determines the significance (salience) of new visual information.

The Salience Network (in more detail)
The following discussion is repeated in the section in the second edition of *The Neurofeedback Book* on **Attention Networks**. Salience combined with parietal, cingulate, and frontal functions, particularly in the right hemisphere for sustained attention, are **major components of attention networking.**

When discussing choosing the 'salience' of new information, regardless of whether it is from internal or external sources, more emphasis should be placed on the role of the anterior portion of the insula and the anterior cingulate gyrus than is done in Bisley's description of visual salience determination. As stated by Menon & Uddin (2010) in their review article "Saliency, switching, attention and control: a network model of insula function." (*Brain Struct Funct,* 214, 655–667): "The anterior **insula is an integral hub** in mediating dynamic interactions between other large-scale brain networks involved in externally oriented attention and internally oriented or self-related cognition." These authors postulate that the **insula is sensitive to salient events,** and that: "Its core function is to mark such events for additional processing and initiate appropriate control signals." These authors reinforce the now-accepted view that the **anterior insula and the anterior cingulate cortex are the major elements in a Salience network.** This network functions to segregate the most relevant among internal and extra-personal stimuli in order to guide behavior. They consider the anterior insula (AI) to be the hub of the salience network. This is particularly important in our work where we combine NFB with HRV and where we have observed that many of our patients who have suffered a traumatic brain injury (TBI), have an anxiety disorder, or have a diagnosis of Autism Spectrum Disorder (ASD) show the left and/or right insula to be outside the database norms. For example, hyperactivity of the right insula might correlate with misinterpretation of the salience of mundane events and lead to anxiety. On the other hand, hypoactivity in ASDs might correlate with a lack of attention to social communication.

In the figure below, the reader can understand that a bottom-up salient event is detected by the anterior insula and ACC. The insula is particularly sensitive to salient events. The insula can then communicate important events to other networks, including those for sustaining attention, executive/cognition, working memory functions and the affect networks. With the posterior insula it will regulate the autonomic nervous system and this will have an effect on HRV and other autonomic nervous system (ANS) functions through connections to the amygdala, locus coeruleus, and the hypothalamus. Thus the **insula is a key link** between incoming bottom-up stimuli and the brain regions such as the ACC that are involved in monitoring this information.

Cognitively demanding tasks have the effect of decreasing activity in areas of the brain that we have previously described as being within the Default network while increasing activity in executive networks. The central executive network (CEN) includes the dorsolateral prefrontal cortex (DLPFC), and the posterior parietal cortex (PPC). The default mode network (DMN) includes the ventromedial prefrontal cortex (VMPFC), posterior cingulate cortex (PCC), medial temporal region, and the angular gyrus. The CEN is important for working memory, and for judgment and decision-making for goal-directed behavior.

The PCC is involved in self-referential thinking and autobiographical memory (Buchner et al., 2008), and the VMPC is important in thinking about self and others (Amodo & Frith, 2006).

The diagram below may assist the reader in picturing Salience network major functions.

This diagram emphasizes the central importance of the Salience network in the dynamic switching between activity generated by the central Executive network (CEN) and the internal self referential activity of the Default mode network (DMN). Menon and Uddin suggest that the Salience network can be conceptualized as having a hierarchy of salience filters that can amplify inputs to different degrees. There are direct connections between the intraparietal sulcus and the insula, and this may be one important link for determining the salience of incoming sensory stimuli.

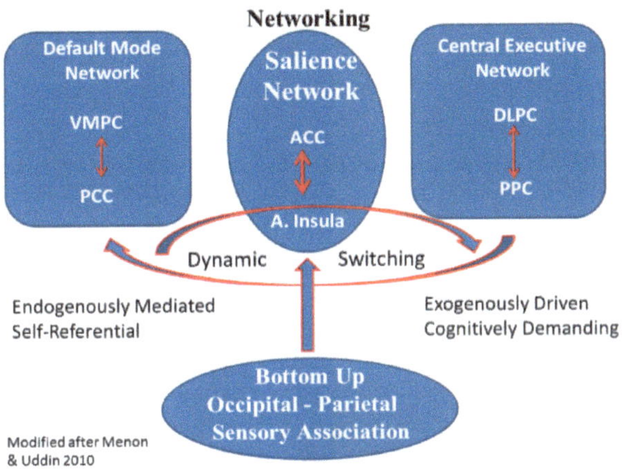

Illustration of major Salience Network connections. VMPC = Ventral Medial Prefrontal Cortex; PCC = Posterior Cingulate Cortex; ACC = Anterior Cingulate Cortex; A. Insula = Anterior Insula; DLPC = Dorsolateral Prefrontal Cortex; PPC = Posterior Parietal Cortex

Why Training at Central Sites Affects 'Networks'

Surface Sites Fz, Cz, Pz, and/or at Deeper Central Midline Structures

The behavioral changes of the client appear to correlate with the client's mental state when doing the NFB with the electrode on a central site; that is, at or between Fz-Cz-Pz. (Cz is the most common single-channel placement for children and FCz the most common site used in adults.) For example, if the patient is doing part of their training on task, and they are using a metacognitive strategy to accomplish the task across a number of sessions, then **the changes that will be reinforced should include** functions associated with the Executive network that is involved in that task. In fact, we do measure marked changes occurring in academics, attention, and IQ measurements. Changes in executive functions have been confirmed in large case series by objective testing done before and after 40 sessions, and can be reviewed in publications by a number of researchers and clinicians. Increases in Full Scale IQ scores of about 10 standard score points, for example, have been reported in four different studies (Linden, 1996; Lubar, 1995; Thompson & Thompson, 1998, 2010).

More about Networks
The thalamo-cortical-basal ganglia loops and connections delineated above underlie our hypothesis regarding how training over the central midline structures (CMS), especially when combined with heart rate variability training, may have such profound effects on complex networks that involve functions related to Affect, Executive, Motor, Salience, and Default networks. When you re-train those loops, it is like re-setting the pacemaker in the brain. Jim Robbin's got the analogy right when he wrote *A Symphony in the Brain.* The thalamus is like the conductor, deciding which sections of the brain are needed for a particular task, how loudly each one should play, and how they interact. It may also be a reason why coherence and phase training, which influence thalamic outputs and cortical communications, may become increasingly important in EEG biofeedback.

Importance of Heart Rate Variability (HRV) Training – Connections to Nucleus of the Solitary Tract in the Brain Stem

The Affect network that we have discussed in the cortex is also connected to important structures in the brainstem, such as the locus coeruleus in the pons and the nucleus of the solitary tract (NST) in the medulla. (You may also see the Latin, *nucleus tractus solitarius* or NTS in some texts.) The NST receives direct afferents from the aortic and carotid baroreceptors. This is one reason why heart rate variability (HRV) training may have such a profound effect on the Affect network and, in particular, on controlling anxiety. HRV, however, is covered in some detail its own section and, therefore, it will not be described here. We mention it to underscore the great importance of combining HRV training with training using NFB. The combination allows you to influence the same structures from two different directions, hitting both afferent and efferent connections. Recall that afferents go *to* the CNS (prefix from the Latin preposition *ad*) and efferents come *from* the CNS (prefix from the Latin preposition *ex*.)

The next two figures are given to help orient the reader to structures that may help the reader to understand why NFB and HRV trainng can act synergistically to improve patient functioning.

The reader can find a description of these important connections in the section of *The Neurofeedback Book* on heart rate variability training.

Brainstem, Pons, Midbrain, and Basal Ganglia-Thalamic Regions.

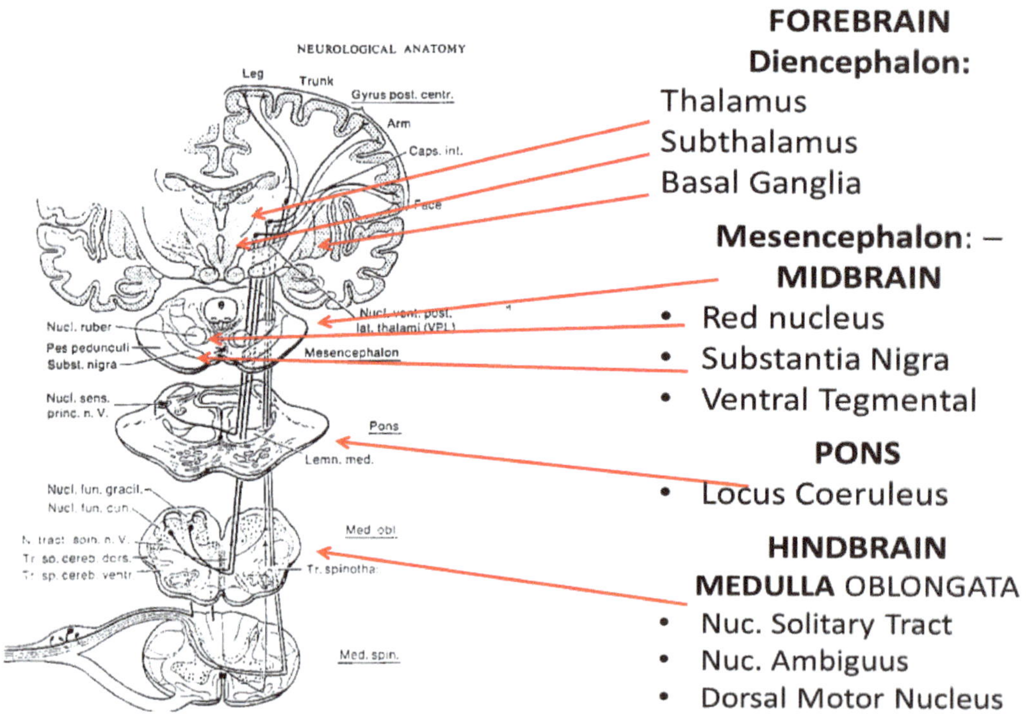

Modified after Smith 1962 (slightly modified from Rasmussen 1932).The above figure is given to help the reader get oriented with respect to the brainstem, pons, midbrain, and the basal ganglia-thalamic regions.

Heart – Brain Connections

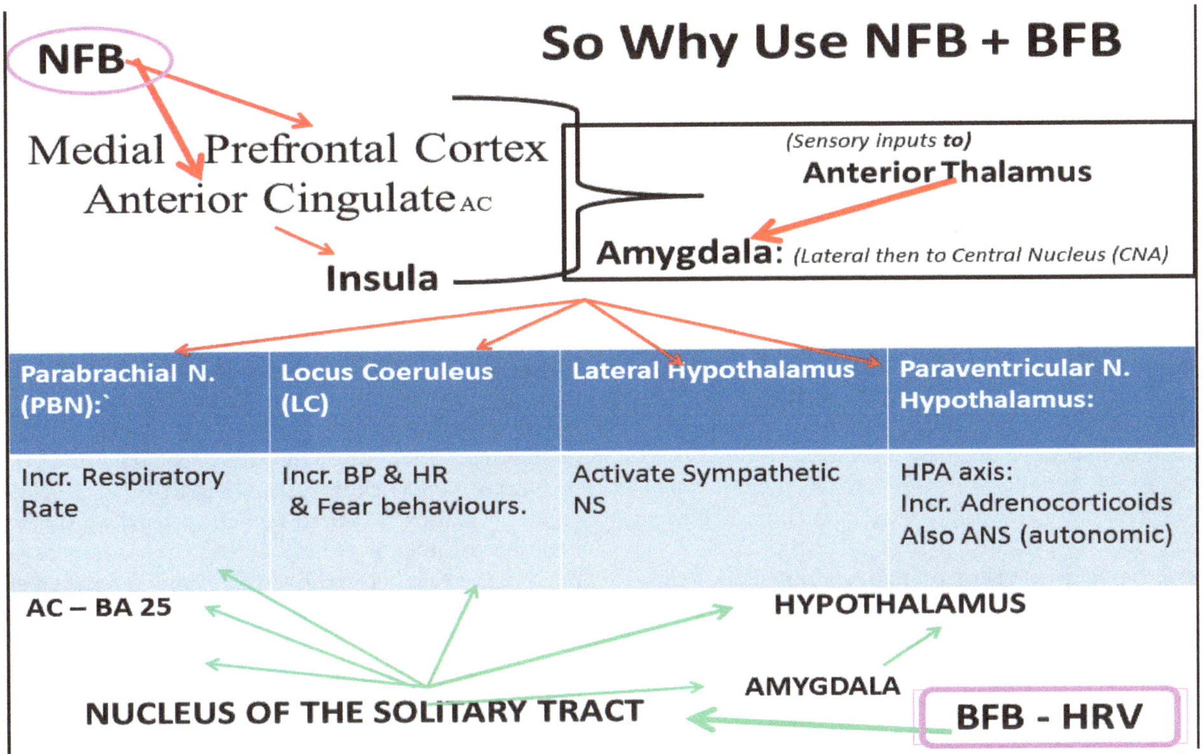

Figure: This figure illustrates how NFB applied as training from the 'top-down,' and HRV given as training from the 'bottom-up' can both affect the same central structures. (Note that our use of the terms 'top-down' and 'bottom-up,' for the past 20 years, is different from the more recent use of these terms in cognitive psychology, economics, and other disciplines. Indeed, in other areas of this book we have used these terms differently when describing parietal sensory bottom-up versus frontal modulation top-down when illustrating the salience network.)

Brodmann Areas and Networks

Brodmann Areas and Networks

Our working definition of a ***network***, for purposes of doing neurofeedback (NFB) and biofeedback (BFB), is **a 'net' of interconnected, functionally related groups of neurons.** In the cortex, these 'groups of neurons,' for convenience of thinking about cortical functions, may be broadly viewed as corresponding to Brodmann areas. Brodmann posited that if the cytoarchitecture of cells is the same, then the function must be the same. This is called a 'structure-function' point of view and is summarized as 'structure dictates function.'

As previously noted, the functions that will be listed in this book for each BA emphasize just the principle functions for that area, but remember that each function also involves many other areas. The reader is asked to understand that our emphasis in training has, accordingly, moved from being primarily concerned with functions at individual Brodmann area sites to an emphasis on training networks that involve a number of Brodmann areas, plus cortical connections to subcortical structures.

Phase-Reset

Thatcher argues that **when different functional systems are working together they are 'phase-locked.' Coherence is a measure of phase-locked activity.** Phase-locked areas produce a relatively high amplitude and synchrony of EEG activity. When there is a shift in task, there is a shift in the sets of neurons involved. This shift involves cortex-thalamus-cortex linkages. The **'shift' will recruit a different set of neurons** that then become phase-locked. During this change-over, called a 'phase-shift' (or **'phase-reset'**), the EEG amplitude drops and there is 'asynchrony.' In this book we use the rather simple overview term 'network' to refer to a set of sometimes distant cortical areas that are functionally connected and interrelated. Thatcher notes that phase shift and phase lock in the coordination of large masses of neurons in functional modules and hubs is what gives rise to the variations in the electroencephalogram (Thatcher, 2012, p 329).

Cortical Connectivity – Modules, Hubs and Nodes Maximize Efficiency

Robert Thatcher has noted that the brain is organized into a relatively small subset of modules or hubs that represent clusters of neurons with **high within-cluster connectivity and sparse long distance connectivity**. This means that there are fewer long distance links for each neuron, which **maximizes the efficiency** of the brain (Buzsaki, 2006; Thatcher, 2012, p305). In routine clinical work, we do not often use the more complex terms such as 'functional modules' (Achard et al., 2006; Hagmann et al., 2008; Thatcher, 2012) or 'node,' though others speak of a **network being a number of nodes connected by links** (Bullmore, Ed & Olaf Sporns, 2012; Thatcher 2012). For our work with NFB, it is sufficient to understand that if one has an effect on a central point within a functional neural network, one will have a reasonable probability of affecting that entire functional network, even though some of the areas within that network are in distant areas of the cortex. We have used this as an argument to explain the positive effects of NFB done over the FCz site on Affect and Executive networks, as seen in the changes in functioning of clients who have symptoms of Asperger's and autism (Thompson and Thompson, 2010).

Nevertheless, because the reader will find the terms 'module,' 'hub,' and 'node' appearing in the literature, we will briefly explain these terms with diagrams. To do this we have used information gleaned from the publication by Patric Hagmann, Leila Cammoun, Xavier Gigandet, Reto Meuli, Christopher J. Honey, Van J. Wedeen, and Olaf Sporns (July, 2008). This was a major cooperative effort between University of Lausanne in Switzerland and the University of Indiana, along with Harvard Medical School, in the USA. We recommend that our readers consult the original paper for more details. These authors made a comprehensive analysis of cortical connectivity. They state: "In the human brain, neural activation patterns are shaped by the underlying structural connections that form a dense network of fiber pathways linking all regions of the cerebral cortex." These authors used diffusion imaging techniques, which allowed the noninvasive mapping of fiber pathways. They **constructed connection maps** covering the entire cortical surface.

Computational analyses of the resulting complex brain network revealed regions of the cortex that were highly connected and highly central. These areas form a structural core of the human brain. They note that key components of this core are portions of posterior medial cortex that are known to be activated when the brain is not engaged in a cognitively demanding task. We have referred to this as the Default network. These authors state that, because they were interested in how **brain structure relates to brain function**, they also recorded **brain activation patterns** from the same participant group. They found that structural connection patterns and functional interactions between regions of cortex were significantly correlated. They concluded that, "Based on our findings, we suggest that the structural core of the brain may have a central role in integrating information across functionally segregated brain regions."

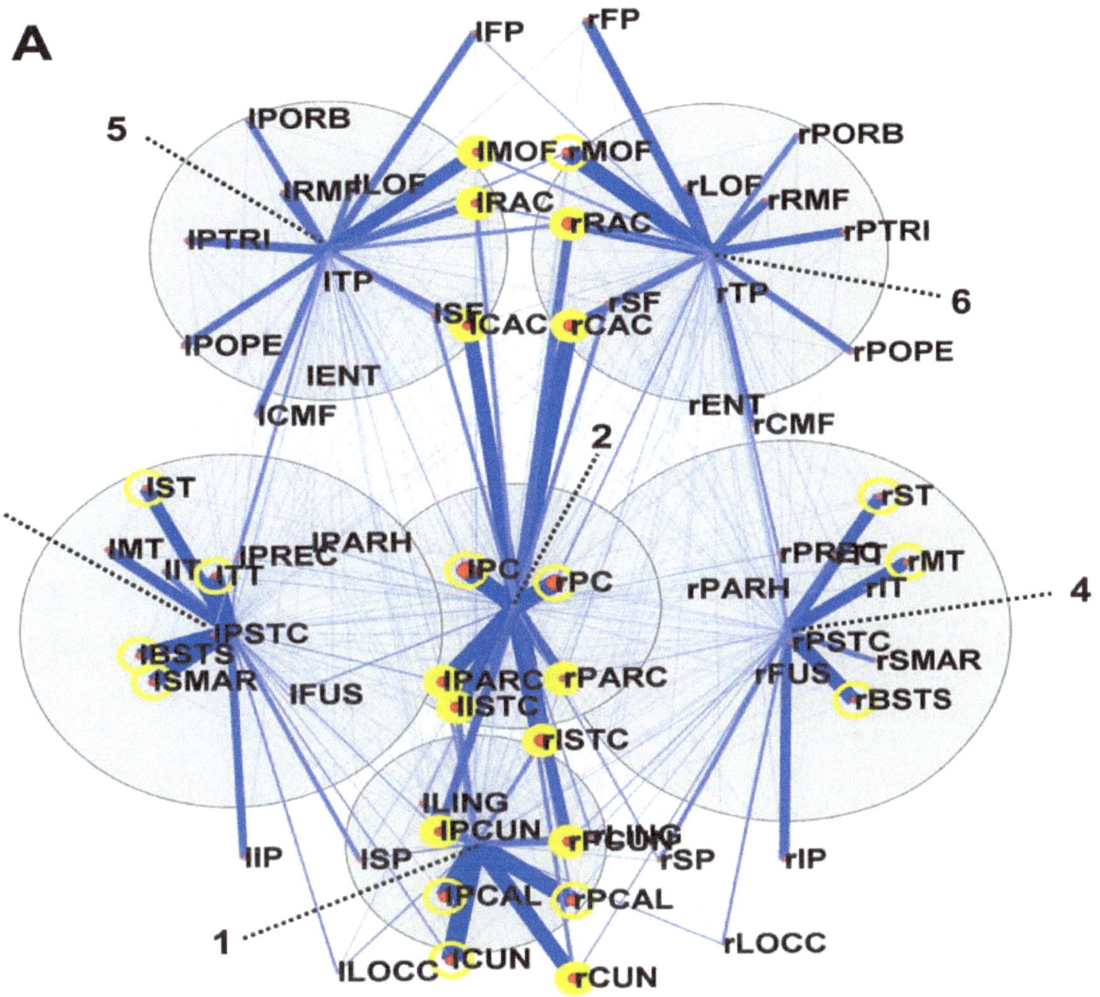

Hagmann et al. (2008). Mapping the Structural Core of Human Cerebral Cortex. (freely available online).

Abbreviations Used Regarding Regions of Interest

*The regions shown are **those that demonstrated the highest connection weight, or connectivity**, between each pair of regions of interest. The diagram thus shows a weighted network of structural connectivity across the entire brain. The 66 cortical regions have two-part labels: a prefix for the cortical hemisphere 'r' (right hemisphere), or 'l' (left hemisphere), and one of 33 designators listed below, largely in alphabetical order.*

BSTS (bank of the superior temporal sulcus), CAC (caudal anterior cingulate cortex), CMF (caudal middle frontal cortex, CUN (cuneus), ENT (or elsewhere labelled ERC is entorhinal cortex), FP (frontal pole), FUS (fusiform gyrus), IP (inferior parietal cortex), IT (inferior temporal cortex), ISTC (isthmus of the cingulate cortex), LOCC (lateral occipital cortex), LOF (lateral orbitofrontal cortex), LING (lingual gyrus), MOF (medial orbitofrontal cortex), MT (middle temporal cortex), PARC (paracentral lobule), PARH (parahippocampal cortex), POPE (pars opercularis), PORB (pars orbitalis), PTRI (pars triangularis), PCAL (pericalcarine cortex), PSTC (postcentral gyrus), PC (posterior cingulate cortex), PREC (precentral gyrus), PCUN (precuneus), RAC (rostral anterior cingulate cortex), RMF (rostral middle frontal cortex), SF (superior frontal cortex), SP (superior parietal cortex), ST (superior temporal cortex), SMAR (supramarginal gyrus), TP (temporal pole), and TT (transverse temporal cortex).

Hubs

The connector 'hubs' have **above average strength** and a high proportion of cross-module connectivity; these are marked as yellow circles. Provincial hubs have above-average strength; they are marked as unfilled yellow circles. In their analysis of connectivity between areas of the cortex, six areas emerged. Four contra-laterally matched modules were localized to frontal and temporal-parietal areas of a single hemisphere. The two remaining modules comprised regions of bilateral medial cortex, one centered on the posterior cingulate cortex and another centered on the precuneus and pericalcarine cortex.

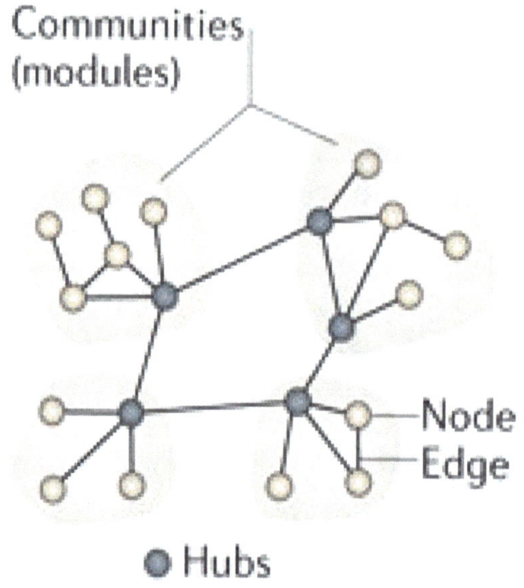

Diagram from: Ed Bullmore & Olaf Sporns (2012)
The economy of brain network organization, Nature Reviews Neuroscience

Functional Module

A **'functional module'** (Achard et al., 2006; Hagmann et al., 2008; Thatcher, 2012) consists of related nodes. A **node** is a large group or **cluster of neurons with high interconnnectivity**. A **Hub** is the key central connecting link for a group of Nodes. A neural **network is** a number of **nodes/modules with functions in common,** connected by links (Sporns, 2011). A neural network may, therefore, also include interconnected modules. It's a bit like travel between airports. There are links to regional airports (nodes) and then there are links to international airports (hubs). To go a long distance, you connect from a local airport to a regional one in order to get to the international airport in the next hub. Interestingly, a German neuroscientist by the name of Poppel posited some years ago that any two neurons can connect with no more than three synapses, which makes sense in terms of connections organized in nodes and hubs. **Phase shift & phase lock** act in the coordination of large masses of neurons in functional modules containing nodes and hubs and, according to Thatcher, this is what gives rise to the electroencephalogram (Thatcher, 2012, p329).

As mentioned above, Thatcher notes that the brain is organized into a relatively small subset of modules with hubs that represent clusters of neurons grouped in nodes with high within-cluster connectivity and sparse long distance connectivity. He notes that this means less in the way of long-distance links for each neuron and maximizes the efficiency of the brain (Thatcher 2012, p305; Buzsaki, 2006).

Part 2
Functions Related to Lobes of the Brain, International 10-20 Sites, and Brodmann Areas

Introduction

Part 2 is organized by lobes of the brain because that is how most practitioners will initially approach their work with NFB. The sections on the Cingulate Gyrus and the Frontal, Temporal and Parietal lobes will each begin with a general introductory overview of important functions and then describe the Brodmann areas (BAs) contained within that region.

A great deal of repetition is to be expected because the functions of a number of different Brodmann areas overlap. The reader can reasonably assume, for the most part, that areas with similar functions are connected in networks. The repetition is intended to help readers find details concerning functions of particular BAs, networks, and lobes of the brain without needing to jump back and forth.

Neurofeedback (NFB) practitioners, when doing training on surface sites with one or more channels of EEG, usually utilize the standard International 10-20 electrode placement sites established for use by neurologists. Therefore this section will initially order the BAs according to their location in lobes of the brain and will also relate them to the standard, 19-channel 10-20 sites, beginning with those over the frontal lobes.

Some practitioners may do LORETA z-score NFB; they will find the list of BAs correlated to the primary functions of each area particularly helpful. That section is followed by summaries concerning the major functional networks in the brain combined with a listing of the BAs that relate most strongly to the functions of each network.

Suggestion Regarding How to Use This Section
This section has been written to provide NFB practitioners with a useful reference guide. After you do a 19-channel assessment with LORETA source identification, you will know that certain 10-20 sites (and, with LORETA, certain BAs) are outside database norms. We suggest that you can then use this section of the book to look up those 10-20 sites and Brodmann areas that are outside the database norms in order to consider what networks and functions are most likely involved, given your patient's major symptoms. From there you may then make informed decisions regarding the placement of your electrodes or, for LORETA NFB, the most important sites and parameters (amplitudes, coherence, phase, etc.) to target with your feedback.
For purposes of doing either surface site NFB or LORETA NFB, the following functional areas are grouped according to their proximity to the International 10-20 sites wherever possible. This was done because most NFB practitioners use surface sites for training purposes and only a smaller number of practitioners have the knowledge, experience, and equipment necessary for carrying out LORETA z-score NFB training.

Reminder: BA Functions Overlap!
Keep in mind, as previously noted, that functions of Brodmann areas listed here are only highlighting some aspects of each area's functions and that any given function likely involves a large number of different areas that operate as a network to achieve that function. Moreover, Brodmann areas themselves are not as precise across different individuals as those depicted in diagrams. One Brodmann area, as drawn below, may overlap another, and a Brodmann area may overlap more than one gyrus.

Summary of Locations of Brodmann Areas

(Remember that BAs can overlap more than one gyrus and a gyrus can have more than one BA associated with it.)

- Areas 1, 2 & 3 – Primary Somatosensory Cortex (frequently referred to as Areas 3, 1, 2)
- Area 4 – Primary motor cortex
- Area 5 – Somatosensory association cortex
- Area 6 – Premotor cortex and supplementary motor cortex (also called secondary motor cortex or supplementary motor area)
- Area 7 – Somatosensory association cortex
- Area 8 – Includes frontal eye fields
- Area 9 – Dorsolateral prefrontal cortex
- Area 10 – Anterior prefrontal cortex (most rostral part of superior and middle frontal gyri)
- Area 11 – Orbitofrontal area (orbital and rectus gyri, plus part of the rostral part of the superior frontal gyrus)
- Area 12 – Orbitofrontal area (used to be part of BA11, refers to the area between the superior frontal gyrus and the inferior rostral sulcus)
- Area 13 (& 14) – Insular cortex
- *Areas 14, 15 (anterior temporal lobe) & 16 – Not found in humans*
- Area 17 – Primary visual cortex (V1)
- Area 18 – Secondary visual cortex (V2)
- Area 19 – Associative visual cortex (V3)
- Area 20 – Inferior temporal gyrus
- Area 21 – Middle temporal gyrus
- Area 22 – Superior temporal gyrus, memory comparison area of auditory cortex, the posterior part is considered to contain a portion of Wernicke's area
- Area 23 – Ventral posterior cingulate cortex
- Area 24 – Ventral anterior cingulate cortex
- Area 25 – Subgenual cortex (part of the ventromedial prefrontal cortex)
- Area 26 – Ectosplenial portion of the retrosplenial region of the cerebral cortex
- Area 27 – Part of piriform cortex
- Area 28 – Posterior entorhinal cortex
- Area 29 – Retrosplenial cingulate cortex
- Area 30 – Part of cingulate cortex
- Area 31 – Dorsal posterior cingulate cortex
- Area 32 – Dorsal anterior cingulate cortex
- Area 33 – Part of anterior cingulate cortex
- Area 34 – Anterior entorhinal cortex (on the parahippocampal gyrus)
- Area 35 – Perirhinal cortex (on the parahippocampal gyrus)
- Area 36 – Parahippocampal cortex (on the parahippocampal gyrus); fusiform gyrus
- Area 37 – Fusiform gyrus, occipitotemporal gyrus
- Area 38 – Temporopolar area (most rostral part of the superior and middle temporal gyri)
- Area 39 – Angular gyrus (part of Wernicke's area in Dominant Hemisphere)
- Area 40 – Supramarginal gyrus (part of Wernicke's area in Dominant Hemisphere)
- Areas 41 & 42 – Primary and Auditory Association Cortex
- Area 43 – Primary gustatory cortex
- Area 44 – Pars opercularis. Contains mirror neurons. (part of Broca's area in Dominant Hemisphere)
- Area 45 – Pars triangularis.(Broca's area in Dominant Hemisphere)
- Area 46 – Dorsolateral prefrontal cortex
- Area 47 – Inferior prefrontal gyrus
- Area 48 – Retrosubicular area (a small part of the medial surface of the temporal lobe)
- *Area 49 – Parasubiculum area in a rodent*
- *Areas 50 & 51 – Found in monkeys*
- Area 52 – Parainsular area (at the junction of the temporal lobe and the insula)

Figures: Lobes, Brodmann Areas, Functions (Networks)

Primary Functions Related to General Areas of the Cortex

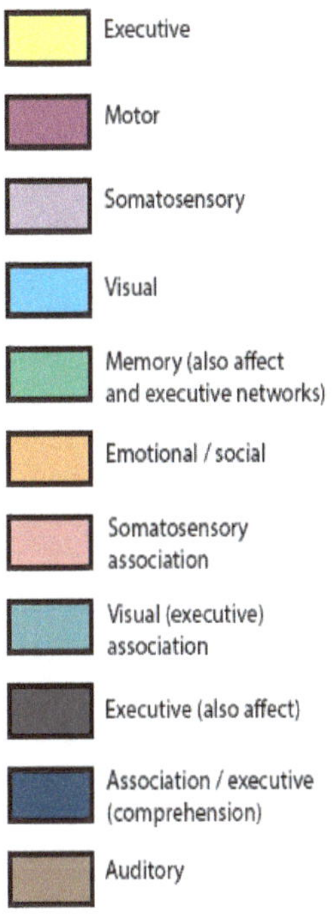

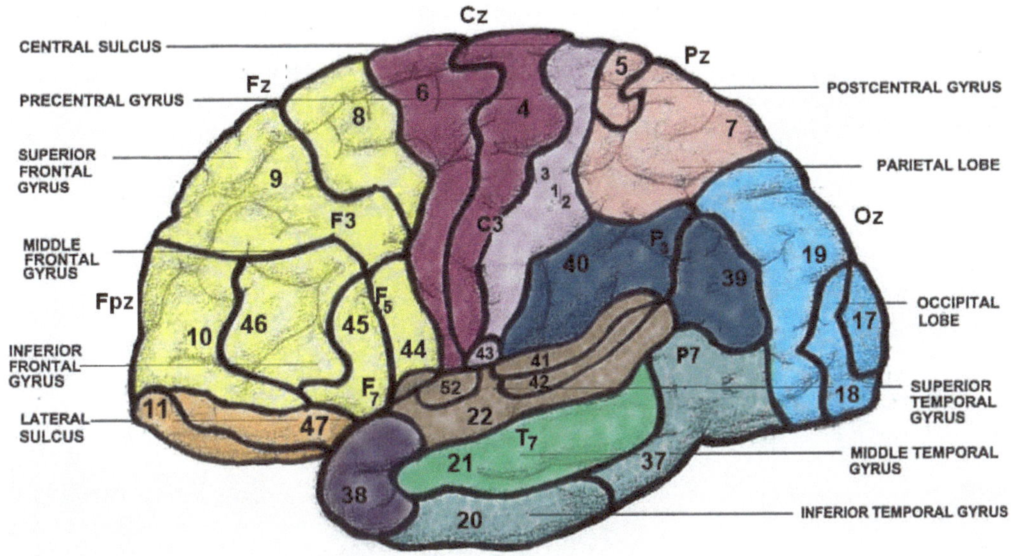

Drawing by Amanda Reeves, Bojana Knezevic, Maya Berenkey;
Functional Areas by Michael Thompson

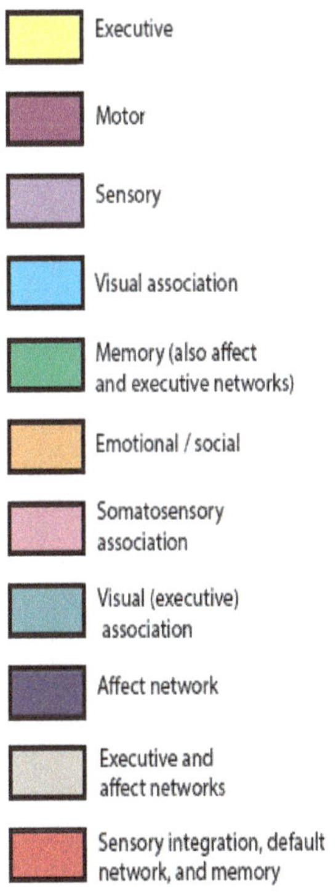

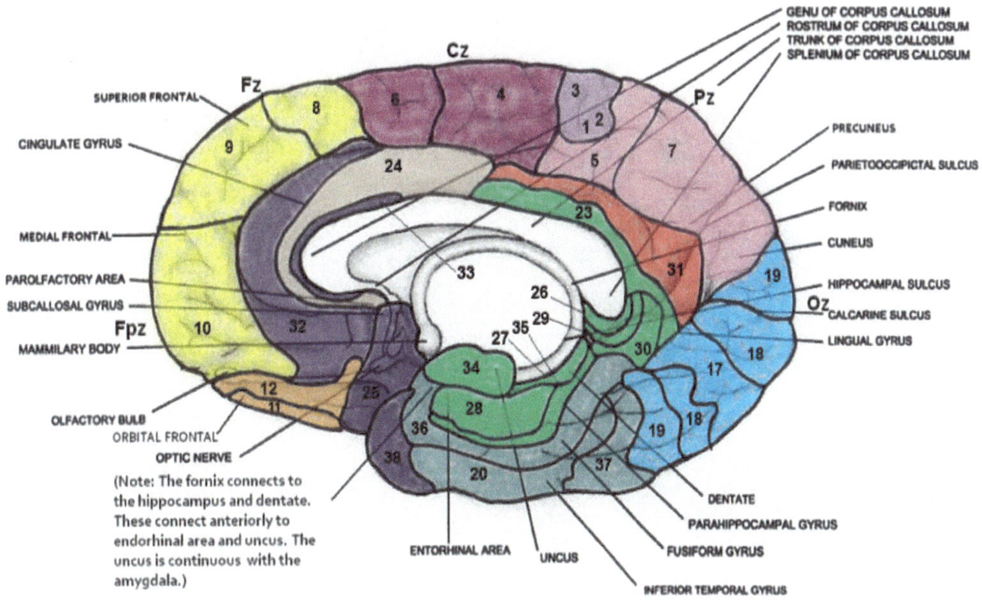

Drawing by Amanda Reeves, Bojana Knezevic, Maya Berenkey;
Functional Areas by Michael Thompson

1. *Attention, Salience, Default, and Memory Networks are too widespread to be usefully illustrated in this diagram.*
2. *Brodmann area 32 is more Executive than Affect but is purple for color contrast in diagram.*

Note that the diagrams above, for purposes of consistency, show just the left hemisphere for the lateral view and the right hemisphere for the midsagittal view. The reader can extrapolate to the homologous sites viewed from the other side of the brain. Keep in mind that an electrode location is on the scalp, not on the actual brain tissue, and thus scalp locations will actually be over slightly different aspects of the brain from one individual to the next.

Note that each region/lobe of the brain has a rather long INTRODUCTION before describing any functions under its Brodmann areas. This is because the same region will function in a number of networks. The individual Brodmann areas do NOT have discreet and unique functions but, rather, have a primary function and also functions that overlap with adjacent BAs and, indeed, they may co-ordinate with other Brodmann areas in distant areas of the cortex to perform some functions. In this manner, each Brodmann area is, for the most part, a component part of complex networks rather than an area that functions independently.

Order of Description of Functions

Lobes or Cortical Areas	Associated Networks	Principle Brodmann Areas	10-20 Sites
Frontal (Lateral & Medial)	Executive Networks Medial: Executive and Affect Networks Medial (BA 9, 10): Default Network	8, 9, 10, 46, 45, 44, 6 47 Lateral and Medial discussed together for each BA --Inferior prefrontal 9, 10, 11, 46, 47	Fz F3, F4 F7, F8 FP1, FP2
Frontal Orbital - Ventral/medial	Affect network – Social (Default network)	11, 12	F9, F10 FPz
Central	Somatosensory Cortex Sensory Network Motor Network	BAs 4, 6, & 1, 2, 3, 5 BAs 1 , 2, 3 Primary (+ 43) Somatosensory Cortex BA 5 Somatosensory Association Cortex BA 4 Primary Motor Cortex BA 6 Motor Association Cortex	Cz C3, C4 Cz C3, C4
Temporal			
- Lateral Aspect	Executive – Auditory	41, 42, 22; 21, (52)	T7 & T8
- Temporal Pole	Executive, Semantic – also Affect Networks	38	T7 & T8 (F7, F8)
Temporal - Medial Aspect - (+ *Amygdala)*	Executive Network – Memory Affect network (+Default)	26, 27, 28 36, 37, (48) 35, 34	(Pz) (P7, P8)
Temporal - Inferior	Object identification; part of the 'what' pathway.	20, 37	T9 & T10
Insula	Affect & Executive	13	C3-T7
Cingulate			
Anterior (ACC)	Affect - Executive - Default	Affect: 24 (also Executive & Default & Salience networks) Affect: 33, 25 Executive: 32 (also Affect & Default)	Cz FCz Fz
Posterior (PCC)	Default Executive – Sensory	23, 31, 26, 29, (30)	Pz
Parietal	Executive, Sensory, Attention, (& Default) Networks; Spatial Awareness, part of the 'where' pathway.	5, 7	PCz, Pz
Temporal – Parietal - Lateral Aspect	Executive Network (& Default) Comprehension/Language Learning Gesture, Emotion, Nuance	39, 40 DH: 39, 40 NDH: 39, 40	P3 & P4
Inferior-Parietal Lateral	Attention & Salience	37	P7 & P8
Parietal Lobes - Medial Dorsal Aspect	Somatosensory Association	7	Pz
Occipital	Visual	17, 18, 19	O1, 02

Important: *The electrodes used for surface EEG NFB may reflect the activity from a number of Brodmann areas. The functions of Brodmann areas overlap with other Brodmann areas. Thus it is inevitable that under each principle BA being discussed, other BAs will be mentioned.*

Notes on Doing Neurofeedback and Heart Rate Variability Training

Please recall that this book is not written to detail anatomy and connections. Rather, it is written to give an overview of some of the sites and neural connections/networks that the practitioner may influence with NFB + BFB training. In part, the importance for most NFB practitioners is to recognize that **NFB applied over one key site within a neural network may affect the entire network**. Also, that NFB may need to be applied to both hemispheres for different effects. For this reason, and also to (theoretically) directly influence some deep midline structures while also affecting coherence and phase relationships between different areas of the cortex, LORETA NFB may be more efficient than surface NFB.

LORETA gives source localization, naming both the Brodmann area and the cortical area (such as BA 24, Anterior Cingulate) that is related to the EEG measured on the surface. When combined with a database, such as NeuroGuide, one also has information about the degree of deviation from the mean for people in the normative sample of the same age and sex for particular frequencies. However, always remember that you must choose the sites for doing LORETA NFB very carefully so as not to adversely affect sites that are deviant but for a positive reason, either related to a person's strengths or activated to compensate for sites that are not functioning normally. For example, when we found significant deviations in the auditory cortex of a physician who was also a musician with perfect pitch and no symptoms related to functions of the temporal lobe, we certainly did not want to normalize those deviations.

In addition, BFB and, in particular, HRV training, because they influence connections between the solitary nucleus and many higher nuclei, including those in the thalamus, cingulate gyrus, and the hypothalamus, may also have effects on a number of neural and endocrine systems and networks. Understanding connections and networks is helpful for doing careful, effective work with clients.

Frontal Lobe

Introduction – Functions Related to the Frontal Lobes

Due to the important involvement of the frontal lobes in the symptoms of many patients who are being treated with NFB, this introduction to the functions of the frontal lobes is more comprehensive than the introduction to other cortical regions. What follows here is a general overview of some of the functions subsumed by the frontal lobes. Most of these functions can be influenced by neurofeedback training. In addition, the functions related to different BAs in the frontal lobes overlap to such a large degree that this section will discuss **functions in general terms before specific functions of the individual BAs** are discussed.

Rather than always using right and left designations, we will often refer to the dominant hemisphere (DH) and the nondominant hemisphere (NDH). In most people the DH is the left hemisphere and they are usually right-handed. However, it is also true that many left-handed people and most ambidextrous people have their DH on the left. The NDH is the right hemisphere in the majority of people. In most individuals, language and verbal functions primarily involve the DH.

The **prefrontal** cortex makes up about one third of the human neocortex. On the lateral surface it corresponds to the superior, middle, and inferior frontal gyri anterior to the premotor region (BA 6). The prefrontal region includes BAs 8, 9, 10, 11, 44, 45, 46 and 47. On the medial surface it includes the anterior cingulate gyrus and the medial prefrontal area comprising BAs 24, 32 and BAs 8, 9, 10, 11, 12. In the orbital/inferior surface it includes BAs 10, 11, 47, and a portion of BA 13 (Augustine, 2008, pp 356, 357).

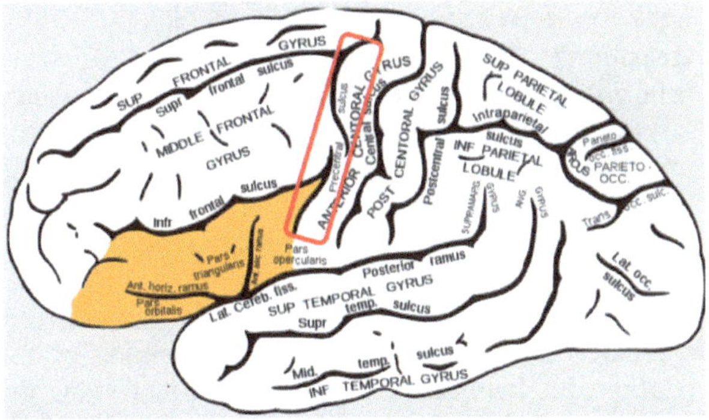

Figure from *Gray's Anatomy* (public domain) to show a lateral view of the prefrontal cortex, inferior, middle, and superior gyri with a red rectangle around the posterior border at the precentral sulcus.

The prefrontal cortex has major connections to the dorsal aspect of the anterior cingulate cortex (ACC). The ACC is a central structure in the ***Executive network,*** and it connects with all functionally related structures, including the dorsolateral prefrontal cortex. The frontal lobes are crucial for all executive functions, such as the evaluation of incoming stimuli, planning an appropriate response, and inhibiting inappropriate responses (Knezevic, 2010).

Definition of Executive Functioning

Executive functioning is one key function of the frontal lobes. It is broadly defined as the overall capacity to manage perception, attention, selection, decision making, inhibition, memory, planning, problem solving, logical thinking (deductive and inductive), sequencing; to monitor, evaluate, and self-correct outputs; and to respond verbally/nonverbally, motorically, and socially for the purpose of the attainment of defined goals.

Although the frontal lobes are crucial for all executive tasks, including the voluntary control of attention, the inhibition of inappropriate and/or unwanted behavior, the planning of actions and executive decision making, these lobes also have many other important functions.

These functions include:

- A role in the maintenance of arousal.
- Temporal sequencing of complex entities such as compound sentences (mainly the dominant hemisphere (DH).
- Hand-writing (Exner's area in the DH).
- Speech articulation (Broca's area: DH BAs 44, 45).
- Frontal mirror neurons (mirror neurons were first observed in monkeys in the Left Frontal Operculum (F5) close to Broca's area).
- Auditory and verbal representation.
- Object naming and word recall (usually DH).
- Representation of visual images evoked by auditory input.
- Letter and word perception and recognition (with input from the occipital and parietal regions).
- Representation of abstract verbal forms.
- Perception of complex relationships.

Some of the Functions of the DH (Left) Frontal Lobe

The **dominant hemisphere** (left) frontal lobe is crucial in the regulation of speech production and syntax. It is important in sustaining and regulating attention, inhibiting actions, and switching responses. It is critical to **analytic, sequential** processing. It is where we utilize inner speech (inner dialogue) to regulate our behavior. The DH's frontal lobe is the location of operations that require sequencing, such as one can test by asking the client to recite a series of numbers or count backwards by 7s. It is involved in regulating routines, **recognizing patterns,** and deciding what to do in different situations.

As a very broad overview, **left hemisphere dominance** is usually thought of as being characterized by a lack of emotion, introversion, goal-directed thinking and action. It is also involved in having an internal locus of control. Mental processing may tend to be relatively slow and serial in keeping with the tendency to be concrete, careful, and sequential. The dominant neurotransmitter is **dopamine.** On the one hand, one may recognize in this description, if taken to the extreme, the pattern displayed by some of your patients who have a diagnosis of Asperger's syndrome. On the other hand, you may also recognize that, **as we grow older**, we move more into this type of functioning and away from the more right-brained functioning that will be described below.

Frontal Lobe Injury

In very general terms, patients who have damage to their frontal lobes show a decrease in spontaneous facial movements and speak fewer words than they did previously. These patients demonstrate **difficulties with flexibility, problem solving, attention span, and memory**. In addition, frontal lobe damage appears to have **more of an impact on divergent than convergent** thinking. This may result in the person appearing to be unmotivated or even lazy, lacking initiative, and appearing rather inflexible and unable to consider alternative options or strategies for solving problems. Despite these deficiencies, in some cases, there is minimal effect on IQ testing, which may be due to the fact that **IQ testing places more emphasis on assessing convergent** rather than divergent thinking. In addition to these general findings, each patient will have specific difficulties that relate to their specific injury.

Some patients with **left (dominant) hemisphere injury** will show more **problems in verbal** areas, be rather apathetic, **depressed**, and have right-sided motor deficiencies particularly with respect to fine motor movements. On the other hand, a patient with more damage to the **right, nondominant, hemisphere** may demonstrate more problems in **nonverbal abilities, lack social graces**, act without tact, lack restraint, and have left-sided motor deficiencies.

In all cases, to varying extents, there may be symptoms related to problem solving, spontaneity, judgment, impulse control, and both social and sexual behavior. People close to the injured patient may comment that the **patient's personality has changed.** These patients show a relative inability to correctly interpret feedback from their environment. They may be noncompliant and show risk-taking behavior (Thatcher 2012). They **may perseverate** (repeat or prolong an action, thought, or utterance after the stimulus that prompted it has ceased). **Orientation** in space may be compromised. Mood can be affected. From the standpoint of general emotional demeanor, as is discussed elsewhere under disorders of affect, activation in the left dominant frontal region has been associated with positive thoughts and approach behavior while right nondominant frontal region activation is more often associated with negative thoughts and avoidance behavior (Davidson, 1995, 1998). So left frontal damage may put one at particular risk for depression.

Reasoning: Deductive & Inductive

Since it is a quintessential frontal lobe activity, reasoning is going to be discussed in detail as an example of how complex and interrelated brain function is within the cortex. You will see how many areas are involved, though the frontal cortex is the main player.

The left/dominant frontal lobe is critical for cognitive work that we generally call reasoning skills. **Reasoning is the cognitive process of drawing inferences from given information.** All arguments involve the claim that one or more propositions (the premises) provide some grounds for accepting another proposition (the conclusion). Arguments may be broadly divided into deduction and induction.

Deductive arguments are arguments that can be evaluated for validity. Validity is a function of the relationship between premises and conclusion and involves the claim that the premises provide absolute grounds for accepting the conclusion: e.g., All men are mortal. Socrates is a man, therefore Socrates is mortal. With **deductive reasoning the conclusion drawn must be true if the premises, whatever they may be, are true.** Thus deductive reasoning takes pieces of evidence and then comes to a valid conclusion from this material.

Inductive arguments are never automatically valid. They must be evaluated for plausibility or reasonableness. The premises provide only limited grounds for accepting the conclusion: e.g., Socrates is a man. Socrates is mortal, therefore, all men are mortal. The conclusion may or may not be true. The premises of an inductive logical argument indicate some degree of support (inductive probability) for the conclusion. **Thus the premises suggest truth but do not ensure it**. A clear example of a false conclusion based on inductive reasoning would be: All crows are birds. All crows are black, therefore all birds are black. Inductive reasoning generally proceeds from detailed facts to general principles. It is commonly construed as a form of reasoning that makes generalizations based on individual instances. In this sense it is often contrasted with deductive reasoning.

Anatomical Relationships in Reasoning
Anatomically, both induction and deduction activate a similar left frontal-temporal system. Induction differs from deduction in greater activation of the medial dorsal prefrontal cortex (BAs 8 and 9). Induction may also have somewhat more right-hemisphere involvement. Deduction is a little more akin to dependence on known patterns and absolute proof, which is a left-hemisphere function. As an example of how complex reasoning networks become, here are some details summarized from research by Goel and his colleagues (2004).

Deductive reasoning (compared to baseline) is associated with activation in the left cerebellum, bilateral inferior occipital gyrus (BA 18), left inferior temporal and occipital gyri (BAs 37/19), left middle temporal gyrus (BA 39), right superior parietal lobule (BA 7), bilateral middle frontal gyrus (BA 6), bilateral putamen, and left inferior frontal gyrus (BA 44, Broca's area) (paraphrased after Goel et al., 2004).

Inductive reasoning (compared to baseline) activates a similar network consisting of the right cerebellum, right lingual gyrus (BA 18), right middle occipital gyrus (BA 18), bilateral superior parietal lobule (BA 7), left inferior parietal lobule (BA 40), right middle frontal gyrus (BA 6), putamen, and left middle frontal gyrus (BAs 8/9/45). This rather complicated 'localization' underscores how a single BA is almost never acting alone!

In the above detailed analysis, **deduction** appears to be associated with activation that is somewhat more left/dominant hemisphere-based, **whereas induction** is somewhat more right/nondominant hemisphere. However, reasoning is definitely a dominant-hemisphere attribute and only the dominant hemisphere is capable of making final inferences (inductive reasoning). There is greater left inferior frontal gyrus (BA 44/Broca's area) activation for deduction than induction. Conversely, the left dorsolateral (BA 9) prefrontal cortex (along with right superior occipital gyrus, BA 19) show greater increases for induction. There are several possible reasons posited for the greater involvement of **Broca's area (BA 44) in deduction** than induction. Broca's Area is part of the phonological loop of working memory, and deductive reasoning has greater working memory requirements than inductive reasoning. Broca's Area is also involved in syntactic (order of words) processing involving logic. Thus enhanced activity in Broca's Area during deduction may be a function of greater engagement of syntactical processing and greater working memory requirements.

Inductive reasoning, on the other hand, is sensitive to background knowledge rather than logical form. The increased activity in the left dorsolateral prefrontal cortex may thus be due to the use of world knowledge in the generation and evaluation of hypotheses (Goel et al., 2004; Grafman, 2002), which is the basis of inductive inference.

In summary, both kinds of cognitive reasoning, deduction and induction, do not just activate left and right prefrontal cortex, respectively. Both forms of reasoning involve the left prefrontal cortex. Consistent with its greater requirements for syntactic processing and working memory, **deduction is characterized by increased activation in Broca's Area while induction involves greater activation in the left dorsolateral prefrontal cortex,** consistent with its need to access and evaluate world knowledge.

The important observation for our work with NFB is that both types of reasoning involve extensive overlapping networks of cortical areas. At the ADD Centre, we will do single channel NFB to activate these networks while the subject is doing cognitive tasks using appropriate strategies. We hypothesize that, by doing some of the training on task, we are reinforcing an optimization of the networks necessary for the particular task, namely, attention, focus, and the specific cognitive functioning necessary for that task. Our combination of NFB with BFB assures that this is carried out in a calm, relaxed state. Published results of large case series of people with ADHD (n=111) and with Autism Spectrum Disorders (n=159), which document improvement on academic and intellectual measures as well as on behavioral ones, support the effectiveness of this approach (Thompson & Thompson, 1998, 2010). The addition of anodal transcranial direct current stimulation (tDCS) for a few minutes prior to doing regular neurofeedback may prove to give added benefit/more rapid results.

The nondominant (usually right) cerebral hemisphere

The right frontal cortex is involved in the regulation of **attention**. The right hemisphere, frontal, anterior cingulate, and parietal, in conjunction with cholinergic activity from the basal forebrain (nucleus basalis of Maynert and the substantia innominata) are important in **sustained attention** performance (Sarter et al., 2001). This hemisphere is also important in the **inhibition of old habits**. The nondominant frontal lobe is involved in understanding metaphors. **Autobiographical 'Sense of Past Self'** may reside primarily in the right frontal NDH. This is in spite of the fact that memory for most verbal functioning is considered to be in the dominant hemisphere with an emphasis on frontal lobe functioning for remembered item retrieval.

Most item retrieval is carried out in the dorsal medial prefrontal cortex (DMPC and left PFC) with links to the hippocampus (Northrop, 2006) and the anterolateral temporal lobes (we will describe under the temporal lobe, connections that involve the uncinate fasciculus, which links these areas to the orbital frontal cortex [OFC]). Researchers such as Seger (2004) note that there are numerous studies that emphasize predominately the right temporal cortex (RTC) and right prefrontal cortex (RPC) (and right uncinate fasciculus) for both autobiographical memory – self in the past (Damasio, 1999, 2003) and for recognition of one's own face vs. faces of others (medial AC and LPC).

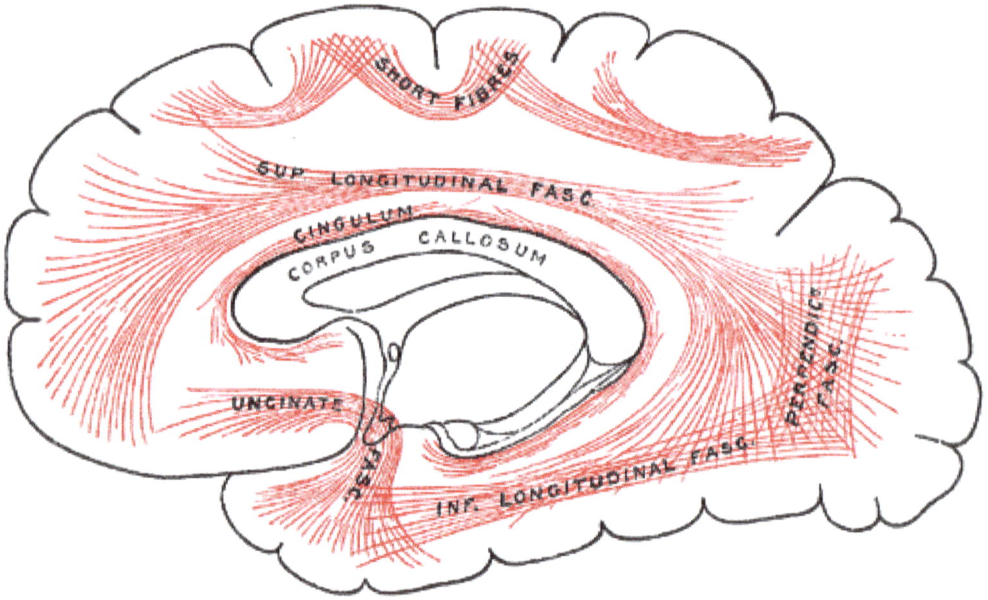

Figure to show Uncinate Fasciculus from Gray's Anatomy *(1918) (public domain). This figure illustrates the Corpus Callosum, which connects the left and right hemispheres, and Fasciculi that connect areas within the hemispheres. These myelinated pathways contain both excitatory and inhibitory pathways, though it has been argued that they are predominantly excitatory.*

Memory

Memories of experienced events have sensory and perceptual components and are therefore, in part, stored in the occipital cortex and related networks. On the other hand, memories **for imagined events are stored frontally**, probably because they contain imagery that is generated in the frontal lobes. As memory declines in some older persons, it is episodic memory with the encoding of new events that deteriorates first. This can leave retrieval of old memories intact, for the most part, including autobiographical memory.

Encoding New Images

It is the networks that involve the right parietal (cuneus, precuneus) with the left temporal regions that encode specific new images, along with the hippocampus, that are most **affected in early memory loss** associated with aging.

In addition, it has been observed that the right prefrontal cortex can show an increase in both alpha and beta activity during anger memory as well as during negative memories concerning self experience (Cannon, 2012).

Other Functions, Nondominant (Right) Frontal

The right frontal areas are **heteromodal** (versus the left, which demonstrates more modality-specific associations). The right frontal lobe integrates sensory information from many sensory channels. It *synthesizes information* from many *distant cortical areas,* like a fleet of airplanes vs. a fleet of taxis (left hemisphere) (Goldberg, 2001). In addition, there is more white matter in the right hemisphere and there are also more spindle cells in the right hemisphere. These spindle cells relay information from distant areas.

The right hemisphere **comprehends novelty**. It may convert novelty to stable familiar patterns or routines that are then part of left hemisphere functioning. Searching for novelty implies dissatisfaction. Seeking newness appears to be **driven more by norepinephrine** than dopamine and may be associated with restless and hyperactive, exploratory behavior. This decreases as we age. As people **grow older, they move from right to left dominance** both cognitively and emotionally.

In very general terms, **verbal IQ** is usually attributed more to left hemisphere (DH) activity while **performance IQ** is attributed more to right hemisphere (NDH) functions. Performance IQ involves some timed tests. Speed on these tests declines with age in adults. This is one of the reasons that norms for IQ are age-adjusted. (In children, speed increases with age, in part because more fibers become myelinated.) **Right hemisphere dominance** is usually thought of as being characterized by distractibility, stimulus-seeking behavior, seeking novelty and change, being emotionally involved, expressive, and extroverted. There may tend to be an external locus of control. There may be more of a tendency for **hysterical, impulsive, and even manic behaviors.**

Processing may tend to be fast and simultaneous in keeping with the Gestalt or holistic tendencies of the NDH. The dominant neurotransmitter is **noradrenalin**, which is associated with speeding up activity, and **serotonin**, which has long been associated with slowing down activity (Tucker, 1984). However, it is also true that decreased serotonin levels may be associated with inflexibility and reliance on known patterns (left hemisphere) as is found in obsessive compulsive disorder (OCD).

In addition, there are a number of other functions that show **predominantly nondominant,** right hemisphere, activation. These include:

- Sensing the Gestalt
- Parallel processing
- Attending to spatial relationships
- Representation of geometric forms
- Speech intonation, musicality, and vowel sounds
- Expressing emotions
- Orientation in space
- Holistic perceptions
- Responding to novel situations
- Intuition
- Eureka-like insight

Lesions in the right prefrontal region may affect any of these functions. The patient may exhibit **constructional apraxia** (inability to copy drawings or to manipulate objects to form patterns or designs). There may be difficulties with learning a maze or with nonverbal visual memory. Psychiatric syndromes, such as **manic behavior**, may be observed.

Comments Regarding Frontal Lobe Lesions

In very severe lesions the patient may not react to environmental instructions or cues and may react to irrelevant stimuli. There may be either echolalia or loss of voluntary speech. Agraphia is common and, in general terms, the patient appears confused.

Orbital Frontal Cortex and Links to the Temporal Lobe

The basal forebrain area is involved in **sleep-wake** regulation. **Concept organization** is also a function of this area of the hemispheres. The orbitofrontal cortex is critical for both **value-based behavior** and learning when value must be inferred. We have already noted that the orbital frontal cortex may be involved in **understanding the effect of one's own behavior on others.** The patient who has a lesion involving this area may be **emotionally labile** with decreased impulse control. **Loss of control** of anger, inappropriate laughter, crying, or inappropriate sexual behavior may be observed. However, with respect to these functions, a slightly different emphasis may be observed in the right and left hemispheres. **Impulsivity**, for example, may be more associated with dysfunction in the NDH orbital prefrontal cortex. Note that both these areas are discussed in further detail under Brodmann area 11 below.

Inferior/Basal Areas of the Dominant Hemisphere (Left)

The orbital/basal surface of the frontal lobe is connected to the temporal lobe by the **uncinate fasciculus**. Structures connected by the uncinate fasciculus from the temporal pole to the orbital surface of the frontal lobe have functions, in the left hemisphere, that include associations with general intelligence, verbal and visual memory, and executive performance. **Damage to the uncinate fasciculus on the left** side may be related to social anxiety and to symptoms of schizotypal personality disorder. These functions may be due, in part, to its connections to the limbic system.

Connections of the Uncinate Fasciculus

The uncinate fasciculus connects the entorhinal-uncus area, amygdala, and hippocampal region in the temporal lobes with frontal areas and, in particular, the orbitofrontal cortex and orbital-medial frontal cortex. The left uncinate fasciculus can relate to proficiency in both declarative and auditory-verbal memory (Mabbott, et al., 2009).

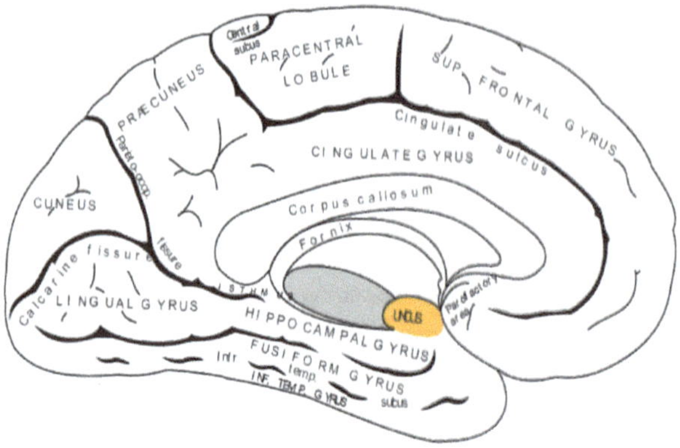

Diagram from Gray's Anatomy *showing uncus of Parahippocampal Gyrus*

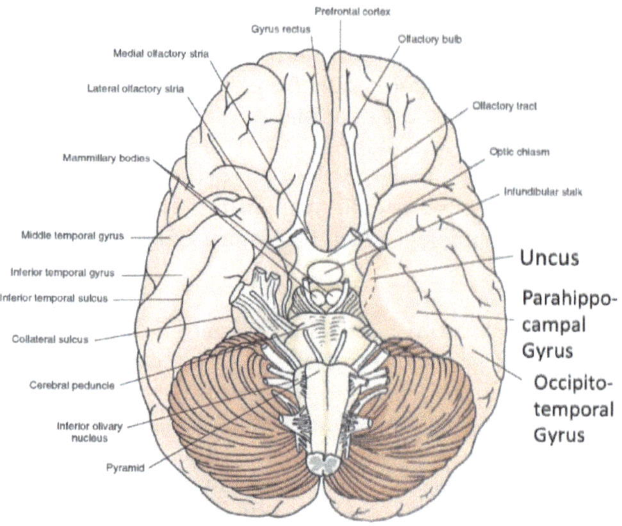

Inferior view adapted From Gray's Anatomy 1918.
To illustrate location of Uncus.

Connections of the Uncinate Fasciculus in the Right, Nondominant Hemisphere

Similar areas on the right side may have somewhat different functions. The right temporal cortex (RTC) and the right prefrontal cortex (RPC) are connected by the right uncinate fasciculus. As noted previously, one related function on the right side is **autobiographical memory**, memories of one's self-in-the-past (Damasio, 1999) and recognition of one's own face versus the faces of others. This last function also involves the medial aspect of the ACC and the dominant (left) parietal cortex (LPC).

Deficiencies in the uncinate fasciculus connections in both hemispheres may correlate with symptoms that are found in autism spectrum disorders.

Lateral and Medial Aspect – Executive Network Fz, F3 and F4: BA 8

BA 8

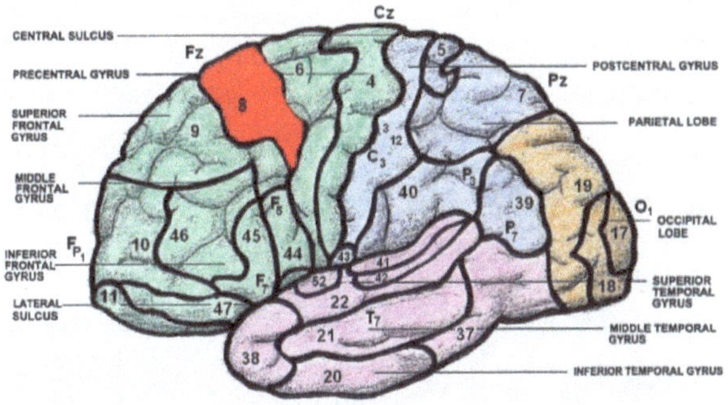

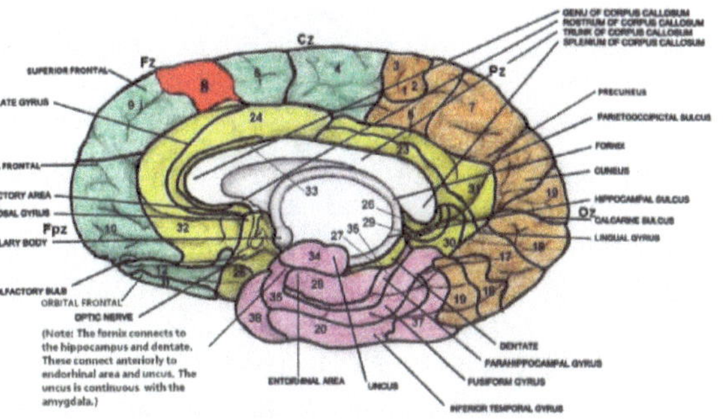

This area is **executive cortex** located in the prefrontal association cortex. As previously outlined, it is involved in **deductive and inductive reasoning**, monitoring, planning, calculating, sequence learning, working memory, speech and language processing, translation, generating sentences, and processing uncertainty. It is important in **memory retrieval**. It contains the frontal **eye-fields** and is involved in horizontal saccadic eye movements. It is a key area in **executive attention** (particularly visuospatial and visuomotor), self monitoring, and executive control of behavior. It is also important in self-image processing. Possibly related to an effect on these areas, it has been shown that LORETA z-score NFB directed to this area can be effective to improve executive attention (Cannon, Congedo & Lubar, 2007, 2009). It is involved in motor learning and imagery.

Lesions affecting this area can result in tonic deviation of the eyes towards the side of injury. Along with other BAs in the premotor association cortex, lesions can affect motor planning, and coordination of complex sequences of movements, in addition to affecting working memory, executive attention, and some aspects of reasoning and planning. (See previous comments on inductive and deductive reasoning.) Because in the **dominant hemisphere** it overlaps with Broca's area, there may also be an effect on speech including an inability to **initiate speech** if there is damage in this area. It is also said to have some involvement in networks for **generating sentences,** language translation, and lip reading. Less often noted are possible changes in the **anticipation of pain** and in motor aspects of imagery.

FP1-F3, FP2-F4: BAs 9 and 10

Functions related to Brodmann areas in the regions between Fp1 and F3 and between Fp2 and F4: Note that the diagrams, for purposes of consistency, show just the left hemisphere for the lateral view and the right hemisphere for the midsagittal view. The reader can extrapolate to the homologous sites viewed from the right side of the brain. Keep in mind that an electrode location is on the scalp, not on the actual brain tissue, and thus scalp locations will actually be over slightly different aspects of the brain from one individual to the next.

Superior Frontal: BA 9

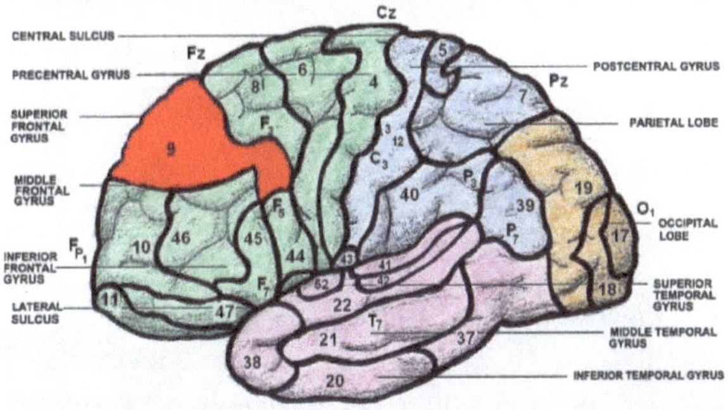

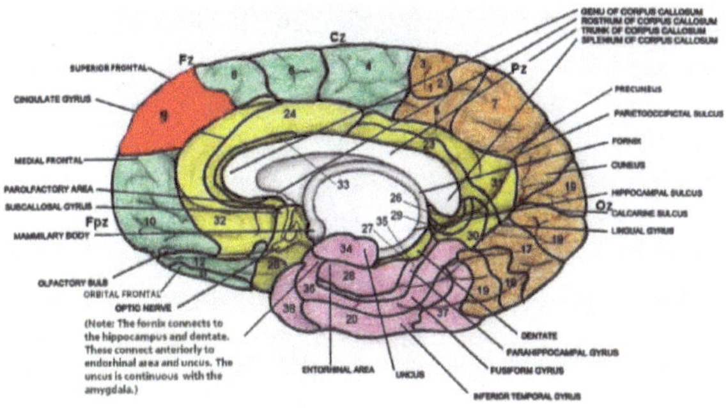

Right, Nondominant Hemisphere

Brodmann area 9 in the right hemisphere may be affected by NFB training that is carried out over the Right Superior Frontal area between Fp2 and F4. It is part of what is often referred to as the dorsal-lateral-prefrontal cortex (DLPFC). Together with BAs 45, 46, and the superior part of 47, it takes in much of the lateral aspect of the superior frontal gyrus and middle frontal gyrus. As will be clear to the reader from the diagrams, this is not a well defined area in the sense that it comprises a number of Brodmann areas. It may be considered to take in parts of areas 8, 10, 44, and, even more broadly, BA 11 and other areas. It is a very important area for most executive functions.

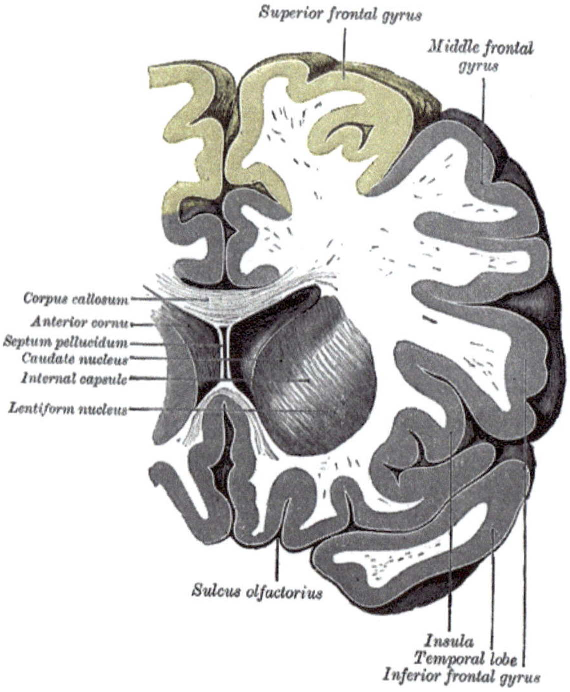

Figure from Gray's Anatomy

It is the executive control area for motor planning and organization. It is involved in the integration of sensory and mnemonic information and in the categorization of data. It is a key area in networks involved with working memory. It is important in networks that are involved in the interpretation of the emotional states of others and in empathy and forgiveness. Inference is a high level executive function that involves this area. Metaphors are liable to be a problem after a lesion in the right DLFC. An example of a metaphor is, "He's a bear in the morning." Understanding this metaphor would be difficult for a person with Asperger's syndrome. Such a patient would be able to interpret more easily a simile such as, "He is *like* a bear in the morning."

The right frontal cortex is involved in word recall and, in conjunction with the parietal operculum and precuneus, in the interpretation of metaphors (G. Bottini, R. Corcoran, R. Sterzi, E. Paulesu, P. Schenone, P. Scarpa, R.S.J. Frackowiak, and D. Frith, 1994). Robert Sapolsky (2010) stated that understanding symbols, metaphors, analogies, parables, synecdoche and figures of speech also involves the insula, the angular gyrus, and the anterior cingulate cortex (ACC). The ACC is part of the network for monitoring and subjective evaluation of stimuli (later noted with respect to pain) and it is an essential part of the process in understanding metaphors. The point is that understanding metaphors involves many brain regions, not just a single area.

The right frontal areas are also among several important areas for people who use sign language. These areas are also among many areas involved in the detection of novelty.

BA 9 Both Hemispheres

Lesions in these areas result in difficulties with most executive functions. These functions include abstract thinking and **working memory,** such as encoding and retrieval functions. For the most part, in the dominant hemisphere, this involves verbal and language functions, whereas in the nondominant hemisphere, this involves visual-spatial information.

In general terms, this area in the prefrontal association cortex is part of the **executive cortex.** It is involved in short-term and working memory and in carrying out arithmetic computations. It is important in error detection and in verbal fluency. It is one of the areas involved in **understanding intentions and regulating behavior.** In conjunction with the cingulate gyrus, BA 9 can also play a role in **sexual arousal.**

In the dominant hemisphere it is involved in verbal fluency including generating sentences and word-stem completion. It is involved in **understanding idioms and categorizing** items.

Many aspects of cognitive executive functioning may be tested using **standardized tests**, such as the Wechsler Intelligence Scale (WISC, WAIS), other intelligence tests, the Tower of London (TOL), and the Wisconsin Card Sort (WCS), to name only a few. It is important to do one or more of these tests of cognitive functioning. It is crucial with patients who have a history of learning difficulties and in patients who have experienced a concussion, even in the seemingly distant past, because the results will help guide your treatment and assist in objectively evaluating the patient's progress in the treatment program. We try to make standardized testing part of the pre-training assessment and it is repeated, free-of-charge, after 40 sessions of training. It is very helpful to be able to demonstrate with objective measures that change has taken place, in addition to having anecdotal reports and questionnaire data. Consider online testing if you want to save time, such as that available through CNS Vital Signs division of Pearson, a publisher and distributor of psychological tests.

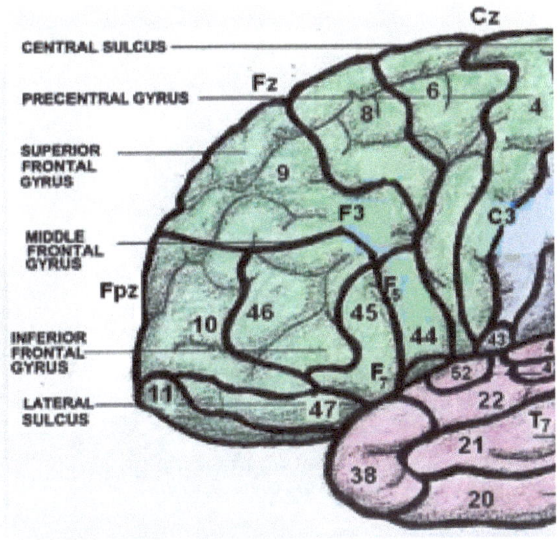

Another important function of this cortical area is governing *attention to and interpretation of* ***emotional and contextual cues***. Although these functions may be more in the nondominant hemisphere, they are found in both hemispheres. In fMRI experiments, Goldberg et al. (2006) found evidence that the superior frontal gyrus when interacting with the sensory system is involved in self-awareness.

The **right, nondominant, prefrontal** cortex is associated with cognitive functions including: working memory, episodic memory, semantic monitoring, and motor imagery (McLeod et al., 1998). Again, however, these functions are not unilateral and both hemispheres are implicated in these functions. This understanding may be important if one is placing the cathode over this area when doing transcranial direct current stimulation (tDCS). The cathode may result in a decrease in activity, and it is often placed over the right orbit in experiments when the anode is placed over an area in the left hemisphere. Although the authors have neither personally experienced nor found any reports of negative effects resulting from this placement of the cathode for tDCS, it is still a possibility that should be recognized.

Left, Dominant Hemisphere, Superior Frontal: BA 9

Brodmann area 9 in the Left Superior Frontal gyrus, between Fp1 and F3, governs **attention to logical** information and to detail. It is also involved in organizing responses. Some liken it to an orchestra conductor. It is also a key area for **phonology** that involves BAs 9, 46, 6, and for **semantics** BAs 9 and 37. It can be involved in the interpretation of **idioms** such as, "It's raining cats and dogs." Patients with Asperger's syndrome often have difficulty with idioms because they take things literally, and idioms, by definition, are turns of phrase that defy literal interpretations because they do not mean what they say.

The **superior frontal gyrus** is also important in producing **laughter** (Fried et al., 1998). Fried found, when exploring to find the source of seizures in a 16-year-old female patient, that stimulation of a two square centimeter area on the left superior frontal gyrus produced laughter consistently. Fried and his colleagues found that increasing the level of stimulation current increased the duration and intensity of the laughter. At low currents only a smile was present, while at higher currents a louder, contagious laughter was induced. The laughter was also accompanied by the stopping of all activities involving speech or hand movements (Fried, 1998). The patient, AK, reported that the laughter was accompanied by a sensation of merriment or mirth. She would attribute it to something in her environment each time, not the stimulation.

Fp1, FP2 (To the left and right of Fpz in the figure)

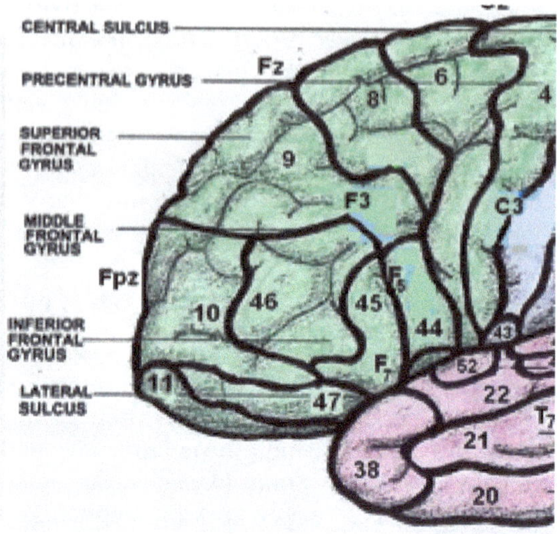

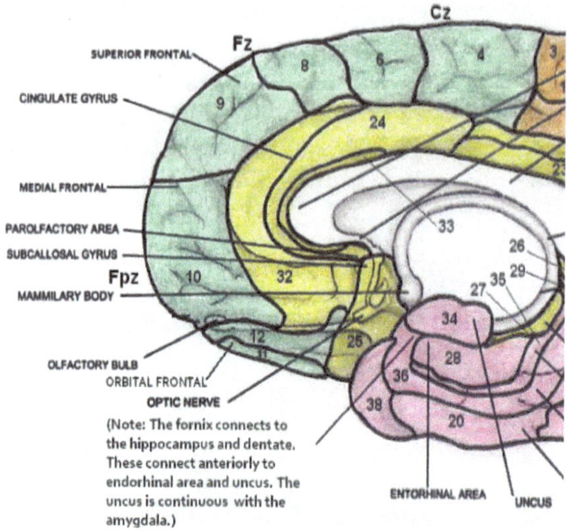

Functions Related to Brodmann Areas Near Fp1 and Fp2: BAs 10 and 11

Fp1, the left prefrontal area: BAs 10 and 11 (see also the Orbital Frontal section for additional discussion of BA 11)

BA 10

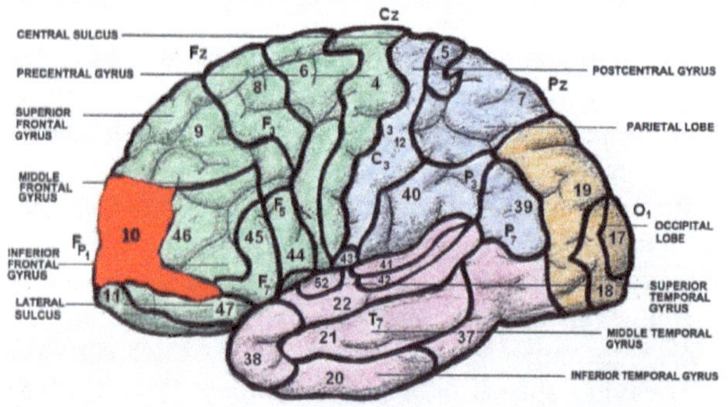

BA 11

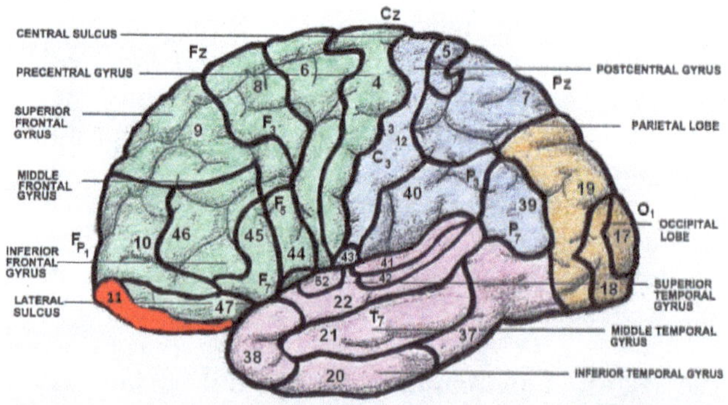

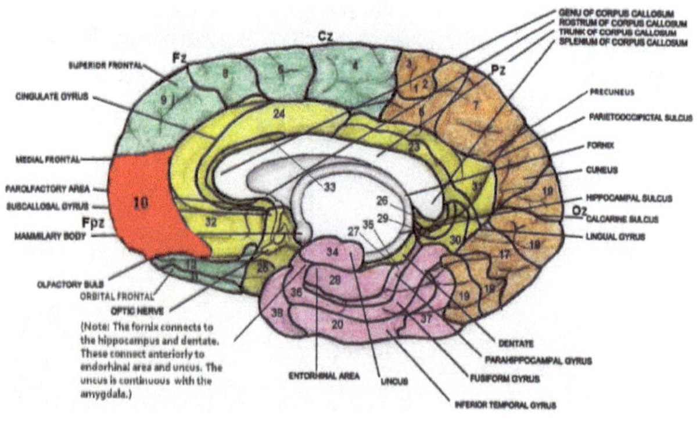

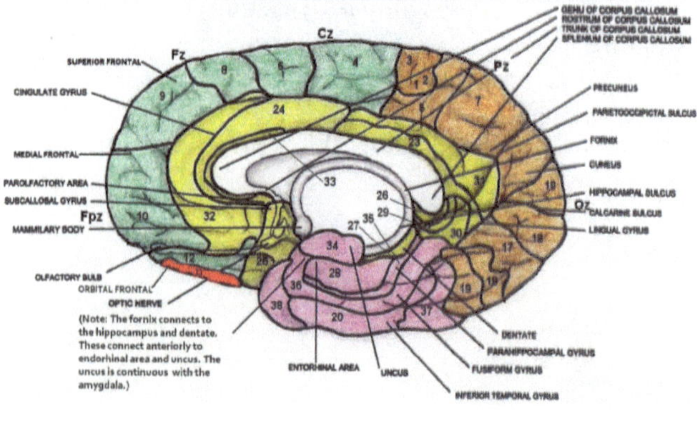

The **middle frontal gyrus** has a fundamental role in **memory** strategies and in controlling memory. Brodmann area 10 is involved in working memory including memory encoding and retrieval. The NFB practitioner understands that these are network functions and even at Cz one may observe an increase around 5.5 to 6.5 Hz when memory encoding and retrieval is taking place. Professionals who are beginning NFB work should watch/record their own spectrum while doing an EEG recording when they are concentrating on mental arithmetic problems or memorizing material. You may be as surprised as the first author was when his 5.5 Hz average amplitude was found to be very high, measured at FCz, compared to the rest of the spectral values at this site when doing math in his head.

BAs 10 and 11 are key areas for **executive functions** including planning and evaluating complicated goal-directed behavior (sometimes called 'executive control of behavior'). These areas are essential for **understanding complexity** in pictures, text, and behaviors. They are involved in high level cognitive reasoning including **making inferences** about other people. These areas are critical to categorizing and, in particular, to **semantic categorization.** They are important in the ability to stop one's course of action and take a different direction or approach, and are thus involved in **shifting mental set**. Deficiencies may result in impulsive judgments.

When this general area is not functioning normally there may be difficulty with abstraction. **Abstraction** is the act of considering something as a general quality or characteristic, as distinct from concrete realities, specific objects, or actual instances. For example, "Mary is laughing." is a concrete observation, whereas describing her as being happy is more abstract. This area is also important for drawing **analogies** (finding a similarity in some respects between things that are otherwise dissimilar). This area is involved in networks related to making decisions that concern emotions.

As previously described in more detail, this dominant (left) frontal area is also important in networks for **language processing**. This includes verbal strategies such as syntactic processing, generating sentences, and, perhaps more in the NDH, metaphor comprehension.

Interestingly, this area may also involve quite diverse functions that include attention to baroreceptor stimulation and to painful thermal stimuli.

Brodmann areas 10 and 11 of the prefrontal cortex are functionally **linked to BA 46**, particularly on the left. They are involved in executive cognitive functions including working memory, and the ability to **plan, reflect, make decisions**, **shift mental set**, initiate response, evaluate response, correct one's response, and to modulate and **inhibit impulses**. These areas are important for the highest levels of cognition involving careful **analysis, judgment**, and decision making involving complex problems or situations and inferential reasoning.

Detection and **processing of errors** involves the cingulate gyrus in addition to these frontal executive areas. The EEG can correlate with the complexity of the context of cognitive activity (Kurova et al., 2007). As previously noted, standard intelligence testing such as with the Wechsler Intelligence Scales, will help to assess many of these cognitive functions.

The **dominant (left) cerebral hemisphere near** Fp1, Brodmann areas 11, 10 and 46, is also involved in verbal analytic cognition and **approach behaviors**. Richard Davidson's work on emotions showed that left frontal activation was associated with positive thoughts and approach behavior. In the dominant hemisphere the anterior cingulate and dorsal-medial PFC is important in **theory of mind** functions (Amodio & Frith, 2006). Calculations and numerical processes are also carried out in these areas.

Fp2, the Right, NDH Prefrontal Area

BAs 11, 10 and 46 on the right side share many of the higher level functions described above. The **nondominant** hemisphere may differ from the dominant hemisphere, however, in that dysfunction may result more in **overactive behavior and this may correlate with irritability, impulsivity, tactless**, and even manic behavior. Other patients may demonstrate **panic, and avoidance** behavior. Davidson found right frontal activation in association with a focus on **negative thoughts and social avoidance**. These areas have important **links to the amygdala**. The right prefrontal area involving BA 10 is also involved in inhibiting action. Elsewhere we have noted that the medial aspect of the prefrontal cortex exerts tonic inhibition of the central nucleus of the amygdala (Thayer, 2012).

BA 10, NDH

Brodmann area 10 in the right prefrontal cortex is involved in aspects of memory recall including spatial memory, **working memory, calculations, and attention.** It is also involved in networks for the recognition of emotions and understanding of **metaphors** and in analyzing **risk versus benefit**. In the nondominant hemisphere, increased activity may be linked to unpleasant emotions, **avoidance behavior** and **anxiety**. Increased activity can correlate with increased activity in the anterior cingulate, posterior cingulate and cuneus, and also increased activity in the insula and in the amygdala-hypothalamic-pituitary-adrenal axis. BA 10 also **responds to baroreceptor stimulation** and may have a role in the regulation of the autonomic nervous system. This finding may be important in understanding the effects of HRV training.

F3: BAs 46 (8, 9)

BA 46

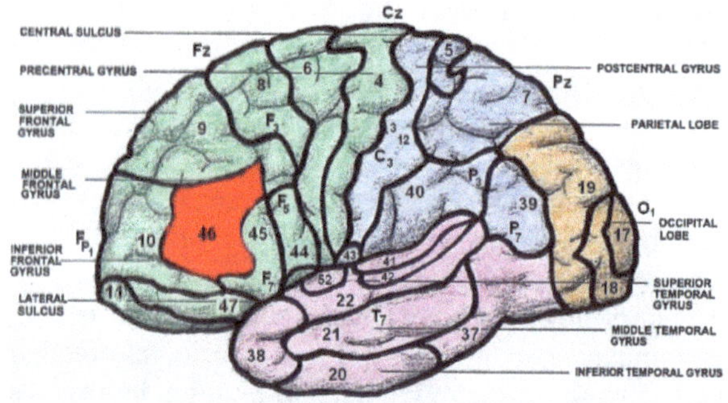

BA 8

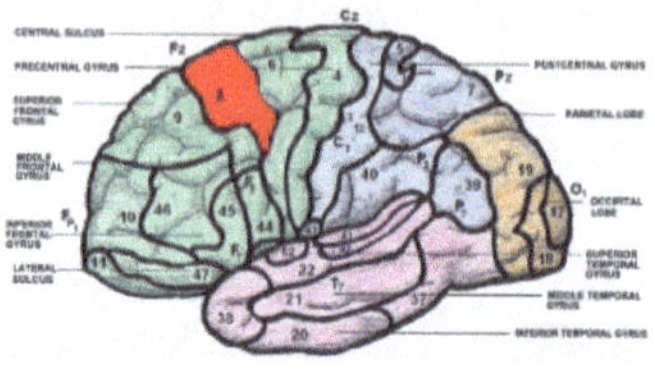

BA 9

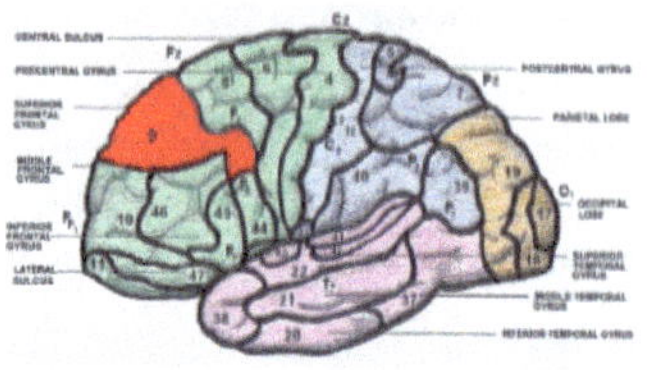

As previously noted under the general discussion of the prefrontal cortex, the functions related to BA 46 (also involving BAs 8 and 9), in the prefrontal, dorsolateral cortex, include making **judgments, planning, monitoring**, revising, **sustaining attention**, working memory, inhibition of responses, and verbal and episodic **memory retrieval. Spatial information is processed** through both the **parietal and dorsolateral frontal cortex** areas. All of these functions are part of networks that involve, as previously outlined in Part 1, specific cortical-basal ganglia- thalamic-cortical circuits.

BAs 46, 8, 9, DH

Functions related to BAs 46, 8, 9 in the **DH (left) hemisphere** under F3 include problem solving, **sequencing, concrete thinking** (extreme in Asperger's), and **deductive** reasoning. Left frontal lobe activation is also considered to be associated with positive emotions and **approach behavior** (Davidson, 1995).

F4: BAs 46, 8, 9, NDH

As previously noted under the general discussion of the prefrontal cortex, the functions related to BA 46 (8, 9) in the **NDH (right)** hemisphere include evaluating the **Gestalt** and **the context** of information and situations. In the past it was felt that inductive creative thinking was right hemisphere. Although this is important, both deduction and induction have major components in the left (dominant) hemisphere, as previously discussed. Important, however, is the **shift** that takes place from youth where creative thinking and novelty seeking – **right hemisphere functions** – **shift** more and more **with age** to the more concrete and pattern-dependent thinking of the dominant (left) hemisphere. The right frontal lobe, when more active than the left, has been found in association with negative emotions and **avoidance behavior**. The nondominant (right) hemisphere is involved in **metaphorical** thinking, short term retrieval of **spatial-object memories**, vigilance, and both selective and **sustained attention**.

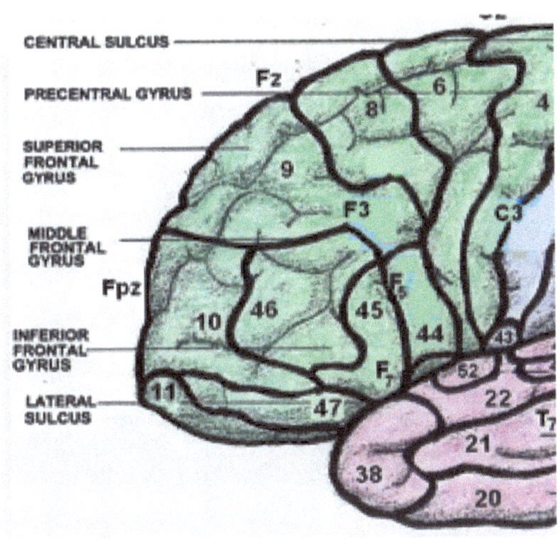

Frontal Cortex

Lateral and Medial views

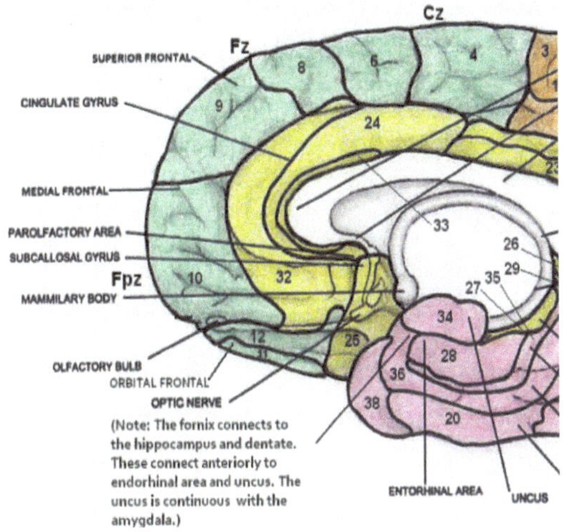

F5: BAs 44 and 45

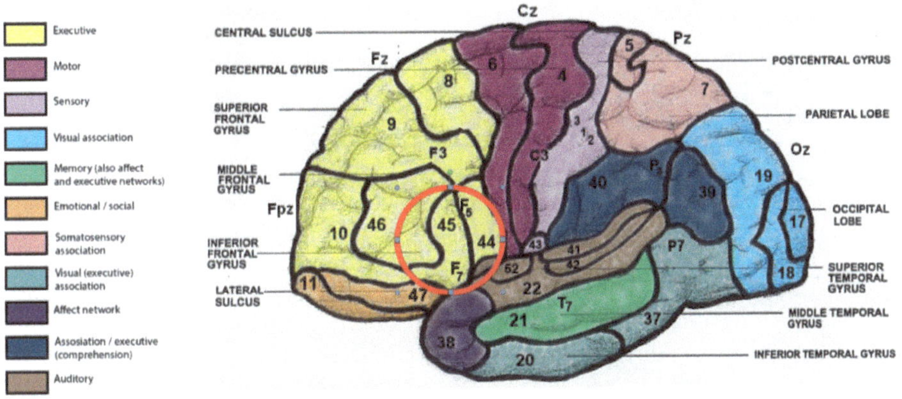

F5 – F7; BAs 44, 45

BA 44

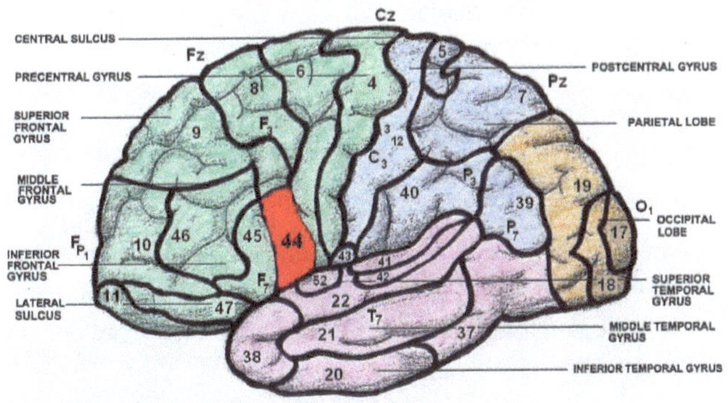

BA 45

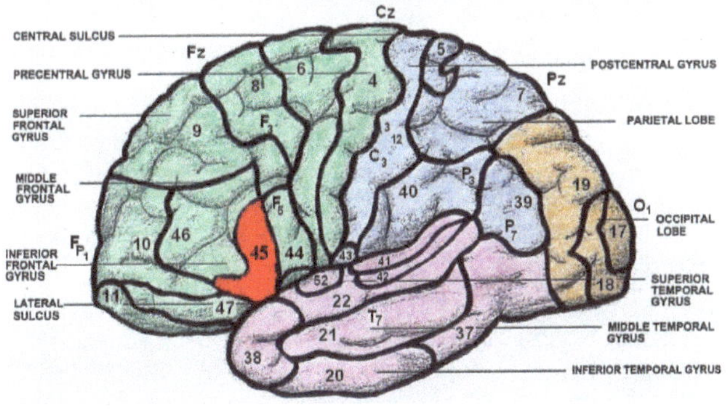

BA 44, Dominant Hemisphere

Brodmann area 44 is called the pars opercularis ("part that covers"). It **covers a portion of the insula**. It was previously mentioned as being important in **deductive reasoning**. Brodmann areas **45 (Pars Triangularis) along with BAs 44 and 46**, in addition to their importance as being part of **Broca's** area in the dominant hemisphere, contain neurons related to the **mirror neuron system** (MNS). The MNS is postulated to be involved in the imitation of movements, and perhaps also in copying appropriate social interactions, as well as being critical to understanding and predicting the behavior of others.

Although **mental rotation** involves the nondominant parietal regions including the angular gyrus, frontal BA 45 is also involved. Important **MNS areas** in the left hemisphere (there are corresponding areas on the right) include frontal near F5, the temporal pole, the temporal-parietal junction, and activities in the anterior insula and the anterior cingulate gyrus. Each area is postulated to have mirror functions that correspond to the functions of that area of the cortex. **Mirror neurons have strong connections to the limbic system including the anterior cingulate (AC)** (Iacoboni & Dapretto, 2006). The cingulate and the insular cortices both contain mirror neuron cells (Ramachandran & Oberman, 2006).

A functional magnetic resonance imaging (fMRI) study demonstrated that activity of the MNS is **correlated with empathic concern** and interpersonal competence (Dapretto, Davies, Pfeifer, Scott, Sigman, Bookheimer & Iacoboni, 2006; Pfeifer, Iacaboni, Mazziatta & Dapretto, 2005). It has also been shown that children with autism spectrum disorders (ASD) have reduced activity in MNS regions during tasks that require the child to mirror facial expressions of different emotions (Dapretto et al., 2006). Findings at the ADD Centre using 19-channel QEEG and LORETA source locations show these areas to be quite consistently outside the database norms (> 2SD) for same age children in clients diagnosed with autism spectrum disorders (Thompson & Thompson, 2010b). There is also a reduction in the volume of gray matter in BAs 44 and 45 in children who have a diagnosis along the autistic spectrum.

BAs 44, 45, DH

The **dominant** frontal cortex under F5 includes Brodmann areas 44 and 45. As previously noted, **Broca's area** is a name that has been applied to this general region, especially when one is discussing verbal language functions including semantics, phonetics, verbal understanding, categorization, speech articulation, selection of information from competing sources, grapheme to phoneme conversion, grammatical processing, and fluency of speech.

Paul Broca

Paul Broca (1824 – 1880) was the French physician and anthropologist who published the first anatomical proof of localization of brain function.

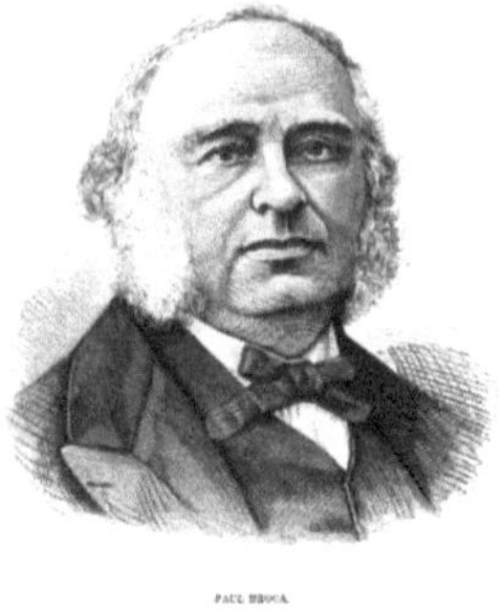

Paul Broca (1824 – 1880)

Broca's evidence, presented in 1861, was based on autopsy findings in a man who had lost the ability to produce speech. He confirmed his initial finding with a dozen more autopsies on the brains of similarly afflicted patients performed in the next two years.

Anterior Insula & Speech

Interestingly, the **anterior insula** may also be involved in some of these **motor-speech functions**. It is essential for processing sequential sounds and for lexical inflection. BA 44 of the dominant hemisphere, as mentioned above, includes frontal **mirror neurons** whose activation is important for empathy and for **understanding the intention of others**. These areas have mirror neuron functions for expressive speech. The mirror neuron areas may also be important in **internal speech** and in the internal rehearsal of information. It is one part of the working memory networks and is important in episodic, syntactic, semantic, and declarative memory encoding. BA 45, the pars triangularis, has a role in the cognitive control of memory. It is a key area in **selective attention to speech**. It is important in sign language, too. When reading aloud, written language needs to be **decoded and correctly pronounced** and this is another function of Broca's area. The role played by these areas in **deductive** reasoning (dominant hemisphere) and inductive reasoning (dominant and nondominant hemispheres) has been previously discussed.

BAs 44, 45, NDH

In the **nondominant** hemisphere, **BAs 44, 45** are involved in expression of **vocal tones and prosody.** Along with the supramarginal and angular gyrus area at the temporal-parietal junction, this area may be involved in the perception of nuance, innuendo, and intonation in speech, though these frontal regions are more involved in language production (putting emotion into speech) and the parietal regions are more involved with language understanding (interpreting tone of voice). It is one part of a network necessary for sentence comprehension and grammar. It is involved in the generation of **melodies** in addition to music enjoyment. It is necessary for arithmetic calculations and sequencing of data. It is involved in **networks for the inhibition of actions**. It is important for word generation and working memory including **syntactic working memory,** episodic and declarative memory, encoding of words and of faces. It is important for arithmetic and **music appreciation**. In conjunction with the dominant hemisphere, it is important for inductive reasoning.

When there is **dysfunction** in these areas **in the non-dominant hemisphere,** the patient may present with a **motor aprosodia** where vocal tones are flat or they do not seem to be emotionally appropriate to the situation, although the patient may understand emotions perfectly. Clinicians who work with people with Asperger's syndrome will not be surprised to learn that LORETA analysis for 19-channel EEG data often identifies abnormal findings with NDH BAs 44 and 45 as the source location. Those with Asperger's symptoms often talk in a monotone without any apparent emotional expression. The seemingly flat affect communicated by the monotone voice occurs even when they are experiencing emotions, as shown by other physiological measures. This **lack of emotional expressiveness** in a person's voice is also found in people who have suffered a stroke affecting this area; it is referred to by neurologists as motor aprosodia.

It is important to repeat that the nondominant inferior frontal cortex that includes these areas of BAs 44 and 45 has been found to be important for the **inhibition** of behaviors (Aron, 2004).

BA 45

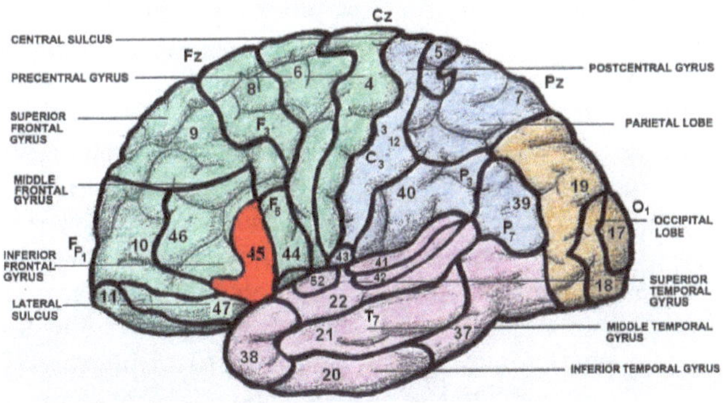

BA 46

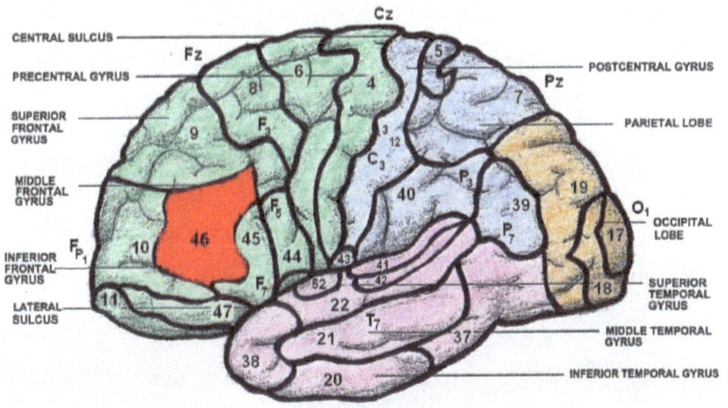

F7 (and between Fp1, F3, and F7): BAs (38), 44, 45, 46, (47), DH

F8 (and between Fp2, F4 and F8): BAs (38), 44, 45, 46, (47), NDH

F7 (and between Fp1, F3, and F7): BAs (38), 44, 45, 46, (47), DH

NFB over the F7 site can influence **Brodmann areas 38, 44, 45, 46, and 47** on the left side. In general terms, think of the functions previously described under the dorsolateral prefrontal cortex and the **executive system** as being influenced by training done at the F7 location. These include visual and auditory **working memory, selective attention**, word retrieval, and functions related to Broca's area including generating words, **verbal fluency, lexical functions, phonemes, grammar, categorization,** syntax. These areas are involved in episodic, declarative, and working memory. As previously mentioned, these areas are a keystone in most aspects of executive functioning.

F8 (and between Fp2, F4 and F8): BAs (38), 44, 45, 46, (47), NDH

Training at the F8 site can influence Brodmann areas 38, 44, 45, 46, and 47 on the right side. In general terms, think of functions previously described concerning the area in the right hemisphere that is homologous to Broca's area. These include spatial & visual working memory, sustained attention, prosody, sensing the Gestalt, and conscious processing of facial recognition information and of information related to emotions. Sensing the **Gestalt** refers to seeing the pattern or the whole picture. **Mood regulation** involving emotion-contextual information can be related to this area, too. The area between F8 and T8 (formerly T4) may be found to be outside database norms in rare cases where **labile mood** with sudden mood changes, such as sudden anger, and impulsivity may be found. The right ventral prefrontal cortex is involved in **anxiety** associated with psychological stress and the ventral lateral prefrontal cortex may be involved in the **activation of cortisol** release (Wang et al., 2005).

This area of the cortex has **strong links to the medial prefrontal cortex, insula, and anterior cingulate**, which are areas involved in increasing cortisol secretion in response to stress. Although the ventral lateral prefrontal cortex does not have strong connections to the hippocampus, these other areas do. Functions related to structures connected by the right uncinate fasciculus may be influenced by NFB over an area between F10 and T8. These can include the capacity for **autonoetic self awareness,** which refers to the ability to **re-experience previous events** from one's past as a continuous entity across time (Levine et al., 1998).

Anger, however, may be primarily related to the Affect network and the stress response system in general, with both left and right ventral prefrontal areas being involved. Some research has demonstrated that **motivational direction** in 'dispositional anger' is an approach-related motivational tendency with a negative valence. It is associated with greater left- than right-anterior activity. This suggests that the anterior asymmetry with emotions may vary as a function of motivational direction rather than affective valence (Harmon-Jones et al., 1998). This is a somewhat different emphasis than that utilized in the NFB alpha-asymmetry protocol developed by Peter Rosenfeld and put into practice by Elsa Bhaer (Rosenfeld, 1996, 1997) that was based on the work of Richard Davidson (Davidson, 1995, 1998) showing left frontal activation was associated with approach behavior and positive mood. The lesson for practitioners is a fundamental one. In clinical practice, do not immediately apply any protocol without doing a careful clinical assessment and EEG assessment. Then follow the findings to design an intervention for the individual patient.

BA 46

Brodmann area 46 roughly corresponds to a portion of the **dorsolateral prefrontal cortex (DLPFC**). The DLPFC comprises the lateral aspects of BAs 9, 10, 11, 12, 45, 46, 47. The DLPFC plays a key role in executive functioning including sustaining attention and working memory. As previously mentioned, we **define executive functioning** as the overall capacity to manage perception, attention, selection, decision making, inhibition, memory, planning, problem solving, logical thinking (deductive/inductive), sequencing; and to monitor, evaluate and self-correct outputs; and to respond verbally/nonverbally, motorically, and socially for the purpose of the attainment of defined goals.

Lesions in this area have been associated with what is sometimes termed **'dysexecutive syndrome'**. Lesions to the DLPFC **impair short-term memory** and cause **difficulty inhibiting responses**. Lesions may also eliminate much of the ability to make judgments about **what is relevant** and what is not. Lesions will also cause problems in the ability to organize. In addition, the DLPFC has been found to be involved in exhibiting **self-control**. The Tower of London Test **(ToL)** is one example of a test that can help the practitioner to **evaluate** many aspects of executive functioning that are primarily related to **BA 46, particularly in the dominant hemisphere**. The ToL involves ten trials of changing the position of colored rings by placing them on three pegs in order to copy a pattern shown by the examiner. It requires the subject to inhibit immediate responses, plan, shift mental-set, use working memory, initiate a thought-out response, and then monitor and evaluate the results of that response. The required cognitive functions all depend on good prefrontal lobe functioning. Part of this functioning involves the dorsolateral prefrontal cortex near F5 and extending downward to F7.

F9 and F10 & Orbital Surface

Neurofeecback using these sites may have an effect on BAs 11, 47, 38. These sites, which are not included in the usual 19-channel 10-20 system sites, may sometimes be used in NFB training due to the need to influence important functions of the orbital surface of the frontal lobes. These functions include understanding the effects of one's own behavior on others.

The orbital surface of the left frontal lobe was the area pierced by the 13 lb. iron tamping rod in the sad case of **Phineas Gage**. This railway worker displayed a total change in personality after the brain injury and, in the words of his physician, became "fitful, irreverent, impatient, vacillating." In general, he became extremely difficult for anyone to get along with and he often got into fights. Though Phineas Gage had a very dramatic injury to his **left orbital frontal** cortex, less extreme but similar difficulties are now being reported in athletes and veterans who have suffered concussions involving this area of the cortex.

The orbital surface of the frontal lobe has connections to the temporal lobe and other structures by way of the uncinate fasciculus. The **left uncinate fasciculus** includes functions relating to proficiency in **auditory-verbal memory** and declarative memory (Mabbott et al., 2009).

As noted above, the **right uncinate fasciculus** is involved in the capacity for **autonoetic self-awareness;** that is, re-experiencing previous events from one's past as part of a continuous entity across time (Levine et al., 1998). (Synonyms for autonoetic consciousness are self knowing and self awareness.)

BA 47

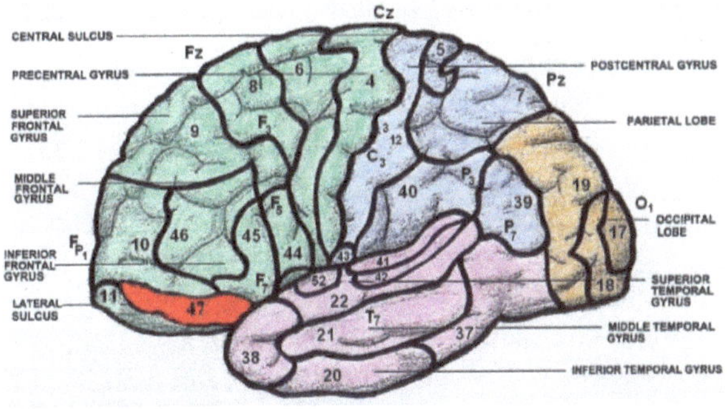

Brodmann area 47 is the part of the frontal cortex in the human brain that curves from the lateral surface of the frontal lobe into the ventral (orbital) frontal cortex and is therefore involved in many functions related to **deductive reasoning, language, and emotions.** It is below **BA 10 and BA 45,** and parallel to **BA 11.**

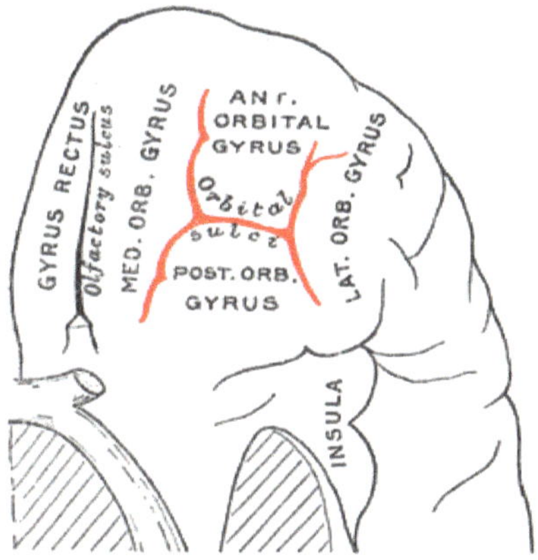

Gray's Anatomy *to show Orbital Sulci*
Public Domain via Wikimedia Commons –

In the human, **on the orbital surface,** it surrounds the caudal portion of the orbital sulcus from which it extends laterally into the orbital part of the inferior frontal gyrus. Like nearby areas previously described, including Brodmann areas 45 and 46, it is part of the **Executive network**. In the dominant hemisphere it is important for **categorization and aspects of language** and speech, and is also important in episodic and **working memory**. It is one of the key areas for **deductive** reasoning. It is important for making inferences. In conjunction with other cortical areas, it helps in **monitoring** actions and incoming information. It is activated when inner speech is used during the performance of tasks. With the insula it may be involved in processing **temporal coherence in music** (Cannon, 2012, p160). It is important in monitoring behavior.

Inferior Frontal Gyrus in the DH

The posterior medial parietal cortex and left prefrontal cortex (PFC) have both been implicated in the recollection of past events. The posterior precuneus and left lateral inferior frontal cortex are activated during episodic source memory retrieval. The **precuneus and the left inferior PFC are important for regeneration of rich episodic contextual** associations. The left ventro-lateral frontal region/frontal operculum is involved in searching for task-relevant information (BA 47) and subsequent monitoring or scrutiny (BAs 44 and 45). Regions in the dorsal inferior frontal gyrus are important for information selection (BAs 45 and 46) (Lundstrom et al., 2005).

Semantic memory comprises general word knowledge, such as word meaning and word use, and it functions to store, retrieve, and associate this information in conjunction with environmental stimuli. On the other hand, **working memory** refers to the short-term maintenance and manipulation of information during processing; keeping something in mind long enough to do something with it, like remembering a telephone number long enough to write it down. Finally, **episodic memory** is employed for long-term storage and recall of previous experiences or episodes, and it allows people to reflect upon their personal past. Entailing more than just event memory and event recall, **episodic memory** includes a special awareness for subjective time known as autonoetic consciousness; it enables people to mentally travel backwards in time and knowingly **retrieve information** from a given personal experience (Lundstrom, 2005). Episodic memory allows current knowledge to be associated with past experiences.

Connections to the Default Network

Several areas of the brain show decreased activity during cognitive tasks and increased activity in the so-called resting state. These include parts of the posterior cingulate cortex (PCC) and medial frontal region incorporating portions of the medial frontal gyrus (MFG) and ventral anterior cingulate cortex (vACC). These areas are part of the **Default mode network** that is engaged during rest and disengaged during cognitive tasks. A decrease in activity is usually inferred when theta increases.

'Hippocampal' Theta and Memory

With the **engagement of working memory, 4 - 7 Hz** (sometimes more specifically around 6 Hz or 5.5 - 6.5 Hz) **synchronized activity may increase and be related to a decrease in hippocampal metabolism** (Hampson et al., 2006; Uecker, 1997). It is detected over the frontal midline. This is sometimes termed **hippocampal theta** and thus the source is different than the excess theta produced in the thalamus that is a marker for Attention-Deficit/Hyperactivity Disorder.

Hampson et al. state that an inverse relationship between activation (as measured using functional imaging) and engagement appears to exist in the hippocampus. They give the example of deactivation in the hippocampus (and adjacent regions) during a transverse patterning task and during virtual navigation of a radial arm maze (Astur & Constable, 2004; Astur et al., 2005). They note that these tasks require engagement of the hippocampus but hippocampal activity decreases during these tasks. They posit that coding of information occurs in terms of neural synchrony rather than rate of neural firing. The **theta rhythm reflects this synchronized activity** and is associated with memory and cognitive function (Gevins et al., 1997; Tesche & Karhu, 2000). They relate this to the observed decreased metabolism (Uecker et al., 1997).

Connectivity between regions is increased during these tasks (Hampson et al., 2006). Clinically, Hampson's observations give support to the notion that we must pay attention to low amplitude findings and increase synchronized slow wave activity when it is well below the database norms. In particular, if amplitudes are low, it may sometimes be appropriate to consider enhancing 6 Hz 'hippocampal theta' because it may be associated with memory functions.

NDH Right Inferior Frontal Region BAs 47, 12

Another function that has been observed for the inferior frontal gyrus (IFG) has come from research concerning the **right lateral inferior frontal** gyrus during **go/no go tasks**. In such a task, the participant has to **inhibit** a prepotent response (for instance, not pressing a button when one signal appears after pressing for another signal). This task involves the general area of BAs 47 and 12. (References that give good descriptions of this include Aron et al., 2004; Kringelbach et al., 2005; Menon et al., 2006; Li et al., 2006.)

It seems that the same area is also implicated in **risk aversion**: higher risk aversion is correlated with higher activity in the IFG (Christopoulos et al., 2009; Knoch, 2006). This might be explained as an inhibition of a signal to accept a risky option. Disruption of activity of this area with Transcranial Magnetic Stimulation (TMS) or Transcranial Direct Current Stimulation (tDCS) can lead to a change in risk attitudes, as behaviorally demonstrated by choices involving risky outcomes. Theoretically, dysfunction in this area could lead to dangerous behavior. On a more positive note, it might be possible to decrease such negative behaviors using LORETA NFB.

Orbital Frontal/Inferior Frontal Cortex

Affect Network – Emotional/Social: BAs 11, 12

BA 11

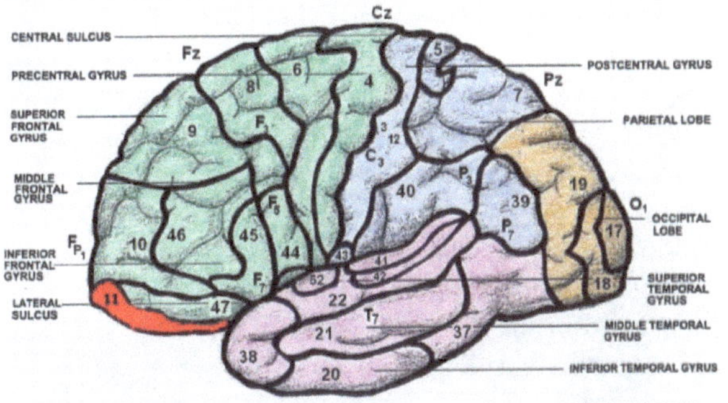

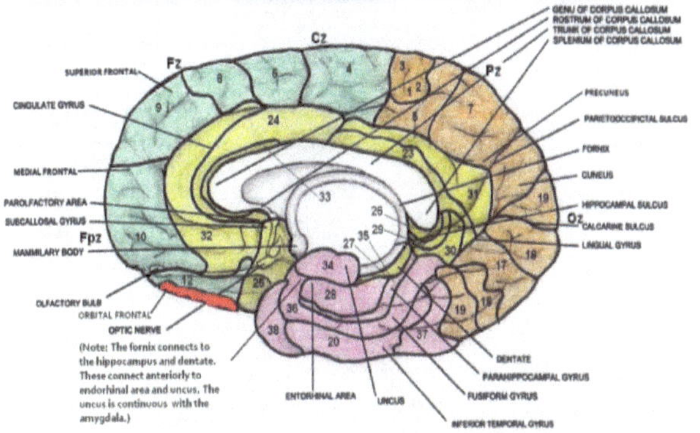

The ventral medial orbital frontal cortex is equivalent to the ventromedial **reward network** (Ongur, 2000). As a reward network, this area is broader than the orbital surface of the frontal lobe and it includes Brodmann areas 10, 11, 12, and areas in the cingulate gyrus 25, 32, and the insula BA 13. However, the term ***ventromedial prefrontal cortex*** is used differently in different articles. In this section we will just discuss BAs 11 and 12.

Brodmann area 11 includes the **orbital frontal association** cortex. BA 11 covers the medial part of the ventral surface of the frontal lobe. It is bounded on the rostral and lateral aspects of the hemisphere by the frontopolar area 10, the orbital area 47, and the triangular area 45; on the medial surface it is bounded dorsally by the rostral area 12 and caudally by the subgenual area 25. These surrounding areas may influence the activity at BA 11 and 12, the orbital frontal cortex. This area of the cortex is involved in the modulation of affect and is an integral part of the **Affect network**. The ventral lateral prefrontal cortex (VLPFC) in both the nondominant (ND) and dominant (D) hemispheres, in conjunction with the ND insula, amygdala, and anterior temporal pole (BAs 21, 38) may, for example, show increased activity with subjective **sadness**.

BA 11 is also important in social and cultural behavior. It is involved in **empathy** and, along with areas in the right parietal-temporal junction, in **understanding what others may be thinking**. Compromised function in the orbitofrontal lobes, an area linked to social and cultural behaviors, will result in the patient demonstrating difficulty with abstract rules, empathy, reflecting on the **effect of their behavior on others** (consequences of actions) and executive functions including self-expression, problem solving, **willpower and planning.** In addition, reward and conflict are analyzed in this area, as are unexpected outcomes to actions or events. **Lesions can lead to personality changes** including **disinhibited behavior** such as swearing, compulsive gambling, drug and alcohol abuse, and hypersexuality. Lesions can lead to disinhibited and aggressive behavior, as was seen in the famous case of Phineas Gage.

Phineas Gage (1823-1860)

As previously mentioned, Phineas Gage (1823-1860) was a foreman with a railway building crew when in 1848, at age 25, he suffered a severe brain injury. A 13-pound iron bar, 3 ft. 7in. x 1¼ in., that he had been using to tamp an explosive charge, flew upwards when the charge exploded prematurely. The bar went cleanly through his cheekbone and skull, exiting from the top of his head. It pierced the orbital surface of his left frontal hemisphere. He was never unconscious. There was, however, an immediate change in temperament and behavior. He had been a wonderful, thoughtful, kind, individual who was well liked by everyone. He was also said to be the most efficient and capable foreman at his company.

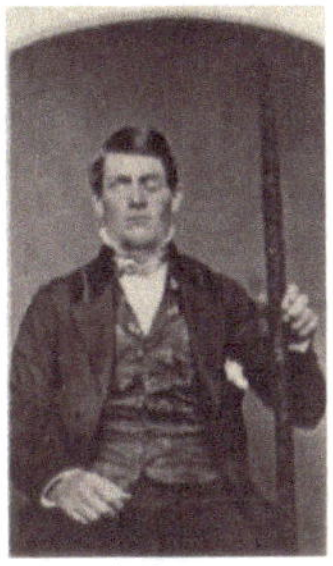
After Accident

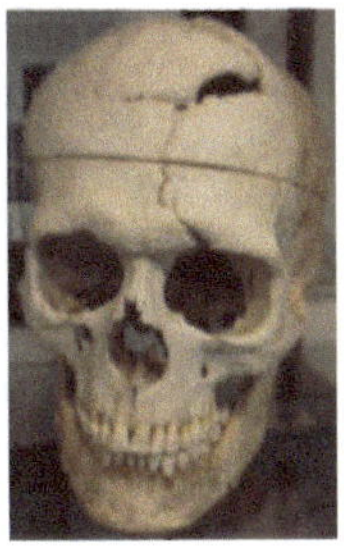
Phineas Gage's skull

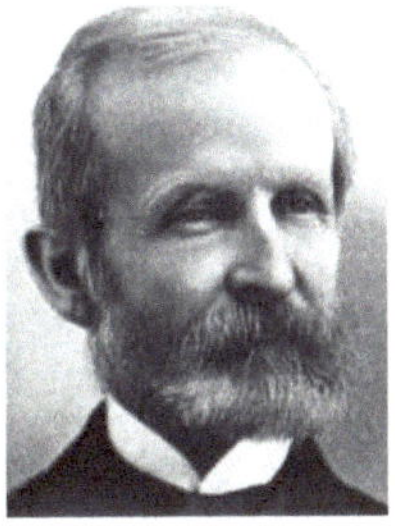
Dr J. Harlow

After the accident he became fitful, irreverent, impatient, and vacillating, showing a very negative personality change. As time went by he worked hard as a stagecoach driver in Chile and did make some recovery. He had figured out how to live even with respect to social interactions. His case was followed until he died in San Francisco, a result of a seizure, by his physician, Dr. Harlow, and Dr. Harlow's notes have become the classic account of the effects of brain damage involving the orbital frontal and ventral medial prefrontal cortex.

This area is involved in the analysis of **idioms,** the encoding of words and, in a network that includes the nondominant fusiform gyrus, putting **faces to names**. As can be understood from these functions, this area of the frontal lobe is considered to be a higher order cortical association area. It is an important part of the **Default network,** which is activated when one considers aspects of 'self' and '**self-in-relation-to-others.**' It plays a key role in feeling **empathy**, an objective understanding of the emotions of another person. In addition, it has areas from an early time of phylogenetic development that are involved in olfaction. This is doubtless because a good sense of smell confers survival value in many species.

BA 12

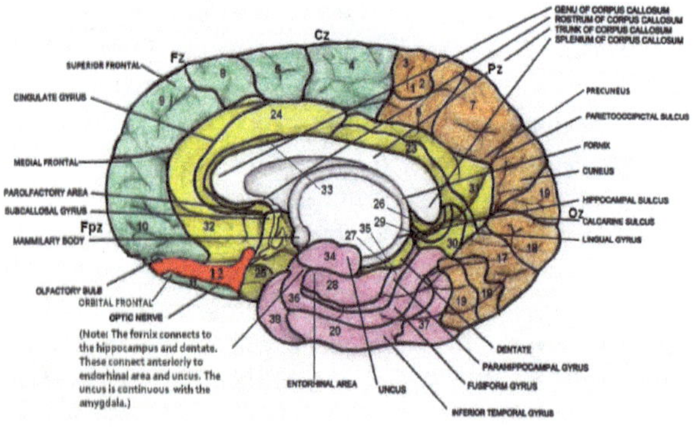

Brodmann area 12 occupies the most rostral portion of the medial aspect of the frontal lobe and includes areas that were originally subsumed under BA 11. This area has been labelled as part of the **paralimbic association** cortex and it is involved in **assessing the affect or emotional value of different reinforcers.** It is also a higher level association cortex that is involved in the **generation of hypotheses,** discrimination of **'same' and 'different,'** making decisions, and in formulating expectations. It has a role in **sensitivity to reward versus punishment.**

Nucleus Basalis of Meynert and Acetylcholine

The nucleus basalis of Meynert (NBM), though it is not located in BA 11 or 12, is **discussed here because of its relation to executive** functions and its connections to executive areas in the dorsal lateral prefrontal cortex, in addition to connections to the basal forebrain and areas within the temporal lobe. The NBM is a diffuse grouping of neurons within the basal forebrain that projects to widespread areas of the neocortex. The NBM is **inferior to the globus pallidus** and within an area known as the substantia innominata. The NBM is immediately inferior to the anterior commissure and superior and lateral to the anterior portion of the hypothalamus. It is the main source of **acetylcholine** (Ach) in the neocortex (Mesulam & Guela, 1988). Neocortical cholinergic innervation principally comes from the Nucleus Basalis of Meynert. It is interesting to note that the **orbitofrontal cortex projects into the nucleus basalis** and thus has the possibility of influencing cholinergic input to the entire cerebral cortex (Mesulam, 1988). This is important in part because Ach is a key neurotransmitter in memory networks.

Anatomical Connections

The other regions **projecting to the nucleus basalis** include the hypothalamus, nucleus accumbens, piriform cortex, entorhinal cortex, temporal pole, anterior insula, septal nuclei, and posterior parahippocampal cortex. We have noted previously that these areas also influence the hypothalamus and the autonomic nervous system. The Nucleus Basalis of Meynert and the cholinergic innervations to the hippocampus and temporal lobes are crucial to laying down new (episodic) memories and are said to be the **first areas to be affected by Alzheimer's** disease. However, there is also an **abnormal connectivity between the posterior cingulate and the hippocampus in early Alzheimer's** disease, which is accompanied by mild cognitive impairment (Zhou et al., 2008).

Alzheimer's and Exercise

We have noted above that the Nucleus Basalis of Meynert and the cholinergic innervations to the hippocampus and temporal lobes are the first to be affected by Alzheimer's disease. However, there are factors that may **influence the degree and speed of progression** of this disorder. Two such factors that should also be considered when discussing deterioration in both physical and cognitive abilities from any cause are diet and exercise. Diet and supplements are of major importance and these will be discussed further in the section on TBI interventions.

Exercise is an important consideration because it has been demonstrated that exercise can **improve neurotrophic factors**, such as the production of brain-derived neurotrophic factor (BDNF) and glial cell neurotrophic factor (GDNF), which are widely distributed throughout the brain and which modulate brain plasticity by **increasing neuritic outgrowth and synaptic transmission.** They are also protective against specific nigral (from the substantia nigra) toxins.

Such toxins include 6-hydroxydopamine (6-OHDA), which destroys neurons and is used to induce experimental Parkinson's in animals. Another such toxin is called MPTP. MPTP (1-methyl-4-phenyl-1,2,3,6-tetrahydropyridine) is a neurotoxin precursor to MPP+, which causes permanent symptoms of Parkinson's disease by destroying dopaminergic neurons in the substantia nigra. It has also been used to study disease models in animal studies related to Parkinson's disease.

In **Parkinson's disease,** nigral BDNF and GDNF expression is diminished (Chauhan et al., 2001). Both these factors cross the blood-brain barrier and levels can therefore be measured in the serum and in saliva. In serum, the level of these neurotrophic factors has been shown to rise proportionally after exercise. It has also been demonstrated that regular **exercise in humans reduces the risk of mild cognitive impairment (MCI)** (Geda et al., 2010), dementia, and Alzheimer's disease (Hamer & Chida, 2009). It has been shown that patients suffering MCI or dementia experienced **significant cognitive improvement with exercise** as compared to subjects randomized to a sedentary intervention (Baker et al., 2010; Kwak et al., 2008).

BDNF is a neurotrophic factor that is critically linked to neuroplastic changes (Lisanby et al., 2000), and might serve to index neuroplastic effects induced by repetitive transcranial magnetic stimulation (rTMS) (Brunoni et al., 2013). In addition, it has been shown that brain-derived neurotrophic factor **(BDNF) may induce the accumulation of AMPA receptors** at synapses previously devoid of these receptors. The α-amino-3-hydroxy-5-methyl-4-isoxazolepropionic acid receptor (AMPA) is a glutamate receptor (Bear, 2004; Cook & Bliss, 2006). These receptors play a **key role in long-term potentiation (LTP)** at the synapse, and are discussed further under the section on LTP in *The Neurofeedback Book.* It is hypothesized that NFB can facilitate LTP through repeated strong activation at synaptic junctions and that this may be one factor responsible for the lasting effects of NFB.

Orbitofrontal and Ventromedial Prefrontal Cortex (VMPC)

At the time of writing this text, the functional differences between the orbitofrontal and ventromedial areas of the prefrontal cortex have not been entirely established. It is known that the areas of the ventromedial cortex **superior to the orbitofrontal cortex** are much less associated with social functions and are **more involved with the regulation of emotions.** Research in developmental neuroscience also has suggested that neural networks in the ventromedial prefrontal cortex are rapidly developing during adolescence and young adulthood. These areas function in conjunction with the amygdala to regulate emotions. This regulation will alter cortisol levels. (See also the section concerning the Stress Response in *The Neurofeedback Book.*) Those with low self-esteem will show high levels of cortisol release in response to tasks that they associate with stress (Cannon, 2012, p70; Holmes & Rahe, 1967; Dedovic et al., 2005, 2009).

The **left lateral and medial orbitofrontal cortex** areas have also been found to be highly active during guessing tasks. An increase in probabilistic scenario complexity is associated with an orbitofrontal cortex activity level increase, suggesting the special role that the ventromedial prefrontal cortex plays in decision making containing uncertainty. In addition, patients with lesions in the ventromedial prefrontal cortex tend to have difficulties when considering the future consequences of their actions when making decisions.

The **right half of the ventromedial prefrontal cortex** is associated with regulating the interaction of cognition and affect in the production of empathic responses. **Hedonic (pleasure) responses** are also associated with orbitofrontal cortex activity level (Kringelbach et al., 2005). These functions suggest that the ventromedial prefrontal cortex is associated with a person's judgment when deciding on preferences. They also suggest that the ventromedial prefrontal cortex has a key role to play in constructing one's **sense of self**. It is one of the links in the Default network.

The ventral medial prefrontal cortex gives **tonic inhibition,** via GABAergic mediated projections, to the central nucleus of the **amygdala**. The amygdala connects to both the autonomic nervous system and to the endocrine system. If there is hypoactivation of the prefrontal cortex, there may be deficient inhibitory control of the amygdala, and it can become active in difficult circumstances, such as with threat and uncertainty (Davidson, 2000; Thayer, 2012, 2006).

Studies with **post traumatic stress disorder** (PTSD) support the idea that the ventromedial prefrontal cortex is an important component for reactivating **past emotional associations** and events, therefore essentially mediating the pathogenesis of PTSD. Treatments geared to the inhibition of the ventromedial prefrontal cortex may therefore be helpful for those suffering from PTSD. It has been shown that the right half of the ventrolateral prefrontal cortex, which is active during emotion regulation, is activated when people are given an unfair offer in an experimental scenario. In other experiments, specific deficits in reversal learning and decision-making have led to the hypothesis that the ventromedial prefrontal cortex (**VMPFC) is a major locus of dysfunction** in the mild initial stages of the behavioral variant of **frontotemporal dementia**.

These are all areas that require further research, but they may give the NFB practitioner a sense of some of the functions that may be affected with NFB directed to these areas, as can be done using LORETA NFB (LNFB).

One particularly notable theory of VMPFC function is the somatic marker hypothesis, accredited to António Damásio. By this hypothesis, the VMPFC has a central role in adapting somatic markers – **emotional associations**, or associations between mental objects and visceral (bodily) feedback – for use in natural decision making. This account also gives the VMPFC a role in **moderating emotions** and emotional reactions. Ventromedial prefrontal cortex lesions have also been associated with a deficit in processing gender-specific social cues.

When we do NFB using surface electrode sites, the VMPFC and orbital cortex are distant from these surface sites. However, we can influence these areas by having an effect on other cortical areas that are within the same neural network. For example, surface NFB at Fz and FCz (between Fz and Cz) may affect the anterior cingulate cortex and, thus, the Affect network. Electrode placement at either F9 or F10 may affect the lateral aspect of the orbital frontal cortex. However, F9 and F10 may also be affected by both muscle and eye-movement artifacts, making it a difficult area to work; thus, the theoretical value of using LORETA z-score NFB (LNFB) to directly influence these deep cortical areas becomes apparent.

As previously noted, in the **nondominant hemisphere, the right inferior prefrontal** cortex includes BAs 44, 45, 47, 12 (noted by Aron, 2004), and the superior frontal sulcus BA 10. These areas are involved in **behavioral inhibition**. This is an important consideration when designing a NFB program in a patient who exhibits impulsivity (Aron et al., 2004; Konishi et al., 2005).

Central Regions

Cz, C3, C4: BAs 4, 6, and 1, 2, 3, 5 – The sensorimotor strip

C3, C4

BAs 1, 2, 3 is the Primary Somatosensory Cortex
BA 4 is the Primary Motor Cortex
BA 5 is the Somatosensory Association Cortex
BA 6 is the Premotor Cortex
When reading this section, the reader will recall that, for sensory and motor functions, the right hemisphere relates to the left side of the body and the left hemisphere to the right side.

BA 6

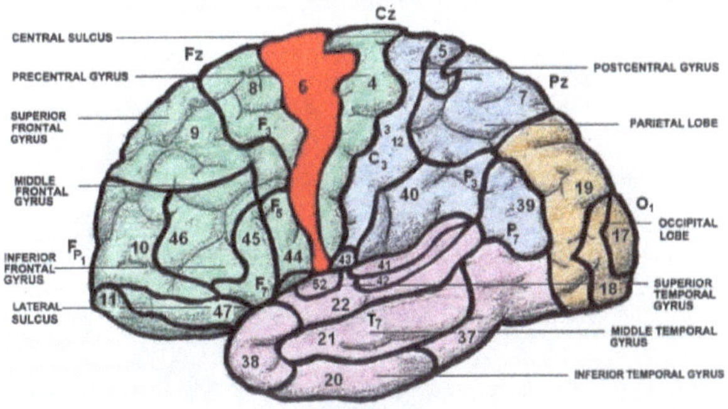

BA 6

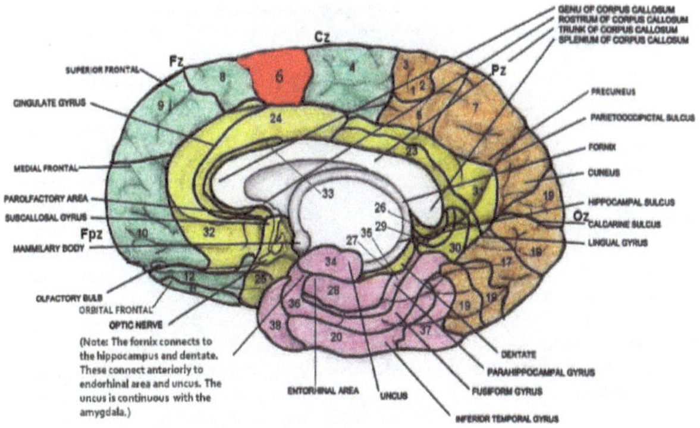

BA 4

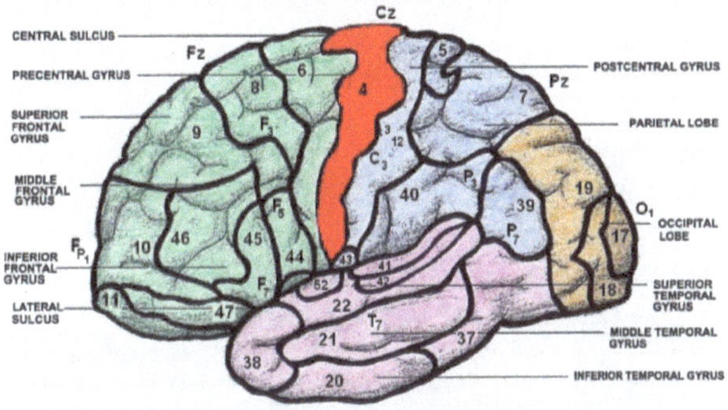

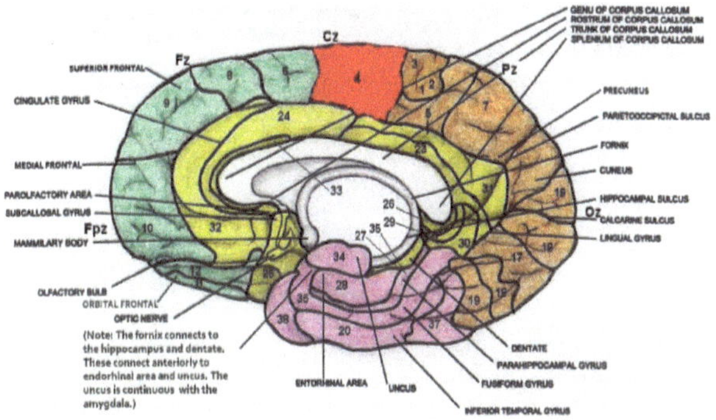

In work with NFB, we use these central sites of Cz, C3, and C4 for enhancing sensorimotor rhythm in the 12-15 or 13-15 Hz frequency range. In seizure disorders, Sterman's approach involves decreasing slow wave activity at the site of the seizure focus, if it is known, combined with increasing sensorimotor rhythm, usually alternating the feedback site between C3 and C4. This training is known to stabilize the cortex and make it more resistant to seizures. We assume when doing this NFB that we are having an effect on the thalamic production of SMR, although we may also, at these frequencies, be having some effect on high-frequency alpha and on cortically generated, low-frequency beta.

The functions of the cortical area immediately beneath our surface electrodes are: **BA 4** Primary Motor (Cz is over the part of the homunculus that connects with the **lower extremities** and C3 and C4 reflect the right and left hands, respectively), **BA 6** Premotor Association and integration, **BAs 3-1-2** Primary Sensory, and sensorimotor integration, **BA 5**

Somatosensory Association cortex, involved in **proprioception.**

Functions include control of voluntary movements, swallowing, blinking, and so on. Functions may include aspects of imagery, and even verbal encoding and motor memory. This motor cortex area may play a role in **hyperalgesia**, which is an increased sensitivity to pain.

Mu activity (brainwaves in the alpha frequency range but with slightly different morphology, namely, pointed at one end) can sometimes be recorded in some individuals at the C3 and C4 sites. Recall that the areas of BA 4 and BAs 3-1-2 under C3 relate to the right hand and under C4 to the left hand. The mu activity simply reflects motor quiescence with respect to the hands; for example, mu at C3 means the right hand is not moving, nor is the person imagining moving the right hand (as might happen if they were doing imagery of something like hitting tennis ball). Mu is a normal variant but does not occur in the majority of people.

We assessed a teenager who received a kick to the left side of his head when sparring in karate who subsequently had trouble in music (playing his trumpet) and in French Language classes at school. A 19-Channel EEG assessment showed high amplitude slow activity at C3 and hypocoherence (disconnect) between C3 and all other sites. NFB training at the C3 site resolved his problems.

Lesions caused by a **stroke or transient ischemic** attack (TIA) affecting BA 4, motor cortex, can result in paralysis of the opposite (contralateral) side of the body in areas such as the face, arm, hand, or leg. The illustration of what is called the homunculus indicates the distribution of motor activity reflected in the cortex. This illustration has been derived from the localization work of Wilder Penfield. Penfield was originally trained in the United States and then went as a Rhodes Scholar to Oxford in Great Britain. He is best known as a neurosurgeon at McGill University in Canada. He worked with Herbert Jasper. Penfield became the first Director of McGill University's world-famous Montreal Neurological Institute.

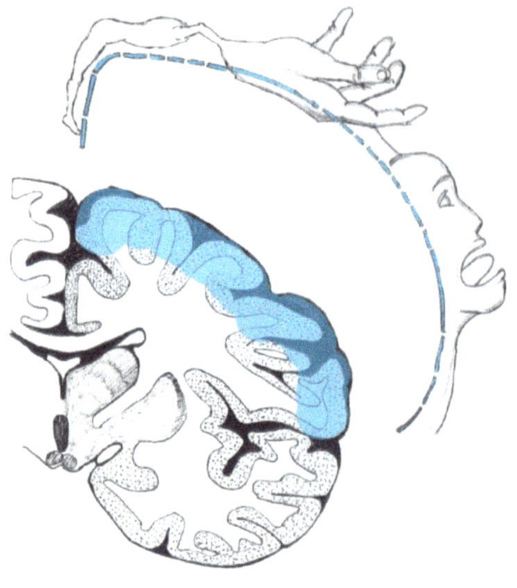

Figure by Maya Berenkey
*The **cortical homunculus** (Latin for 'little man') is a pictorial representation of the anatomical divisions of the primary motor cortex and the primary somatosensory cortex.*

BAs 1, 2, 3: Primary Somatosensory Cortex

BA 1, 2, 3

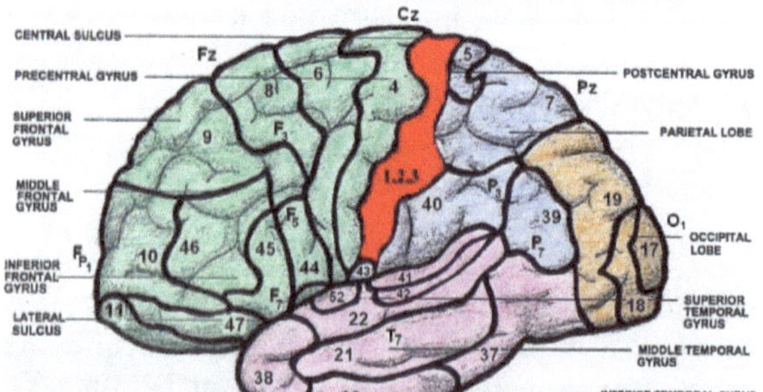

BA 1, 2, 3

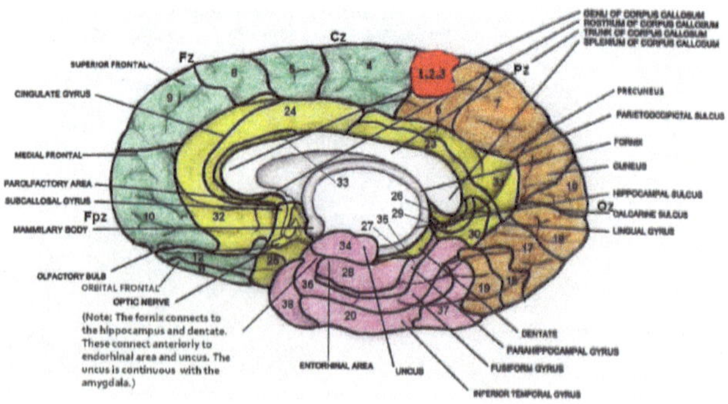

BA 1

Brodmann area 1 is central to a number of functions including **localizing sensations** such as touch, vibration, temperature, proprioception, and pain. The motor components govern hand and finger movements, movements of the tongue and mouth, swallowing. They are part of networks that allow the **anticipation of pain** and other sensations.

BA 2

Brodmann area 2 may be more involved in **agraphesthesia** (difficulty recognizing a written number or letter traced on the palm of one's hand) after parietal damage.

BA 4

Moving **anteriorly to Brodmann area 4**, the functions relate more to **sequences** of muscle movements: hands, fingers, mouth, tongue, eyes, eyelids, limbs. It is involved in **breathing** and complex body actions. The somatosensory cortex is involved in voluntary movements, organization of movements, and it also has mirror neuron functions. These areas contain **mirror neurons that become active when observing the actions of other people**. These mirror neuron functions seem to be impaired in persons with autism; that is, the mirror neurons in the area around C3 may not fire in the person with autism when he watches someone throwing a ball.

In a movement network these areas have important connections that include connections to the thalamus, cerebellum, and premotor cortex. Functions of this network include internal representation of action, and even a role in **anticipating and understanding actions.**

BA 3

Within the primary somatosensory cortex, **near the representation of the face** in the homunculus diagram and at the transition between the somatosensory cortex and the motor cortex, the cells in **Brodmann area 3** respond to proprioceptive and visual stimuli as well as to **vestibular** stimuli. Many of these neurons are activated by moving visual stimuli as well as by rotation of the body (even with the eyes closed), suggesting that these cortical regions are involved in the **perception of body orientation** in extra-personal space (Gray, 2013).

Cerebellum

This area is not being described in this text because it is not a primary site for NFB training. However, it is important in networks that the NFB practitioner is influencing and this brief note may therefore be of assistance:

Cerebellum in Latin means little brain. The cerebellum is the area of the hindbrain that controls motor movement coordination, balance, equilibrium, and muscle tone. Like the cerebral cortex, the cerebellum is comprised of white matter and a thin, outer layer of densely folded gray matter. The folded outer layer of the cerebellum (cerebellar cortex) has smaller and more compact folds than those of the cerebral cortex. The cerebellum contains hundreds of millions of neurons for processing data. It relays information between body muscles and areas of the cerebral cortex that are involved in motor control.

The cerebellum is involved in several functions of the body including:

- Fine Movement Coordination
- Balance and Equilibrium
- Muscle Tone

Of critical importance for some of our patients is the involvement of the cerebellum in **vestibular input** to the cortex. Patients after a concussion often demonstrate difficulties with balance and controlling themselves when walking and doing the tasks of daily living. The vestibular system with its connections to the cortex appears to be dysfunctional in these patients. Assessment of this system has been a major part of the assessment procedures used with concussed athletes that were developed at Penn State University (Thompson & Hagedorn, 2012).

The vestibular network encompasses cognitive and sensorimotor functions including perception of motion, spatial navigation and memory, perception of orientation of oneself (head and body) in the environment, and visual processing related to gravitational cues. The vestibular pathways originate in the vestibular nuclei in the brainstem, and the information goes to the cerebellum, thalamus, and the cerebral cortex. This network provides the brain with signals concerning gravity, such as which direction is up. Vestibular signals are of crucial importance for oculomotor and postural reflexes, and they are also basic to conscious perception and spatial cognition. The **pathways to the cortex apparently go through the ventral posterior nuclei of the thalamus to the Sylvian fissure (usually called the lateral sulcus or lateral fissure), insula, retroinsular cortex, frontoparietal operculum, superior temporal gyrus, and the cingulate cortex** (Lopez, Blanke & Mast, 2012).

Figure to show Operculum: Frontal – Parietal – Temporal – (Insula)

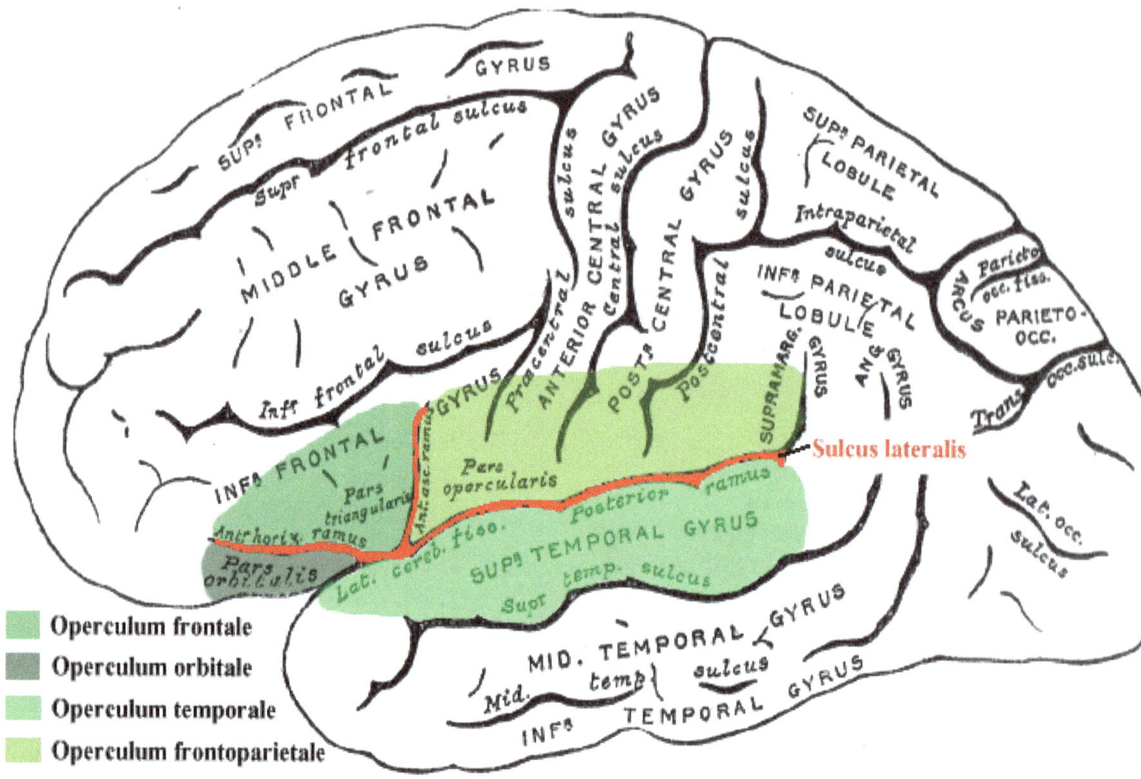

Figure from Gray's Anatomy
Portions of the frontal, temporal and parietal lobes form an 'operculum' (a covering or lid) that covers the insula.

BA 6: Premotor Cortex

BA 6

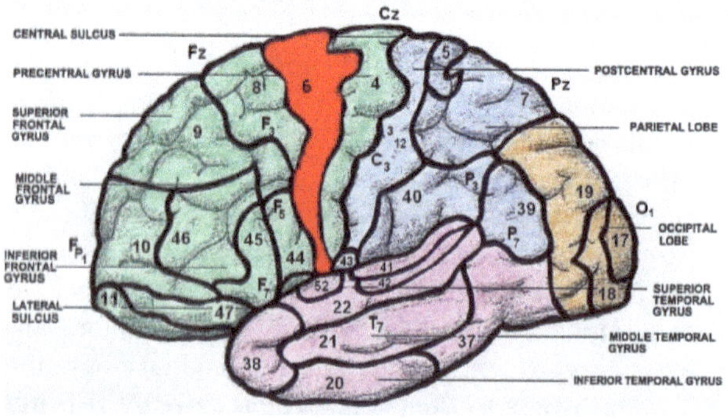

BA 6

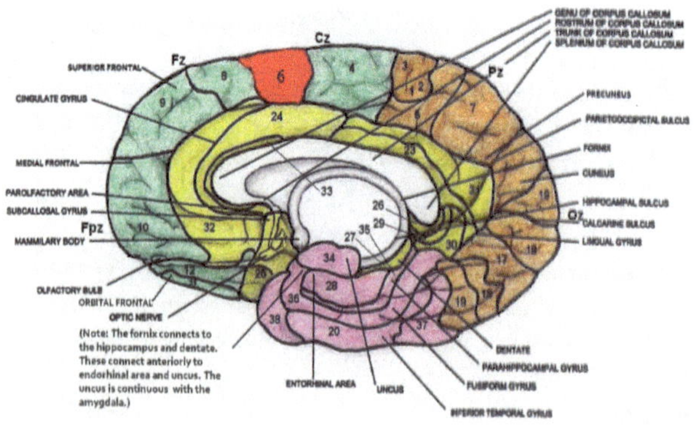

Rostral or anterior to BAs 1, 2 and 3 is **Brodmann area 6**. This region extends forward to the precentral sulcus between BA 6 and BA 8 that forms the **posterior border of the prefrontal cortex**. BA 6 is involved in a wide range of basic functions (motor, language, memory, attention), and in complex functions, such as planning, problem solving, calculations, frequency detection, behavior control, mirror neuron functions, and in the **dominant lobe: deductive** reasoning and the processing of **emotions**

related to reflections on 'self' (part of the Default network). It is the key BA for **planning and initiating** movements and motor **sequencing** during movement. Thus a form of **kinetic apraxia** (problems with skilled movements independent of any motor weakness) will result from lesions in this area. It is important for **sensory guidance** of movement. It may be involved in smiling and laughter. In the **nondominant** hemisphere it is important for same-different discrimination and responding to strong odors.

Brodmann area 6 is a **motor association area** that is involved in **sequential movements** and sensorimotor voluntary action. Control of **trunk** and proximal body musculature resides here. In conjunction with BAs 8 and 9, it is involved in the **smooth sequencing** and flow of movements. It is essential for the ability to do rapid alternating movements (**diadochokinesis**), carrying out complex actions, such as threading a needle, and for rhythmic movements such as finger tapping. Near the midline, along with the cingulate cortices, it is crucial in **monitoring errors** (more right hemisphere) and **inhibiting responses** (more left hemisphere). It is crucial for motor learning, sequencing, complex movements, such as laughing and smiling, and the voluntary control of breathing.

In the **dominant (left) hemisphere** it is involved in networks for mnemonics, phonemes, calculations, **speech**, speech motor programming (overlapping with Broca's area), and handwriting (**Exner's** area). In the dominant hemisphere it controls speech perception, language processing, **language switching**, phonological (sounds of letters) and syntactical processing of the arrangement of words to form a phrase or sentence, object naming, lip reading, word retrieval, and lexical decisions concerning word meanings and pseudowords.

It is a key area for both working memory and episodic long-term memory, and is involved in mnemonic rehearsal. In the **nondominant (right) hemisphere** it is more involved in acoustic **rhythms, melodies**, and topographic memories. It is one of the areas that is involved in both **deductive** reasoning and in **working memory**. It has neurons related to **guiding eye movements** with direct links to both temporal and parietal areas.

BA 6 is also important in **attention to visual actions and in the recognition of objects**. It can be involved in **imagining movements**. This region is **vital for attention**, both visual-spatial and visual-motor. The **frontal eyefields** guide visual movement and are a part of Salience networks for attention to visual and auditory stimuli. This region has a role in attention to human voices and to rhythm and sequential sounds.

As previously mentioned, lesions can result in **kinetic apraxia** with movements that appear rough and uncoordinated due to difficulties with motor sequencing and the planning of movements. (For extreme detail, the reader can go to: http://neuro.imm.dtu.dk/services/jerne/brede/WOROI_325.html).

F3-C3: BAs 6, 40, DH

In the left frontal area, approximately between F3 and C3, is an area of the cortex related to **handwriting** called **Exner's** area. C3 may be closer to BAs 6, 40, and 43, and be related to functions that involve attention and execution of action.

BA 5: Somatosensory Association Cortex

BA 5

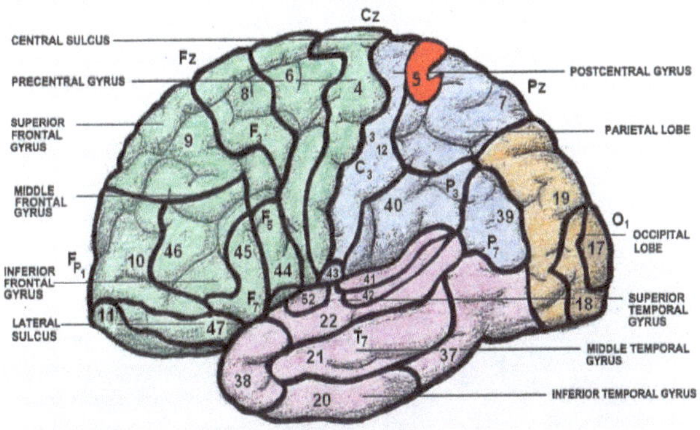

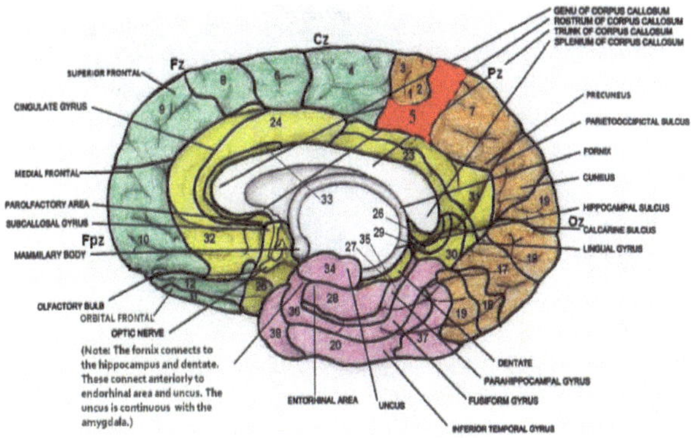

Brodmann areas 5 and 7 are in the superior parietal lobe. The intraparietal sulcus separates them from the inferior parietal lobe, BAs 40 and 39. Between Cz and Pz, in Brodmann area 5, one major function is the **perception of patterns**. This area, particularly in the nondominant hemisphere, is in a network for spatial perception and imagery of movements. It is therefore important in the use of tools and other objects. It may be involved in networks for **mirroring** gestures and movements, and is important in bimanual manipulations. It is involved in networks that are important for **working memory** and the conscious recollection of events. It may be involved in the processing of emotions and **reflections on 'self'** during decision making. It also has some role in spatial mnemonic (memory) processing, semantic categorization, detection of rhymes, temporal context recognition, and saccades (lateral-medial eye movements). It is important in **localizing pain** and in touch. Pain perception could prove to be an important function for NFB work. From all of these roles the reader will understand that it is **critical to the attention networks**.

The **right NDH somatosensory** cortex is more involved in **visual-spatial processing, spatial attention,** spatial awareness, mental rotation, and spatial imagery involved in deductive processing. It can be important in imitation and motor learning. It may also be important in **perception of personal space.**

In the **dominant hemisphere,** it is involved in **temporal context recognition**. **Tactile** localization is important in the superior parietal lobe whereas tactile recognition is a function of the inferior parietal lobe.

Lesions in this area can result in **ideomotor apraxia,** which is the loss of the ability to produce purposeful, skilled movements that are independent of any motor weakness, paralysis, coordination, or sensory loss. Lesions may also result in **astereognosis** (tactile agnosia), which is the loss of the ability to recognize objects by feeling them without being able to see them. (http://neuro.imm.dtu.dk/services/jerne/brede/WOROI_324.html)

Temporal Lobes

Introduction

General Discussion

Functions related to Connections to Orbital and Medial Frontal Areas

Introductory Overview

Homologous structures in the right and left hemispheres have similar intrahemispheric connections, act in the same general networks (such as the Affect and Executive networks), and often have very similar functions. For the areas under corresponding electrode sites for the dominant and nondominant hemispheres, we will therefore describe general functions that may be influenced by NFB over specific sites and **will only give differences in functions** of the dominant and nondominant hemispheres when there appear to be clear differences documented in the literature. By dominant hemisphere we mean the hemisphere in which the primary language functions reside, which is the left hemisphere for people who are right-handed and also for the majority of people who are left-handed. The right hemisphere may be dominant in a small percentage of people who are 'pure lefties,' that is, people who are left-hand, left-foot, and left-eye dominant, and whose language functioning resides predominantly in the right hemisphere.

For example, as previously described, it is clear that **Wernicke's area** in the dominant (usually left) hemisphere is primarily involved in language functions. Deficient function will be experienced as difficulties in language comprehension. The homologous area in the nondominant (usually right) hemisphere is concerned more with emotional aspects of speech, understanding of feelings conveyed by emotional tone, innuendo and nuance, and reading nonverbal cues. Deficiencies in these right hemisphere, parietal area functions, when they occur in people who have had strokes, are referred to by neurologists as sensory aprosodia (Ross, 1981).

On the other hand, T7 and T8 are close to BAs 40, 41 and 22, which are areas within the auditory cortex. Although one might expect the right ear to relate to the left **auditory cortex** and the left ear to relate to the right cortex, this is only partially true. Hearing from both ears goes to both sides with an emphasis on the left side for verbal/language input.

Influencing CMSs with NFB: For central midline structures (CMSs), the authors suggest that the NFB practitioner may be able to influence the appropriate side by doing the feedback while the client is carrying out task(s) that relate to the functions that one wishes to target. For example, if we are working with a student on mental arithmetic, which involves memory, recall, visualizing, sequencing, and manipulation of numbers, we will do these tasks while encouraging activation of the left cerebral hemisphere. We will teach the student a strategy and then have them carry out tasks while simultaneously doing the NFB plus BFB (such as effortless diaphragmatic breathing). On the other hand, we often are working at a central location (Cz) and we may be influencing a whole network that links memory and visualization and spatial reasoning areas. The task may push the brain into involvement of the correct neural network, in this example, the Executive network. We feel that the NFB practitioner's task often involves much more than just placing electrodes over a site and doing operant conditioning to change the amplitude of particular frequency bands. We recommend combining NFB with BFB and metacognitive strategies to have the biggest impact by influencing broader networks, especially networks that are appropriate to the particular needs of each client. Certainly, operant conditioning of SMR is beneficial for many, many conditions. Combining SMR enhancement with HRV training for managing stress has a role to play, too. However, even here, strategies for achieving a calm relaxed state may be important, and the strategies (which might include cognitive reframing or negotiation strategies or other skills related to stress management) represent added value for the client.

The temporal lobes are involved in Sensory networks and in the primary organization of sensory input (Read, 1981). The **lateral aspect** of the temporal lobes includes part of the auditory cortex. Input from both ears goes to both the left and right auditory cortices. **Verbal encoding** results in left-lateralized activation of the inferior prefrontal cortex and the medial temporal lobe (MTL). **Pattern encoding** activates the right inferior prefrontal cortex and the right MTL. Scenes and faces show approximately symmetrical activation in both regions. Lateralization of encoding processes is determined by the verbalizability of stimuli (Golby et al., 2001).

The **medial aspect** of the temporal lobes includes the **hippocampal region.** This region comprises the hippocampus and adjacent structures such as the parahippocampal gyrus, dentate gyrus, and the entorhinal cortex. This region is part of the limbic system and therefore the Affect network. It is also part of the Executive network and has important roles in the consolidation of information from short-term to long-term memory. This region receives **cholinergic input from the medial septum**. Interference with this input results in severe memory impairment. The hippocampal region is also involved in spatial navigation. It is one of the first regions of the brain to suffer damage in **Alzheimer's** with early memory loss and disorientation. Bilateral damage can result in **anterograde amnesia** (inability to retain new memories). Even **déjà vu** is said to be associated with the temporal lobe. Both left and right side lesions can affect recognition of visual content (e.g., recall of faces). Lesions more of the **middle temporal** area may result in an inability to **retain a series**, or just the correct order of a series, of sounds, syllables, or words in memory.

Animal studies have shown that hippocampal damage can result in difficulty learning to inhibit responses that they have previously been taught. In addition to Alzheimer's, damage to the hippocampus can result from oxygen deprivation, encephalitis, and medial temporal lobe epilepsy. Atrophy of this area can also occur with prolonged stress and with depression.

Seizures in the temporal lobe can have dramatic effects on an individual's personality. **Temporal lobe epilepsy** can cause perseverative speech, paranoia, and aggressive rages (Blumer and Benson, 1975). Severe damage to the temporal lobes can also alter sexual behavior, increasing such activity (Blumer and Walker, 1967). **Personality changes** such as loss of libido, loss of sense of humor or sudden religious conversion have been associated with a damaged temporal lobe as well.

Of interest to NFB practitioners is that long-term potentiation was first researched in the hippocampus. In addition, we have noted previously that midline frontal 5-7 Hz (3-10 Hz possible) theta waves are associated with memory encoding and recall, and these waves reflect a pyramidal cell rhythm from the hippocampus that may be controlled by cholinergic output from the septal area.

Left (Dominant) Temporal Lobe

Language can be affected by temporal lobe damage. Left temporal lesions disturb recognition of words and individuals with temporal lobe lesions can have difficulty placing words or pictures into categories. The medial aspect of the temporal lobes that includes the hippocampal area with the parahippocampal gyrus are highly associated with memory skills as previously described. **Left (dominant) temporal** lesions result in impaired memory for verbal material. These lesions result in decreased recall of verbal and visual content, including speech perception. If the left temporal lobe is damaged, perception of language and memory of words will be impaired.

The auditory cortex in the left hemisphere, temporal lobe, communicates **with the left frontal** lobe and has major control over functions that have to do with speech and language, including **speech articulation.**

NFB Over Dominant Hemisphere Temporal Lobe

In summary, NFB over T7 (T3) may influence functions of the left temporal lobe. It may influence the **integration of auditory, visual, perceptual, and memory** inputs, including those necessary for reading. These inputs can include: **phonemic** (letter to sound), **lexical** (sight words), and **semantic** (meaning) inputs. NFB may also have beneficial effects on other problems that relate to temporal lobe functions. These can include, for example, some people who are suffering from tinnitus (de Ridder, 2010) though it should be noted that tinnitus is complex and not necessarily easy to treat. Training over the left temporal lobe may also have some beneficial effects on visual memory and sequencing.

Right (Nondominant) Temporal Lobe

If the right, nondominant, temporal lobe is damaged, **perception of sounds and shapes** is impaired. Right temporal damage can cause a **loss of inhibition of talking.** Right side lesions may adversely affect the recall of nonverbal material, such as **music** and drawings. Right side lesions can also result in decreased recognition of **tonal sequences** and impair many musical abilities. Right anterior temporal lobe damage can interfere with recognition and recall of patterns (both visual and auditory) that are not coded verbally. Visual analysis is generally impaired and there is an impairment of maze learning. There is an inability to recognize faces (**prosopagnosia**). A patient may have difficulty recognizing common objects when they are viewed from unusual angles.

The following case demonstrates some of the effects of ***nondominant temporal-parietal and frontal residual damage*** *after experiencing encephalitis. A*

44-year-old woman had been a brilliant student and top of her class in university until she suffered encephalitis at age 22. Two decades later she still suffered from profound memory loss for visual experiences, had a mild speech impediment, disorientation (stumbled into objects), and the left side of her face drooped slightly. She had a markedly decreased ability to think in abstract terms. Prior to the illness she had been superb at visualization, but damage to right parietal area meant that, since the illness, she needs to have everything presented concretely (left frontal function). She had been highly involved in social events in school and university. Post-encephalitis she was unable to understand innuendo, nuance, and meaning of changing emotional tone in conversation (sensory aprosodia, right parietal temporal damage). She was verbally still bright. She is a very capable woman and she has devised means for interpreting what people mean in social situations. Numerous medical specialists told her that there was nothing wrong, because MRI and CT scans showed no abnormalities and she did well in IQ tests, which are quite dependent on left-hemisphere verbal attributes. She was greatly relieved after her QEEG evaluation that someone could show definite findings in areas of the brain that did precisely correspond to her symptoms. She was so happy that someone could finally confirm the source of difficulties she had experienced for over 20 years that she actually cried with relief. Some of the QEEG findings are summarized in the following two figures.

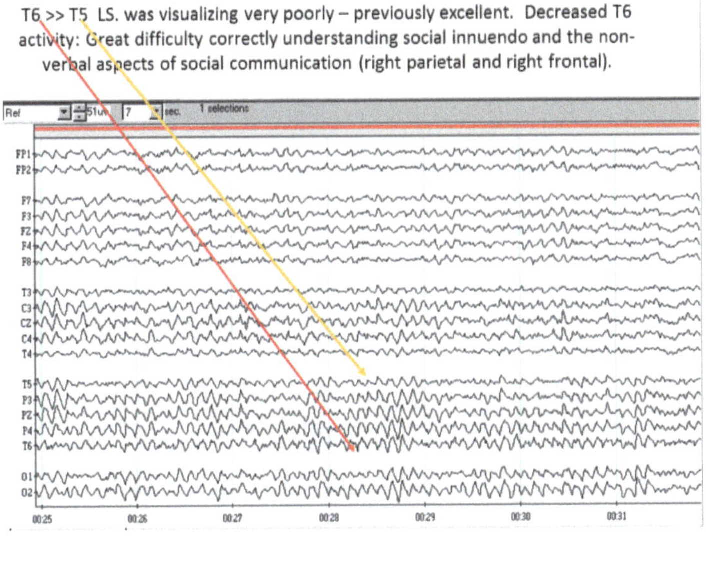

BA 20

T9, Inferior Temporal Lobe

The **inferior temporal lobe** in the dominant hemisphere, along with its connections to the frontal lobes, is involved in **representation of visual images evoked by auditory input**.

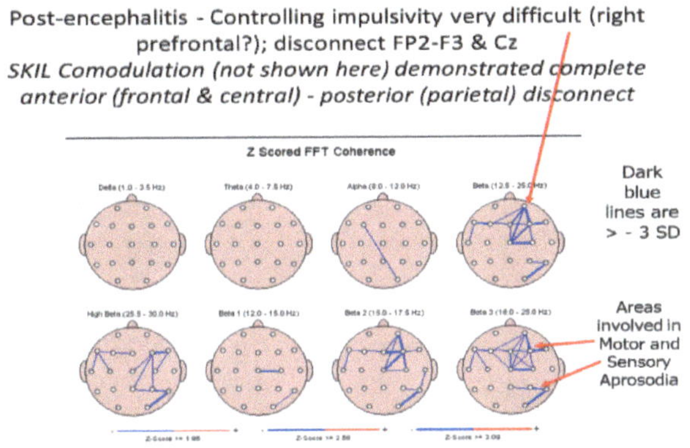

The temporal lobe is a key area in a number of important cognitive functions. The medial aspect of the temporal lobe is an extremely important target for NFB but it may require LORETA NFB to reach some of the structures located deep in the cortex. As suggested above, single channel neurofeedback over T7, T9, and areas between these sites and parietal sites such as P7 may influence a number of different functions. Below we will separate these, discussing first the more superior and lateral portions of the temporal cortex which includes the auditory cortex. This discussion is followed by a connected but somewhat more posterior region in the temporal parietal junction often, in the dominant hemisphere, referred to as **Wernicke's** area. This broad general area includes aspects of the angular gyrus and the supramarginal gyrus which lie in the parietal lobe just superior to the temporal lobe. Dysfunction in these areas may affect a great many functions related to learning. This is followed by a brief overview of functions of the inferior portion of the temporal lobes.

Discussion of Brodmann areas will look at the following areas:

- Lateral Aspect, Superior and Middle temporal lobe
- Lateral Aspect, Inferior temporal lobe
- Lateral Aspect, Temporal – Parietal Junction
- Medial Aspect including BAs 34, 26, 27, 28: uncus, parahippocampal gyrus, hippocampus
- Medial Aspect and Inferior Temporal Lobe, parahippocampal gyrus, fusiform gyrus

Temporal Lobes – Lateral Aspect

T7 (formerly T3); T8 (formerly T4): BAs 41, 42, 22; 21, 43, 52; 20

Overview Illustration

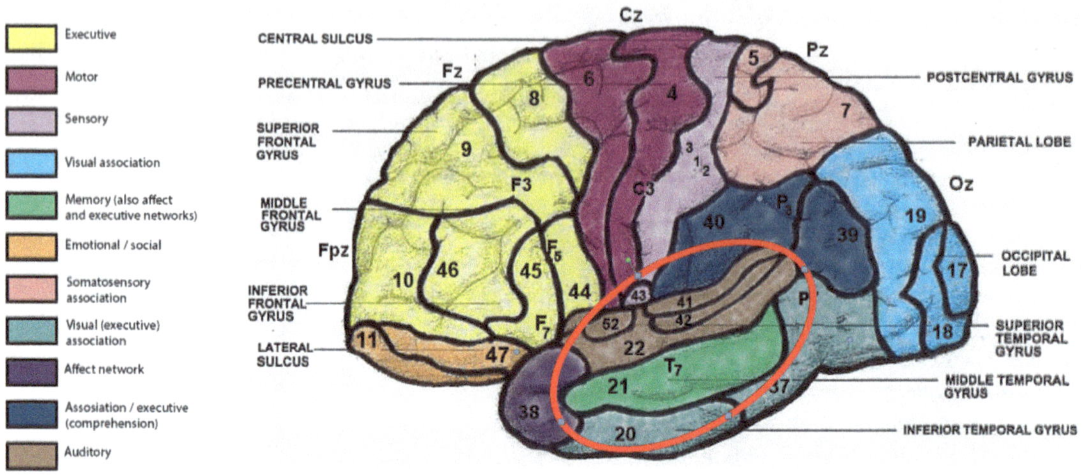

BAs 41, 42, 22 Including the Auditory Cortex

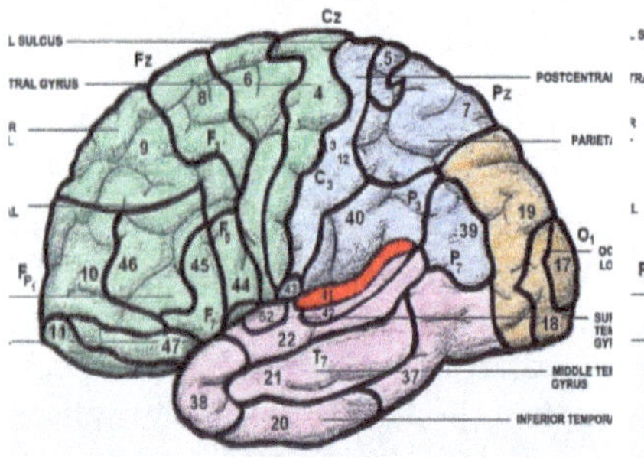
BA 41

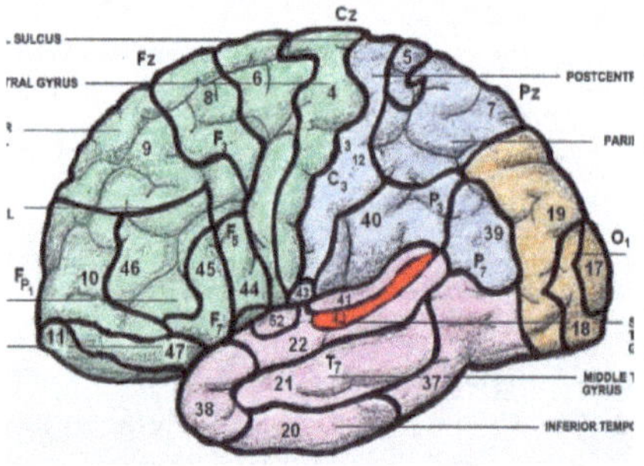
BA 42

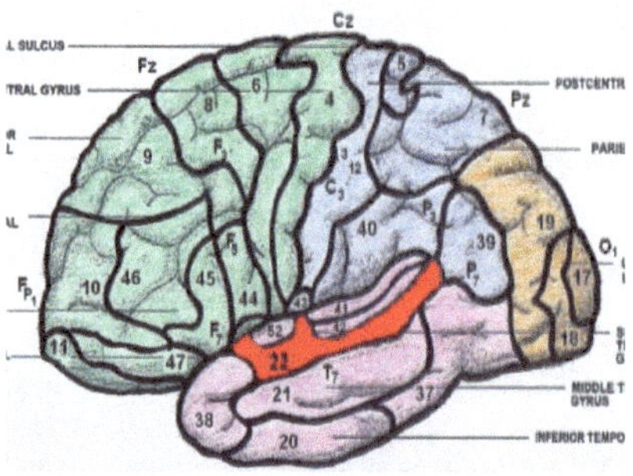
BA 22

Auditory Cortex

The **auditory cortex** is in the posterior portion of the superior temporal lobe. The auditory cortex comprises: **Brodmann areas 41, 42, 22**. The pathway for auditory information, in general terms, is from the ear to the medial geniculate area of the thalamus, then to the temporal lobe. In the superior temporal gyrus, BA 41 and BA 42 comprise the auditory association cortex while BA 22 in the superior temporal gyrus is auditory memory cortex. Complete **bilateral damage** to these areas will result in a **loss of the conscious awareness** of sound even though the ability to react reflexively to sound remains because that is based on subcortical and brainstem functions.

BA 41 & 42

Brodmann area 41 is the first cortical region of the auditory pathway. BAs 41 and 42 are involved in **hearing different frequencies**, pitch, harmonic tones, intensity, acoustic patterns, and volume. It is part of the auditory working memory network. Lesions can lead to a loss of awareness of sound.

Transverse Temporal Gyri

Brodmann area 41 includes the **transverse temporal gyri** that are also called **Heschl's gyri**. This is an area of the primary auditory cortex that is within the lateral sulcus with the gyri running mediolaterally towards the center of the brain rather than front to back as is true for all other temporal lobe gyri (see figure below). This is an area that is activated with sounds, but apparently may **also**

become active during visual word recognition and with auditory short-term memory. It may also activate when observing the face of another person who is speaking, which may be a mirror neuron function.

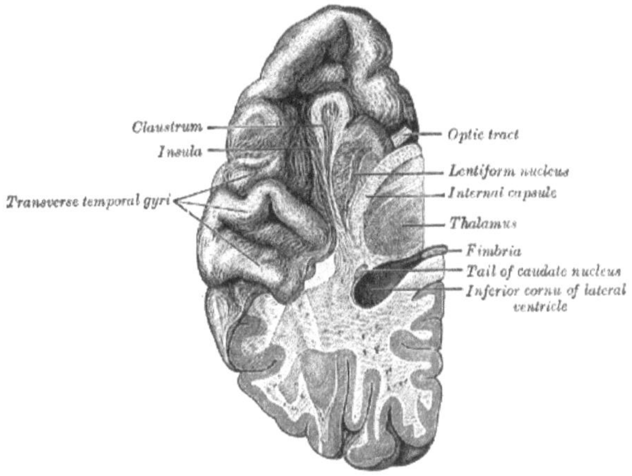

From Gray's Anatomy *(public domain) to show the transverse temporal gyri.*

BA 22

Brodmann area 22 is essential for **auditory working memory.** For example, when measuring evoked responses using an **auditory odd-ball paradigm** (the task might be to count the high tones in a series that is mainly low tones), **a comparison** with previously heard signals is reportedly done in this area and it occurs approximately **175 msec after the stimulus**. This is an experimental example of how BA 22 is important in **comparing present input with past experience**. Functioning in the auditory cortex is also concerned with the relationship of **phonetics** (letter-sound relationships) and in the **categorization** and organization of information. It is also important in normal functioning of both **episodic memory** (remembering events) and **declarative** memory (remembering facts) and with grasping the whole picture as a **Gestalt** versus sensing auditory input in fragments. This last function may be dysfunctional in autism, just as it is with sensing a visual Gestalt.

In some patients, lesions in the left dominant temporal lobe can leave some of the functions noted above intact but leave the patient with other functions deficient. An example is **word deafness**. Dysfunction in the auditory cortex may result in the patient having an increased threshold for some sound frequencies. Older patients may complain of hearing **loss for high frequency** sounds and often have an associated problem with **tinnitus**. In these cases there is an association between the nerve deafness, thalamic connections, and the tinnitus (de Ridder, 2010). BA 22 deficits may also interfere with a person's ability to **localize sounds** and to decode speech sounds (phonemes). As this becomes more severe, auditory comprehension of speech may become quite difficult. Lesions involving BA 22 include **paraphrasias** (incorrectly produced words). In conjunction with the frontal lobe, dysfunction in the left temporal area may contribute to perceptual distortions.

The **superior temporal lobe,** auditory cortex, in both the right and left hemispheres is involved in **auditory perception and processing**. The dominant hemisphere is more involved than the nondominant, but both hemispheres have input from both the right and left ears. The auditory cortex is also important for the processing of meaning (semantics) in both speech and vision. The superior temporal gyrus includes an area (within the Sylvian fissure) where auditory signals come from the cochlea via the medial geniculate. Similar to the cochlea, the primary auditory area contains neurons that respond to particular frequencies, a kind of **tonotopic** organization. Adjacent areas in the superior, posterior, and lateral parts of the temporal lobes are involved in high-level auditory processing. The auditory cortex is important in the integration of stimuli that come from different sources. **Like the inferior lateral areas of the parietal lobe, the auditory cortex connects to the frontal eye fields (FEFs)**. It is possible that dysfunction here could prevent the person from grasping the whole picture and instead view the world in fragments with one stimulus after another vying for attention. As noted above, this may be one of the problems experienced by children with autism. In some children who have a learning disability, their visual perception regarding **discrimination of detail** is not functioning normally and this can relate to malfunction of the dominant (left) parietal-temporal region (between T7 and P7).

Conduction aphasia, characterized by good auditory comprehension and fluent but disordered speech production, is classically viewed as a **disconnection syndrome.** Conduction aphasia may result from damage to cortical fields in the dorsal portion of the **left posterior superior temporal gyrus** which participates not only in **speech perception**, but also in **phonemic aspects of speech production** (Hickok, 2001).

BA 22

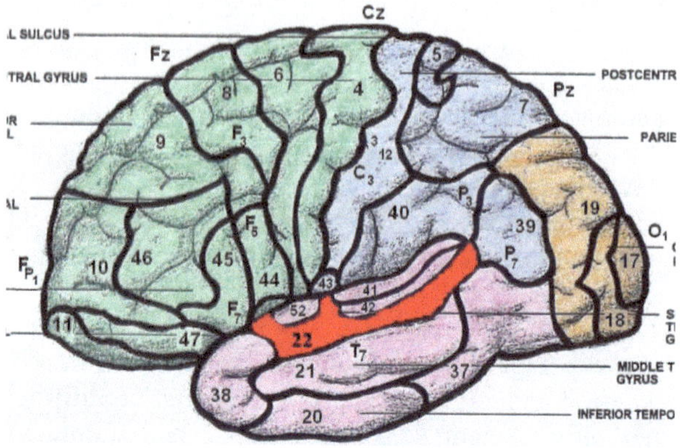

Data from experiments using evoked potentials demonstrates that sound travels from BA 41, then 42, to BA 22. In **Brodmann area 22, the incoming stimulus is compared to memory traces**. If the stimulus does not match memory traces, then one can observe a higher amplitude N1 (negative going wave at about 100 msec after the stimulus) event-related potential, followed by a high-amplitude P2 (positive going wave occurring about 200 msec after the stimulus) in an auditory oddball test, described in more detail under N1-P2 event-related potentials (ERPs). From the BA 22 area of the auditory cortex, auditory information is transferred to the anterior cingulate. Kropotov has given an example of this in his textbook (Kropotov, 2009). Using evoked potentials, he has demonstrated that information travels from the ear to the medial geniculate area in the thalamus in about 116 ms, to BA 42 after about 132 ms, and then to BA 22 within 200 ms. From BA 22, it travels to the anterior cingulate cortex in about 236 ms.

Brodmann area 22, however, is also important in other functions related to language, such as word and **sentence generation in the dominant** hemisphere.

In the **nondominant** hemisphere it is important for detection and **understanding emotional tone** of voice (happy, angry), nonverbal sounds, and affect-prosody. It is important in learning a tone-based language.

Lesions in the dominant hemisphere can result in **Wernicke's aphasia**, which is discussed below in the section **Lateral Aspect, Dominant Lobe, Temporal – Parietal Junction.**

BA 21

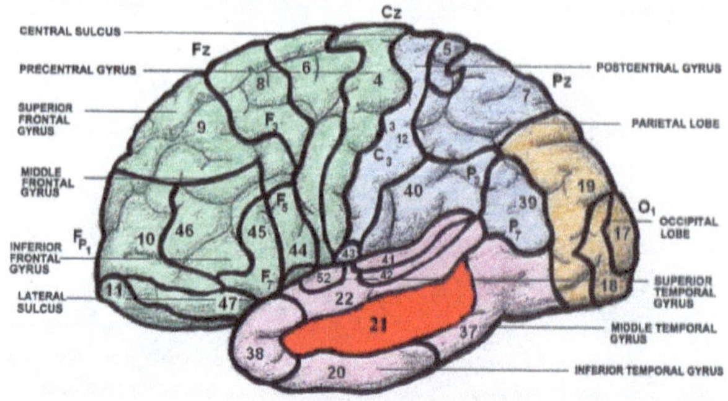

Brodmann area 21, in the middle temporal gyrus, has a role in both auditory and visual **memory and event sequencing**. It is part of the auditory cortex and is involved in processing of complex sounds. It is a key area in monitoring text and speech. It is important in **word and sentence generation.** It is activated during executive functions such as decision making. Lesions here can affect semantic tasks. It is part of the network for **deductive reasoning** and may have a role in categorization.

The **anterior** temporal areas are more involved in **syntactic** (order of words) functions. The **posterior** temporal areas are more concerned with **temporal** relationships **and naming** functions. The **dorsal** areas of the left posterior temporal-parietal lobe are involved in early integration of the **phonological-lexical-semantic features of printed** words. The **ventral** areas of the left occipital-temporal lobes are involved in fast word identification.

In the **nondominant(right)** hemisphere, BA 21 can play a role, along with the supramarginal (BA 40) and angular gyrus (BA 39) areas, in understanding **prosody** (the emotional aspects of speech conveyed by modulation, timing, and tonal qualities of speech), and in attributing intention to other people.

BA 43

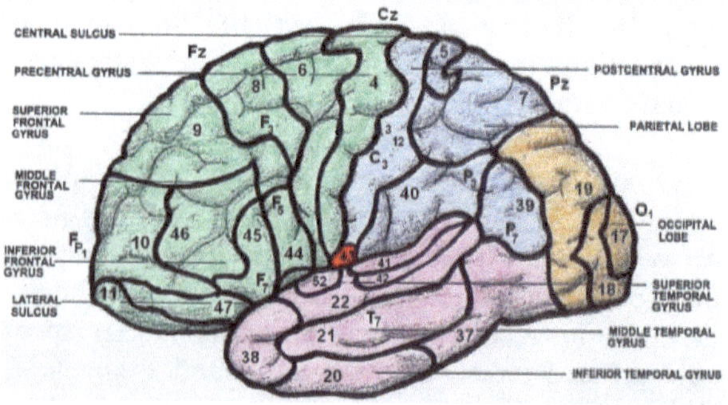

Brodmann area 43 is also referred to as the Gustatory Cortex. BA 43 is at the junction of the insula, frontal, and parietal lobes and occupies the postcentral gyrus and the precentral gyrus between the ventrolateral extreme of the central sulcus and the depth of the lateral sulcus at the insula. It is in a portion of the **sensorimotor cortical area** in the inferior margin of the postcentral and precentral gyri where the frontal-parietal operculum merges with the insula just below the inferior termination of the central sulcus. This area may participate in the sensorimotor representation of the **mouth and taste** reception. It may also overlap with the sensorimotor cortex areas for the **digits**. It can respond to **vibro-tactile** digit stimulation. It can also respond to speech.

The following diagram gives an overview of how the information coming from the medial geniculate to the mid-superior portion of the temporal lobe, auditory cortex, is then conveyed to different areas of the cortex for different purposes. In very general terms, the rostral (anterior) portion of the temporal lobe is related to the **'what'** of auditory information processing, and the superior portion of the parietal cortex is related to the **'where'** (Kropotov, 2009). As noted previously, the time relationships of the movements of information can be investigated using evoked potentials, as has been carried out by Juri Kropotov.

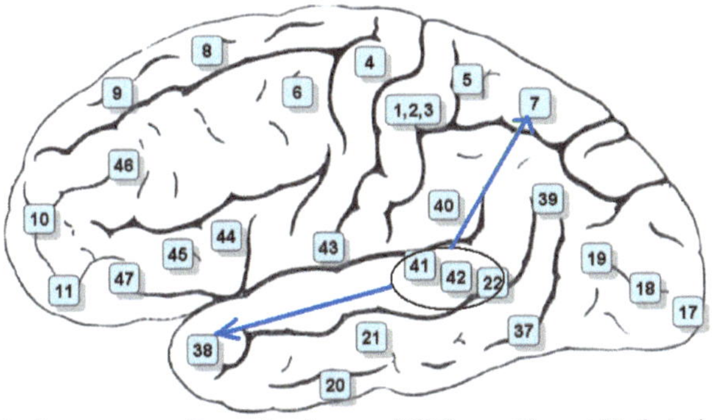

Reference: Quantitative EEG, Event-Related Potentials and Neurotherapy. *Kropotov, 2009. Diagram adapted from* Gray's Anatomy *(public domain).*

The above figure illustrates how the auditory cortex connects anteriorly to the entorhinal cortex (ERC) and BA 38 of the temporal cortex to determine the 'What,' and posterior and superior to BA 7, parietal cortex to determine the 'Where' for incoming auditory information.

BA 52

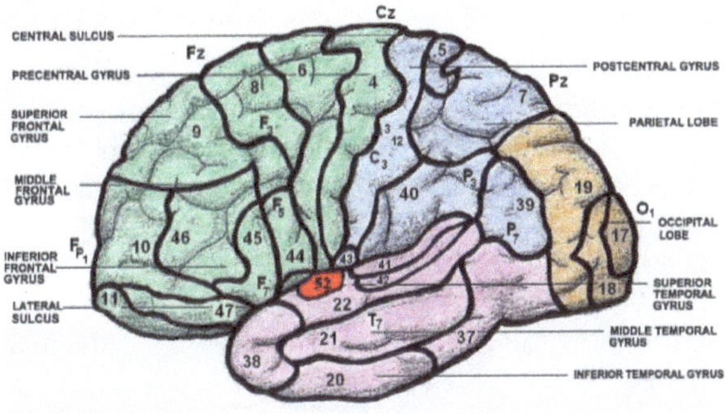

Brodmann area 52 is the parainsular area (at the junction of the temporal lobe and the insula). Functions of this area are assumed to overlap with those of the superior temporal lobe and insula.

BA 20

Inferior to T7 and T8:

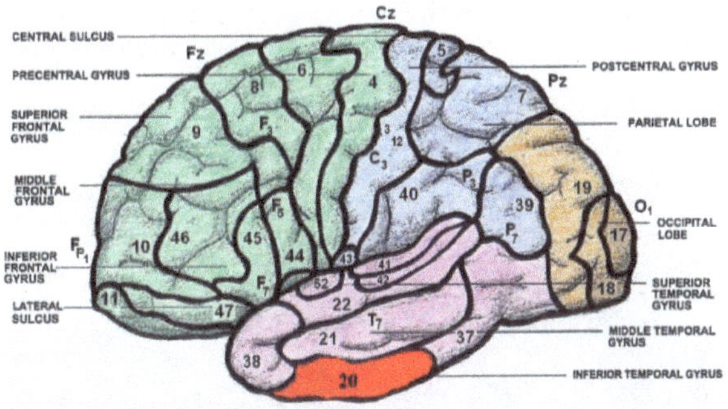

The inferior temporal gyrus, BA 20, is an association cortical area that participates in **higher order visual processing,** including the analysis of visual form, the representation of objects, visual memory, visualization, and visual categorization. In the **dominant hemisphere** it may also have functions related to Wernicke's area. It may play a role in **lexical categorization** (nouns and verbs are lexical categories).

In the **nondominant hemisphere,** it may be involved in the **comprehension of semantic ambiguity.** It is important in **recognition memory, semantic memory, self-recognition,** self-reference, and perhaps also in self-regulation. It may also have a role in networks involved in the **empathic understanding of the emotional states of other** people. Although the nondominant lobe may be more involved in **visual fixation and interpretation,** these functions are present in both hemispheres. However, in the nondominant (right) side, for the most part, it is associated with the representation of **complex object features**, such as global shape. It is involved in face perception. A minor role may be in metaphor comprehension.

Interestingly, this area is also involved in **telling the truth, and having suspicion.** It is involved with other temporal areas of the left hemisphere in language comprehension, **lexical categories,** and in a network that possibly includes the right prefrontal cortex for the comprehension of metaphors. It has a role in identifying intention and, in the right hemisphere, in ambiguity of categories, perceptual closure, and working memory. Also of interest, the inferior aspect of the temporal lobe BA 20 is involved in **creativity and introspection**.

Kropotov has also demonstrated that one can follow the **time sequence after a visual stimulus** using evoked potentials and this is shown in the heavy black lines in the figure below. Visual stimuli can travel from the lateral geniculate nucleus of the thalamus to the occipital lobe and from the lateral posterior nucleus of the thalamus to BAs 1, 2, 3.

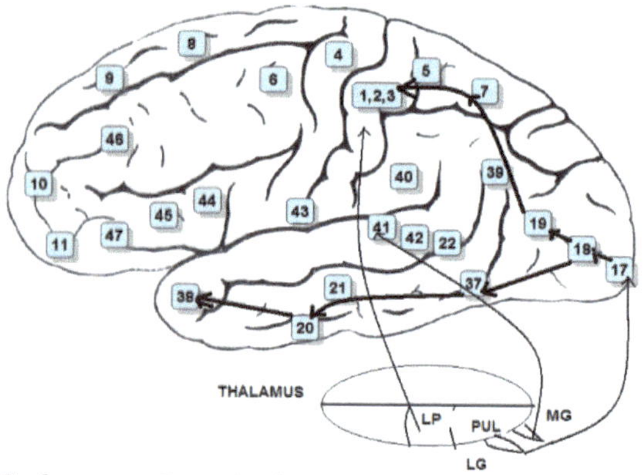

Reference: Quantitative EEG, Event-Related Potentials and Neurotherapy. *Kropotov, 2009. Diagram adapted from* Gray's Anatomy *(public domain).*

To do feedback over this area, the practitioner must be alert to EMG artifact from jaw, neck, or shoulder muscle tension, and be careful not to inadvertently encourage muscle tension with NFB. The practitioner must distinguish between a true increase in beta activity (which is an indicator of activation) and increased beta band amplitude that is due to EMG artifact. It is very easy, given the low amplitude of fast activity, to mistake the effects of EMG for an increase in beta.

Connections

The **inferior temporal lobe** in the dominant hemisphere, along with its connections to the frontal lobes, is involved in **representation of visual images evoked by auditory input**. Patients with frontal lobe lesions have difficulty in the temporal organization of information, such as lists of words. A name can pass through Wernicke's area and then, via the angular gyrus, arouse associations in other areas of the cortex. In this manner, the **angular gyrus is a connecting link** between sensory input and speech production areas. It is an important association cortex that **combines auditory and visual** information that are both necessary for reading and writing. It is involved in the steps between reading and speaking. Damage to the angular gyrus can result in **alexia** (inability to read) with **agraphia** (inability to write).The patient is unable to match spoken letter sounds to written letters. They can only spell the very simplest words.

Right hemisphere lesions in the parietal-temporal-occipital cortex can result in an inability to understand temporal relationships and, thus, future planning. There may also be visual-spatial defects, and problems in retaining a visual image.

Left hemisphere lesions in these general areas result in **aphasia**, inability to evoke a visual image in response to a word, inability to organize sequentially, draw proper angles, and copy designs.

NFB Over the Dominant Temporal Lobe

NFB over T7 (T3) may influence functions of the left temporal lobe. It may influence the integration of auditory, visual, perceptual, and memory inputs, including those necessary for reading. These inputs can include **phonemic** (letter to sound), **lexical** (sight words), and **semantic** (meaning) inputs. NFB may also have beneficial effects on other problems that relate to temporal lobe functions. These can include, as previously noted, some people who are suffering from tinnitus (de Ridder, 2010), though it should be noted that tinnitus is complex and not necessarily easy to treat. It may also have some beneficial effects on visual memory and sequencing.

Amygdala

The amygdala needs to be discussed along with the medial regions of the temporal lobe, and we have chosen to introduce the amygdala before discussing these medial regions.

The Amygdala is not part of the cortex, and thus does not have a Brodmann area number assigned to it. Nevertheless it is a crucial structure when we discuss the Affect network. In addition, the gray matter of the amygdala is continuous with the gray matter of the uncus, and it is therefore an essential structure when we consider the important connections of the uncinate fasciculus. The amygdala lies at the rostral end of the hippocampal cortex. The older corticomedial nuclei of the amygdala are connected to the hypothalamus by the stria terminalis. The newer basolateral nuclei project through the ventral amygdalofugal pathway to the hypothalamus, preoptic region, septal nuclei, midbrain tegmentum, and periaqueductal gray matter.

The dorsal periaqueductal gray matter is related to the sympathetic NS, rostrally for fight and caudally for flight, and the ventral-lateral periaqueductal gray matter is related to functions of the unmyelinated vagus.

Stephen Porges *(2007) notes that the unmyelinated vagus originates from the dorsal vagal nucleus in the medulla. The unmyelinated vagus is the key structure that enables some animals to freeze and feign death. Freezing allows a drop in heart rate and blood pressure and a rise in resistance to pain.*

The **central nucleus of the amygdala** is related to sympathetic drive, fight and flight, and is inhibited by the medial frontal lobe, the superior temporal cortex, and the fusiform gyrus. It is an integral part of the system that controls autonomic and endocrine responses to emotional states. The amygdala receives inputs from many sites within the cortex, including the medial frontal cortex, the cingulate, the temporal lobe, in addition to important inputs from the thalamus, hypothalamus, and midbrain.

The left and right amygdalae serve somewhat different functions in the processing of emotions: the left may respond to a specific stimulus, whereas the right may respond to any stimulus (Glascher & Adolphs, 2003).

In general terms, the amygdala is involved in processing **unconscious memories** and may be involved in bringing back an autonomic nervous system body state which accompanied the emotions that were linked to an event. This is a form of state-dependent learning. It seems to be designed to activate and remember emotional events (Buchanan et al., pp 289–318, 2009; Kim & Gee et al., 2011; Whalen, 2003). These events may include experiences characterized by feelings of fear, disappointment, and horror, but also of joy and celebration. It is also the key area involved in **traumatic memories**. The amygdala's role in unconscious memories lies in contrast to the role of the hippocampus in laying down conscious memories.

The amygdala is a central key in the **stress response,** which is controlled by interaction along a brain stem (locus coeruleus release of nor-epinephrine) - amygdala-hypothalamus (sympathetic system) - pituitary-adrenal axis (AHPA). More detail can be found in other sections of *The Neurofeedback Book*, particularly in the section on HRV and in the discussion of TBI. Not surprisingly, the amygdala may be hyperactive in people with borderline personality disorder (Donegan, Sanislow, Blumberg, Fulbright, Lacadie, Skudlarski, Gore, Olson, et al., 2003).

Although we are discussing each separate cortical area and some subcortical nuclei, the reader should always keep in mind that these structures have major connections that involve basal ganglia to thalamus links.

For decades we have said in our lectures that it is as if the **thalamus is the hub of the wheel** with connections radiating like the spokes of a wheel to every corner of the nervous system. The anterior cingulate cortex, the amygdala and hippocampus are rather like gearshifts, in many ways governing aspects of thinking, feeling, memory, and behavior.

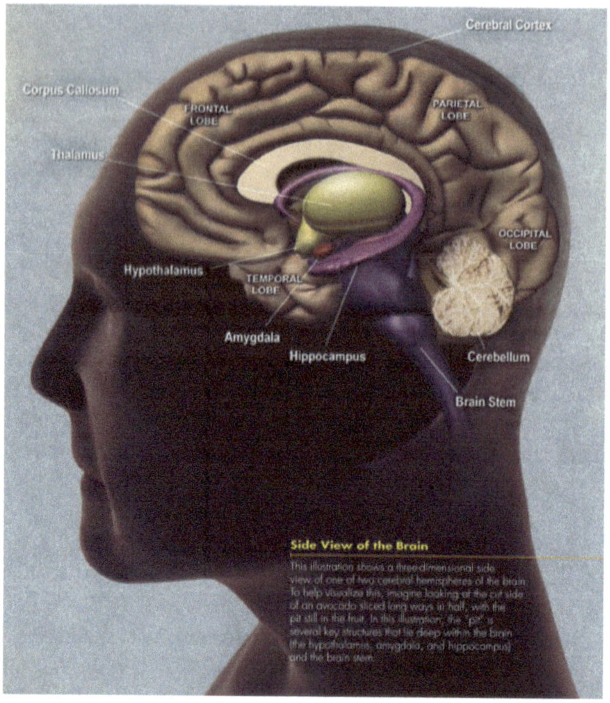

Public domain figure. It is used with great thanks to an unknown US Government employee.

This figure is included to provide practitioners with an overview of the relative locations of the thalamus, hypothalamus, amygdala, and hippocampus. The thalamus location in the brain has been compared to the pit in an avocado. The relationships between these structures can be difficult to visualize using only two-dimensional diagrams.

Figures to Illustrate Amygdala

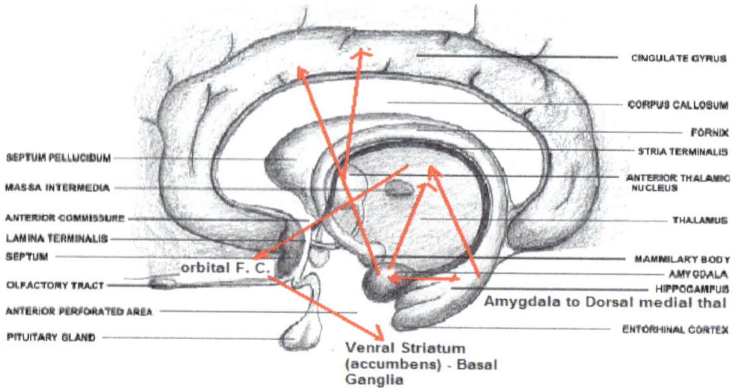

Some serotonin-related connections of the amygdala, hippocampus anterior thalamic nucleus, orbital cortex and the nucleus accumbens Figures adapted from Smith, 1962.

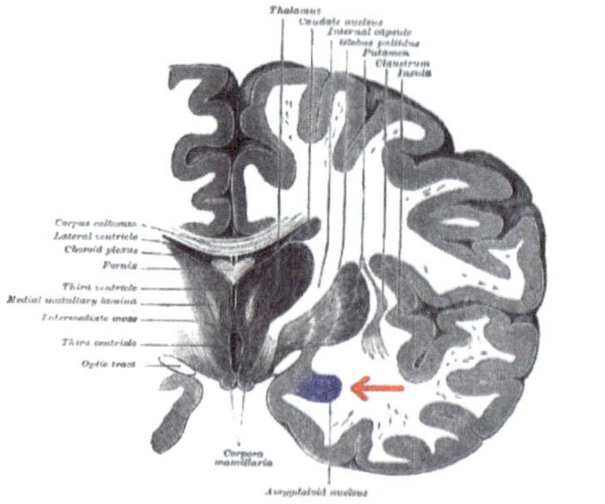

Amygdala is inferior to the globus pallidus

Amygdala

The above figures suggest how the amygdala may be involved in many areas that influence emotional responses. As described previously, the amygdala is involved in far-ranging Affect-related phenomena including appetite, sexual behaviors, fear responses, anger, aggression, reward behaviors and aversion responses. It also has a role in alerting and orienting, and thus in many decision-making processes, in addition to its role in responding to emotionally laden stimuli. Some aspects of its functioning will appear in a number of the following sections of this book.

Temporal Lobe – Medial Aspect

BAs 34, 26, 27, 28

Plus links to uncus, amygdala, parahippocampal gyrus, hippocampus, fornix

Introduction to the Medial Aspect of the Temporal Region

The medial aspect of the temporal region includes the amygdala, hippocampus, medial and inferior temporal lobes, and posterior aspects of the cingulate gyrus. Particularly important in this region are structures within the Executive memory network that are involved in **episodic and declarative memory.**

Deep inside the medial temporal lobes lie the hippocampi, which are essential for memory function – particularly the transference from short- to long-term memory and control of spatial memory and behavior. Damage to this area typically results in anterograde amnesia. **Anterograde amnesia** refers to a loss of the ability to create new memories after the brain trauma that caused the amnesia. With a severe concussion there can also be partial or complete inability to recall the event that caused the damage (retrograde amnesia).

A client was severely injured and rendered unconscious when a truck T-boned his car. This client noted cheerfully that he had no fear of driving because he had no recall whatever of the accident.

Not just structure, but physiology is important, and functions of the hippocampus are controlled, for the most part, by a neurotransmitter, **acetylcholine** (Ach), from the septal area. The septal area and the hippocampus turn out to be only a part of the networks involved in laying down memories.

Papez Circuit

The entire **Papez circuit** is thought to be critical in memory. Thus, in short-term memory, all of the following are involved: the hippocampus, which connects to the dorsomedial nucleus of the thalamus (which projects to the orbitofrontal and temporal cortex) and the mammillary bodies (which project to the anterior nucleus of the thalamus and then to the cingulate gyrus), and the fornix, which connects the hippocampal region with the amygdala. It should also be acknowledged that severe memory disturbance only appears to occur with bilateral lesions of the hippocampus. It makes sense that our brain has some built in redundancy for a function as important as memory.

The **fornix** joins the hippocampus to the mammillary body, which has major connections to the anterior nuclei of the thalamus and this connects to the anterior cingulate. The fornix also becomes the hippocampal commissure that joins left and right medial temporal areas, and is shown in the figure below. The rostral temporal poles are connected by means of the anterior commissure. All of these structures are involved in the Affect networks, as described previously.

To review, affect information goes from the orbital frontal and medial frontal cortex, anterior cingulate, hippocampus, amygdala, and the temporal entorhinal cortex to the basal ganglia, and in particular, to the nucleus accumbens. The nucleus accumbens connects to the ventral pallidum, which is inhibitory. This links to the medial dorsal nucleus of the thalamus and the anterior thalamic nucleus. These thalamic nuclei then connect back to the neocortex to regulate the anterior cingulate and thus all aspects of the Affect network.

The Affect network regulates mood and emotional reactions. It becomes more and more clear that many structures that are primary parts of the Affect network are also critical to laying down new memories. One's earliest memories are nearly always tied to events that were emotionally charged. Thus these two functions of memory and emotional experience are discussed together in this brief overview. It should also be no surprise that the hippocampus is involved in a number of psychiatric disorders (Cannon, 2012, p163).

Figures to Illustrate Commissures
Hippocampal, Anterior, Corpus Callosum

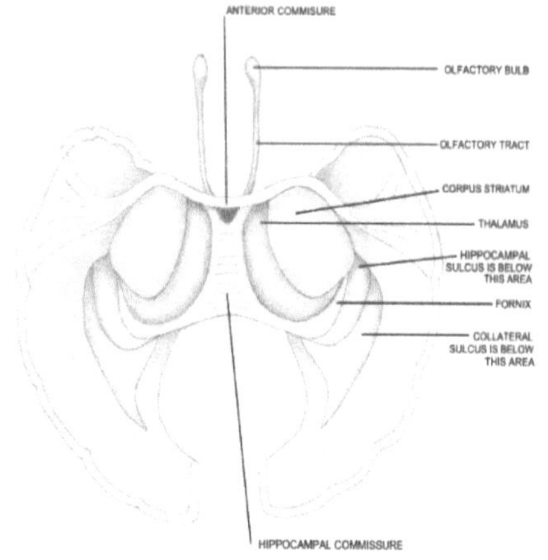

Figures by Amanda Reeves, after Smith (1962)

The hippocampal commissure links the left and right hippocampal areas.

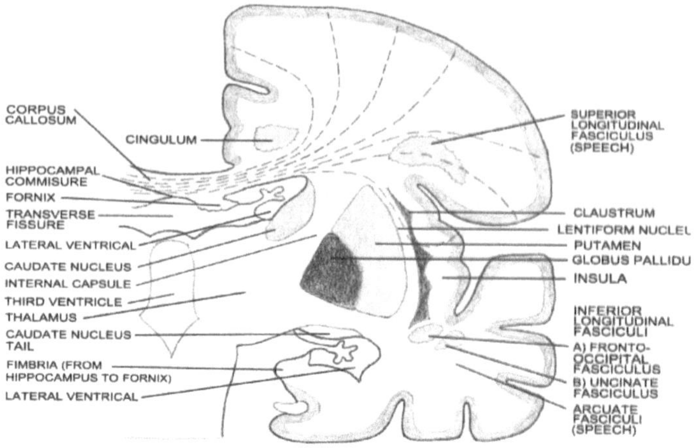

Transverse Section, Right Cerebral Hemisphere. Note the corpus callosum lies over (superior or dorsal to) the hippocampal commissure, which lies above the horizontal fissure. This fissure is above the Diencephalon. Note in cross section the Cingulum and Superior and Inferior Longitudinal Fasciculi.

Cingulum

The **cingulum is a fasciculus** that runs predominantly through the centre of the cingulate gyrus. The cingulum is a large band of association fibers that connects the temporal lobe with the cingulate gyrus, parietal lobes, and the frontal lobes (particularly the orbital surface). It is **connected to all parts of the limbic system.** It is involved in the **conscious perception of emotions**. One can conclude that the hippocampus has connections to the areas concerned with emotions, the autonomic nervous system, the endocrine system, memory, and consciousness.

Seizure Symptoms

Functions of the temporal lobe are complex. One way for the reader to obtain a better understanding of the range of these functions is to **consider symptoms** that may be observed in **simple partial seizures** (SPS) that originate in the temporal lobe. ('Simple' means that consciousness is not altered.) SPS can involve the amygdala and/or small areas of the temporal lobe, such as the hippocampus or other specific areas. A SPS may only cause **sensations** without any overt motor movements. These sensations may be cognitive, such as **déjà vu** (a sense that you have experienced this before), **jamais vu** (the phenomenon of experiencing a situation that one recognizes but that nonetheless seems very unfamiliar), a specific single memory or a set of memories, or amnesia. The sensations may be purely sensory, such as **auditory** sounds or tunes, gustatory, such as a **taste, or olfactory**, such as a smell that is not physically present. Sensations can also be **visual**, or they can involve feelings on the skin or in the internal organs. The latter feelings may seem to move over the body. More unusual possibilities include **psychic** sensations, which can occur as an out-of-body feeling (de Ridder et al., 2007).

Emotions can also occur, such as dysphoric or euphoric feelings, fear, anger, and other emotions. Often, it is hard for persons with SPS of temporal lobe origin to describe the feeling. SPS are sometimes mistaken for the 'aura' that is associated with a grand mal seizure when it is actually an independent event and no generalized seizure occurs.

It is also possible that the temporal lobe may be the origin of complex **visual hallucinations**, including religious ones, such as are attributed to St. Joan of Arc. Hallucinations originating in the temporal lobe become more complex in the more anterior regions, and may include the experience of out–of-world phenomena or even ghosts. The most vivid hallucinations tend to be triggered from the right, not the left, temporal lobe (Penfield & Perot, 1963).

Temporal Pole: A Junction of Inferior Frontal and Temporal Regions through the Uncinate Fasciculus

BA 38

F7, F9-T7; F8, F10-T8;

(T7 in the figure was formerly called T3 in the 10-20 system; T8 was formerly called T4 in the 10-20 system)

BA 38

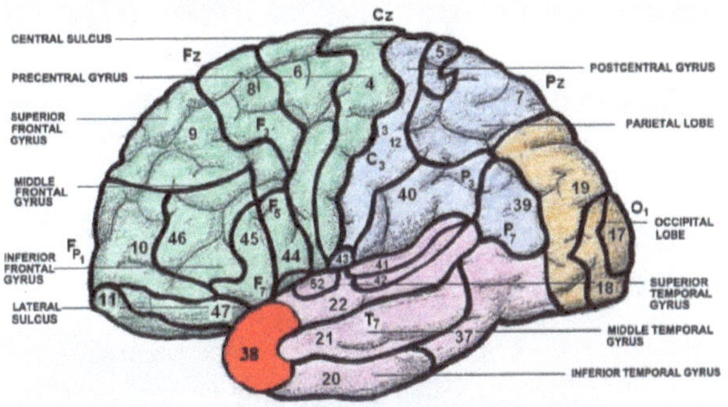

Brodmann area 38 is at the anterior end of the temporal lobe, known as the temporal pole. It is directly connected to the **entorhinal cortex** and thus to the uncus. The neurons of the uncus are continuous with the amygdala. These structures are directly connected through the **uncinate fasciculus** with the orbitofrontal cortex.

This area may be involved in moral judgments. These connections mean that BA 38 is involved in both **Affect and Executive** (memory) networks for experiencing emotional stimuli (fear and threat) and for **experiencing emotional states**. It is one area involved in emotional attachment. It is said to be involved in the visual processing of emotional images. Thus it is not a stand-alone area that functions independently of other areas. Although some functions related to BA 38 have been suggested to be hemispherically differentiated, such as female sexual arousal on the left and male arousal on the right, these kinds of distinctions require more research. It must be considered as networked with the amygdala and the orbital frontal cortex, and functionally considered with these areas.

In the **dominant hemisphere,** it is one of the areas involved in **selective attention to speech**, speech comprehension, semantic processing, long-term memories, comprehension of **narrative**, and word retrieval. It is one of the areas involved in the **comprehension** of both **irony and humor.** and is involved in aspects of **inferential reasoning**. It is involved in responding to **music**. It overlaps with the auditory cortex, and is part of the area involved in attention to speech and tone.

It is an important part of networks related to memory and in particular, to **memory retrieval**. Importantly, BA 38 is one of the first areas to be affected in **Alzheimer's** disease, and it is also one of the areas most **frequently damaged in traumatic brain injuries.** It may be an important area responsible for figure-ground difficulties, such as having difficulty **distinguishing speech from background noise**, which is a problem that some patients with TBI experience.

This area can be important in **visceral-emotional responses,** and thus we can postulate that dysfunction may result in symptoms that occur in depressive disorders.

F9 and T7 electrode sites overlap BA 38, which is found in the rostral portion of the temporal lobe, as can be seen in the above figure. It is likely that electrodes placed in this general area may pick up activity from (and thus be able to influence) more medial structures too, including the uncus with its connections to the amygdala. As noted above, the amygdala has activity related to emotions such as fear, anger, and anxiety, and is important in behavioral reactions to these emotions. The uncus is linked by the **uncinate fasciculus to** other structures, too, including the hippocampus and the orbital surface of the frontal lobe, which includes BA 47 and 11. The **hippocampus** has functions related to short-term memory, but it also is a part of the old Papez circuit for emotions, which more recently has been expanded and called the limbic system. It is therefore related to **mood regulation as well as memory.** Memory functions are facilitated in part by its connections via the uncinate fasciculus, which runs between the uncus on the rostral portion of the temporal lobe, past the amygdala and hippocampus, and then to the orbital surface of the inferior frontal gyrus, BA 11. We have noted previously that this pathway and the orbital surface of the frontal lobe may have a role in understanding the effects of one's own behavior on others. It is, therefore, very important in our work with people who have autism spectrum disorders and deficits in that ability. It is difficult to influence these areas with surface electrodes and, though one can do single-channel feedback with placement between F9 and T7, one may be better able to target these areas with the use of LORETA NFB training if that is available. Otherwise, one might try central training, such as the FCz site, and rely on network properties to influence this area.

Medial Aspect, Inferior Temporal Lobe, Parahippocampal Gyrus, Fusiform Gyrus – Memory and Affect Networks

For surface NFB: Inferior to T7 (around T9) and T8 (around T10): BAs 28, 34; 36, 37, 27, 35, 36

BAs 28

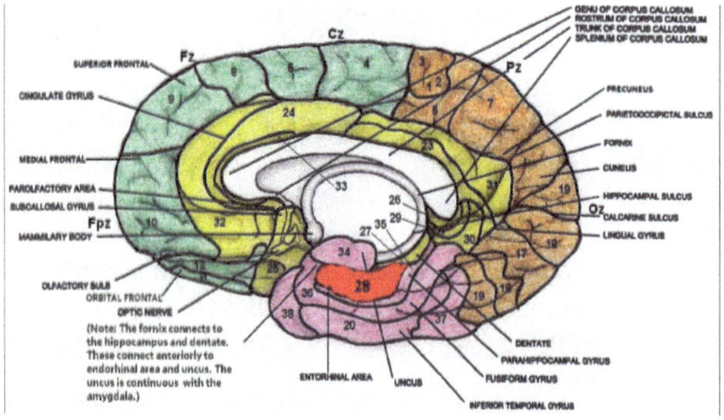

BA 34

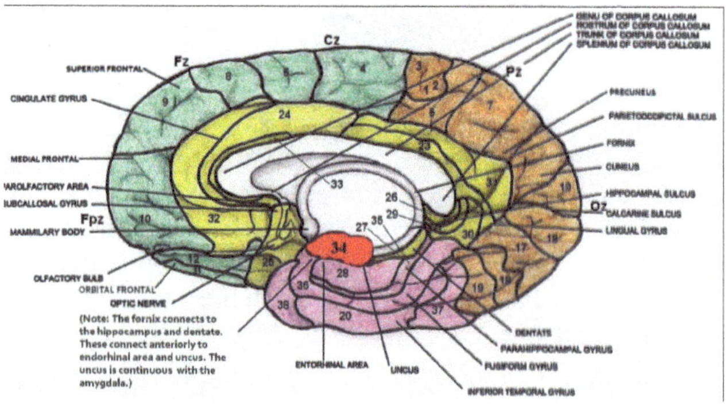

BA 28

Brodmann area 28 includes areas involved in the **paralimbic** cortex on the medial aspect of the temporal lobe, which includes the **entorhinal cortex** (BAs 28 and 34), **uncus** (BA 34, composed of grey matter continuous with the amygdala), and the **parahippocampal** gyrus (BAs 27 and 28). We have noted previously under BA 38 that the **entorhinal cortex (ERC)** is the main interface between the hippocampus and the neocortex.

Particularly in the **nondominant hemisphere**, the ERC-hippocampus system plays an important role in **autobiographical**/declarative/episodic memories and, in particular, **spatial** memories. This includes memory formation, memory consolidation, and **memory** optimization during sleep. The ERC assists in the association of stimuli from the eye and the ear. The ERC receives input from other cortical areas such as the perirhinal and parahippocampal cortices and the prefrontal cortex.

Thus the **ERC receives highly processed input from every sensory modality**, as well as input relating to ongoing cognitive processes. **ERC** neurons process general information, too, such as **directional** activity in the environment, which is in **contrast to functions of the hippocampal** neurons, which usually encode information about **specific places.** This suggests that ERC **encodes general properties about current contexts** that are then used by the hippocampus to create unique representations from combinations of these properties (Jacobs et al., 2010).

As previously noted, the entorhinal cortex is one of the first areas to be affected in **Alzheimer's** disease. In 2012, neuroscientists at UCLA conducted an experiment using a virtual taxi video game connected to seven epilepsy patients with electrodes already implanted in their brains, allowing the researchers to monitor neuronal activity whenever memories were being formed. As the researchers stimulated the nerve fibers in each patient's entorhinal cortex as they were learning, they were then able to navigate better through various routes and recognize landmarks more quickly. This signified an improvement in the patients' spatial memory. With over 30 million people worldwide today suffering from Alzheimer's disease, the study at UCLA was highly relevant. The researchers helped discover that ongoing stimulation of the entorhinal cortex did not necessarily provide a means to boost one's memory. Instead, it was found to be **effective only when trying to learn information** that was **important to that particular individual**. This discovery provides evidence for a possible mechanism that could enhance memory for relevant information. They also observed that entorhinal stimulation resulted in a resetting of the phase of the theta rhythm (Suthana et al., 2012).

In the **dominant-hemisphere BAs 28 and 34**, temporal lobe, the ERC-hippocampus system plays an important role in **declarative and episodic memories** and, in particular, all verbal memories. In **both hemispheres**, these functions include memory formation, memory consolidation, and memory optimization in sleep.

Relation to Dementia

As previously noted, the ERC-hippocampus system is one of the first areas to be affected in **Alzheimer's** disease. Other dementias affect slightly different areas in their early stages: **Picks** disease affects the frontal and temporal poles BAs 8, 12, 38, while **Diffuse Lewy Body** disease affects first the ACC BA 24, Insula BA 13, and parahippocampal gyrus BA 28. Interestingly, cognitive impairment can also occur in older people with no evidence of dementia (Choo et al., 2009, 2011).

Anatomical Connections

With any discussion of memory, one must consider the involvement of a number of important locations. For **long term memory**, these are most often in the central midline structures including the septum, hippocampus, the parahippocampal gyrus and, indeed, the whole Papez circuit. The original **Papez circuit** (hippocampal-mammillo-thalamic tract) comprised reciprocal connections between the hippocampal formation (hippocampus, dentate nucleus), via the fornix, to the mammillary body, anterior thalamic nucleus, cingulate gyrus and, via the cingulum, back to the hippocampal formation.

Other connections have been added to this Papez circuit and the unit is now referred to as the **limbic system,** or emotional brain. These additional areas include the amygdala, hypothalamus, prefrontal cortex, and association cortex. The **amygdala** connects to the entorhinal cortex, which has direct connections to the cingulate cortex. The cingulate projects to the temporal lobe and the orbital cortex.

Now we understand that the **fornix divides**, with some fibers going **to the septal** area (which has direct connections to the hippocampus) and others going to the mammillary body. From the mammillary body fibers go to the anterior nucleus of the thalamus and from there to the anterior cingulate cortex (ACC). This ACC feeds back through the cingulum to the entorhinal area, which connects with the hippocampus from which the fornix emerges. The **septum** turns out to be a key link. It produces **acetylcholine,** which activates the hippocampus and is thus a key in the initial phase of memory production.

Subiculum of Hippocampal Region

The ***subiculum*** *(Latin for 'support') is the most inferior component of the hippocampal formation. It lies between the entorhinal cortex and the hippocampus. It receives input from the hippocampus and entorhinal area and is the main output area of the hippocampus. The pyramidal neurons of the subiculum send projections to the nucleus accumbens, septal nuclei, prefrontal cortex, lateral hypothalamus, nucleus reuniens, mammillary nuclei, entorhinal cortex, and amygdala. The nucleus* ***reuniens*** *within the midline area of the dorsal thalamus links the medial prefrontal cortex with the hippocampus and regulates the amount of neural traffic according to changes in attentiveness* (Vertes et al., 2007). *The pyramidal neurons in the subiculum exhibit transitions between two modes of action potential output: bursting and single spiking. The transition between these two modes is thought to be important for routing information out of the hippocampus.*

Long-Term Memory

The hippocampus, the temporal lobes, and the structures of the limbic system that are connected to them are essential for the consolidation of long-term memory. To be recorded in long term memory, information must pass through the Papez circuit. Any lesion in this circuit, for example, caused by a **stroke or by TBI,** will result in some form of memory impairment.

In **Korsakoff's** syndrome, due to alcoholism with vitamin B1 deficiency, in addition to confabulation, disorientation, and confusion, the patient will have

anterograde amnesia with an inability to store new information in their long-term memory.

Memory is consolidated and made permanent within the Papez circuit. It is then **permanently stored outside of that circuit** in the area of the cortex from which the sensory information originally came, for example, visual information in the occipital cortex and auditory in the temporal cortex. For this reason, these **long-term memories are not lost** when there is damage to the nuclei within the Papez circuit, such as the hippocampus. Only the ability to form new long-term memories is compromised.

Within the **Papez circuit, the hippocampus** is a key structure for encoding new long-term memories. It has the capacity to facilitate associations among various parts of the cortex. It should be no surprise that the Papez circuit is also central to the Affect network and the limbic system as well as being included in the network for encoding memory. The hippocampus can link, for example, a tune that you heard at a concert with the faces of the people who accompanied you to the theatre. Instead of this memory fading, it may be strengthened and eventually etched into long-term memory due to the strength of your interest in that occasion and the strength of the emotions associated with it.

The **parahippocampal gyrus** is a grey-matter cortical region of the brain that surrounds the hippocampus. This region plays an important role in **memory encoding and retrieval**. The anterior part of the parahippocampal gyrus includes the perirhinal and entorhinal cortices. The posterior part is continuous with the medial aspect of the fusiform gyrus. The parahippocampal gyrus is important in the **recognition of scenes** such as landscapes, cityscapes, or rooms (rather than faces or objects). As was previously noted, damage (for example, due to stroke) to the **parahippocampal place area** (PPA), which is a subregion of the parahippocampal cortex that plays an important role in the encoding and recognition of scenes, often leads to a syndrome in which patients cannot visually recognize scenes even though they can recognize the individual objects in the scenes such as people and furniture. The right, **NDH,** parahippocampal gyrus also enables people to **detect sarcasm**.

Intense activation of the temporal lobe, hippocampus, and amygdala may be associated with sexual, religious, and **spiritual** experiences. **Chronic hyperstimulation** is said to be able to induce an individual to become hyper-religious or visualize and experience ghosts, demons, angels, and even God, as well as claim demonic and angelic possession or the sensation of having left their body. There are many references for these and similar kinds of experiences in the literature, but two older articles serve as an introduction to the effects of experimental stimulation of the cortex, namely Bear & Fedio (1977) and Penfield & Perot (1963). **Fear** is one of the most common feelings that can be generated by stimulation of these structures. It can include feelings of panic, terror, or of something horrible about to happen (Chiesa et al., 2007; Gloor et al., 1982; Penfield & Jasper, 1954).

BA 34: Uncus

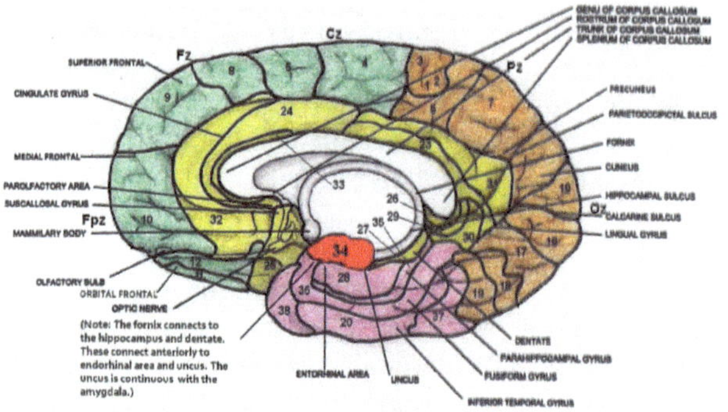

The anterior extremity of the parahippocampal gyrus is recurved in the form of a hook called the uncus. It is a part of the olfactory cortex. The connections of the uncus have been described above in the discussion concerning the temporal pole, entorhinal area, the amygdala and the uncinate fasciculus. Seizures that are preceded by the perception of disagreeable odors may have a source in this area of the temporal lobe. It is also involved in **social and emotional associational processing** functions due to its links to the amygdala, parahippocampal gyrus, and the frontal lobes.

More detail concerning Temporal Lobe Functions
The uncus, in conjunction with the amygdala and hippocampus, is involved in **visual closure**. These structures contain neurons that respond selectively to **faces and complex geometric** and visual stimuli as noted above. The **inferior and middle temporal** lobes are the **recipients of two diverging (dorsal and ventral) streams of visual input** arising from within the occipital lobe and the pulvinar and dorsal medial nucleus of the thalamus. The **dorsal stream** is more concerned with the **detection of motion** and movement, orientation, binocular disparity. The **ventral stream** is concerned with the **discrimination** of shapes, textures, objects, and faces. This information flows from the primary visual to visual association areas and is received and processed in the temporal lobes. It is then shunted to parietal lobe, and to the amygdala and entorhinal cortex (the gateway to

the hippocampus), where it may then be 'learned' and stored in memory (Joseph, 2000).

The **anterior temporal** region is more involved in the initial **consolidation and storage** phase of memory, whereas the **posterior region** is more involved in memory retrieval and **recall**. In addition, the temporal lobes directly interact with the frontal lobes in memorization and remembering. Indeed, the greater the activation of the frontal and temporal lobes (and associated tissues), the greater is the likelihood that subjects will remember, whereas reduced activity is associated with forgetting. Hence, these areas **interact to promote memory and retention**. In consequence, if the frontal lobe is injured, even if the temporal lobes are spared, patients may demonstrate significant memory loss due to an inability to correctly search for and find the memory.

Hippocampal stimulation may be associated with memory-like hallucinations, including feelings of familiarity, and dream-like hallucinations. Hallucinations require interactions between the amygdala, hippocampus, and the neocortex. It is only when the hallucination involves the neocortex of the temporal lobe that the individual becomes conscious of it. **In sleep,** the right hemisphere becomes highly active during REM sleep; conversely, the left brain becomes more active during non-REM sleep.

BA 36

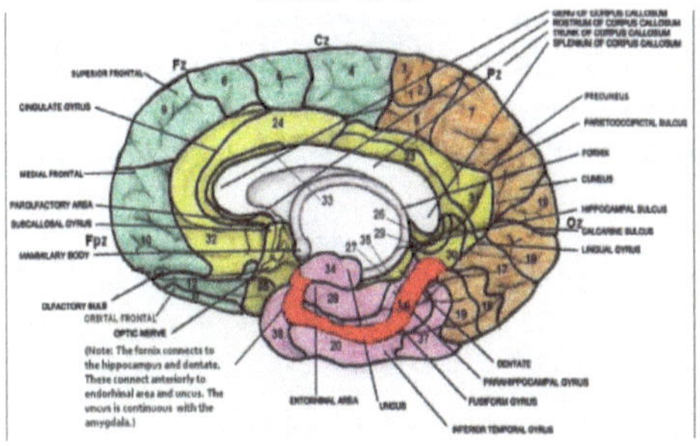

BA 37

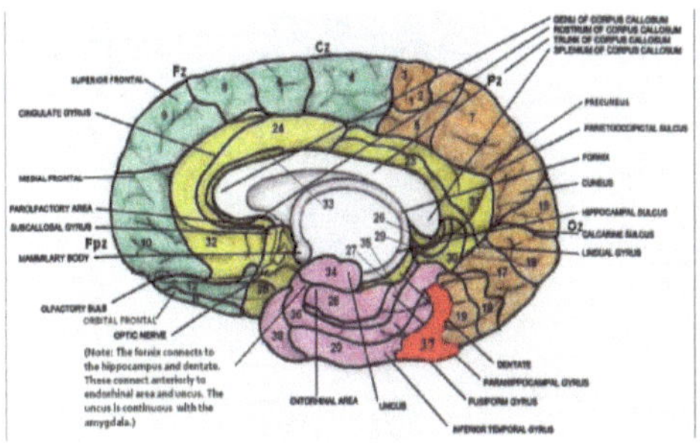

BA 37

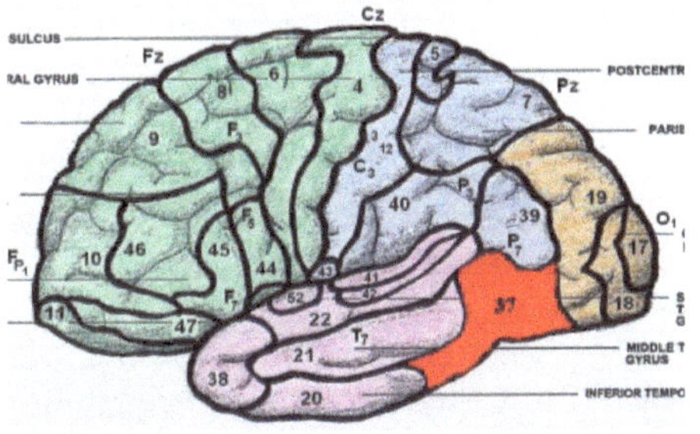

BA 37

Brodmann area 37, which contains part of the fusiform gyrus, is also known as the occipitotemporal gyrus. The underside or **ventral aspect** of the temporal cortices appear to be involved in visual fixation and high-level **visual processing of complex stimuli**. The **visual processing of scenes** involves the **parahippocampal** gyrus. Anterior portions of this ventral stream for visual processing are involved in object perception and recognition.

In the **inferior medial aspect**, this visual processing includes facial recognition in the fusiform gyrus BAs 36 and 37. This includes **face identity** and judgment of familiarity. It is also part of the Executive network related to deductive reasoning.

BA 37, DH

The visual word form area in the dominant (left) hemisphere, the **fusiform** gyrus holds a **prelexical representation** of visual words. The visual word form area responds **only to written stimuli**, not to spoken stimuli, independent of their semantic content (Dehaene et al., 2002). It is an area that is involved in networks for **semantic** relations (meaning of words) and categorization. Face-name associations are carried out in this area, too. It is important in sign language. It is another area that may be involved in the interpretation of metaphors. It is involved in **word retrieval,** and lesions in this area can lead to word finding difficulties. It is involved in **monitoring color and shape** and in drawing. It is part of a network that **relates to intentions**. It is part of networks related to the laying down of new memories and short-term memory, and is involved in episode encoding. It may be involved in true-false memory recognition.

BA 37, NDH

The nondominant (right) hemisphere BA 37, which includes part of the **fusiform gyrus,** is similarly important in the recognition of faces, and lesions can lead to difficulties in face recognition (called **prosopagnosia**), and in face-name recognition. It is important for drawing, too. Lesions can also lead **to constructional apraxia,** which is a visuoconstructive disorder. BA 37 is a part of the right hemisphere network for **sustained attention.** It is also one of the areas that is involved in the attribution of intentions to others.

The fusiform gyrus is involved in inhibiting the central nucleus of the amygdala. When this inhibition is deficient, sympathetic drive may increase. Functioning of this area appears to be deficient in autism spectrum disorders.

BAs 27, 35, and 36

BA 27

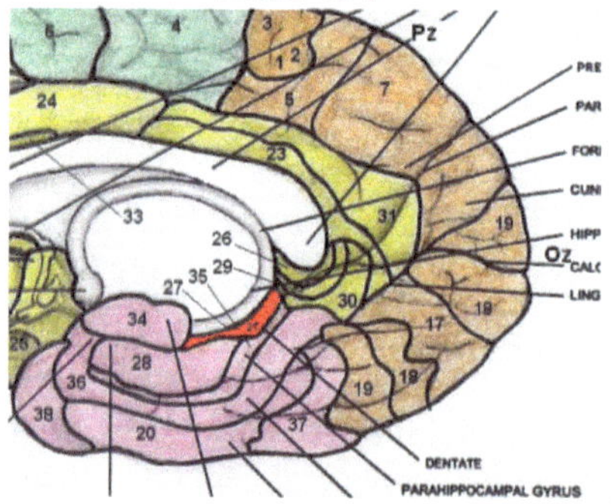

BA 35

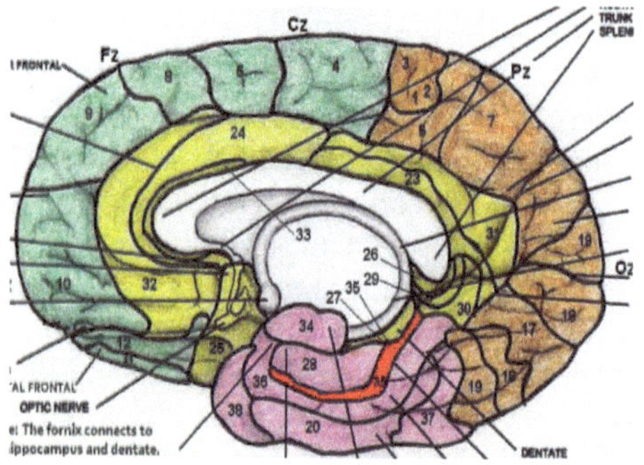

BA 36

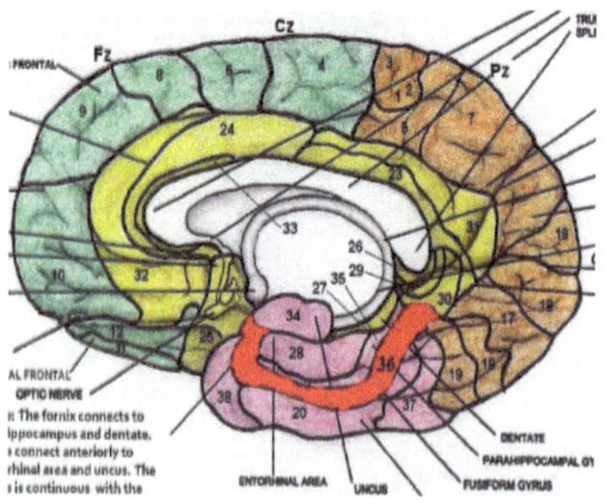

The parahippocampal cortex bilaterally is a key area (along with the hippocampus) for **short-term working memory**. As with other cortical areas, the left hemisphere is more related to verbal and the right hemisphere is more related to visual-spatial functions, but there is a great deal of overlap. BA 27 and parts of BA 35 and BA 36 play an important role in the encoding and recognition of **scenes** (as contrasted to recognition of faces or objects). Part of BA 36 overlaps with the fusiform gyrus. fMRI studies indicate that the hippocampal region of the brain becomes highly active when human subjects view **topographical scenes** such as images of landscapes, cityscapes, or rooms; that is, **images of places**. After a stroke affecting this area, the patient might be able to recognize people and objects but not recognize the scene in which they are being viewed.

In addition, the **right, NDH, parahippocampal** gyrus may play a crucial role in identifying **social context** including paralinguistic elements of verbal communication, such as **sarcasm**. It is also an area that is important in memory including faces, pictures, novelty, negative stimuli, olfactory, and gustatory experiences, as well as auditory and visual memories. It is involved in **procedural memory** consolidation and in recognition and recall. It is in a **network for autobiographical** memory and for insight. In addition, it is part of the limbic system and is involved in the Affect network and modulation of emotions. It is important in emotions that include **embarrassment and regret**. It may have a role in hunger and craving. It is part of the **Executive network for both categorization** and for decision making. Interestingly, the right parahippocampal area is activated when a person who is known to be accurate with **telepathy** is engaged in such activity (Persinger & Saroka, 2012). **BA 35** is important in the retrieval of words, acquisition of new memories, short-term memory, and spatial mapping. It is also involved, along with other areas, in the detection of novelty.

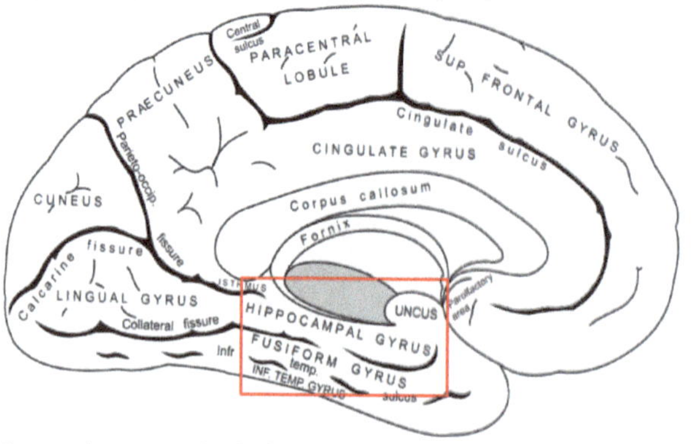

Reproduction of a lithograph plate from Gray's Anatomy, *Medial surface of left cerebral hemisphere. Image is in the public domain.*

NFB to Target Central Midline Ventral Structures

Practitioners with LORETA NFB may prefer to use that program to target activity in the central midline areas in order to be more precise in training for normalization. On the other hand, many practitioners appear to have been successful in altering activity involving Brodmann areas on the medial aspect of the temporal lobes and the temporal-parietal areas using single-channel NFB on the surface of the scalp. In the Neuroguide Manual, Robert Thatcher has outlined which surface electrode sites can be expected to reflect activity from these deeper structures. Indeed, in this Neuroguide QEEG assessment program, if you right click on any of the 19-channel sites, the BAs reflected in activity at that site are shown. The next figure illustrates this point. In this figure the arrows point to BA 30. If activity were outside the database norms at this site using LORETA, then this activity might be reflected, for example, in the surface EEG at Pz, P3, P4, T5, and T6.

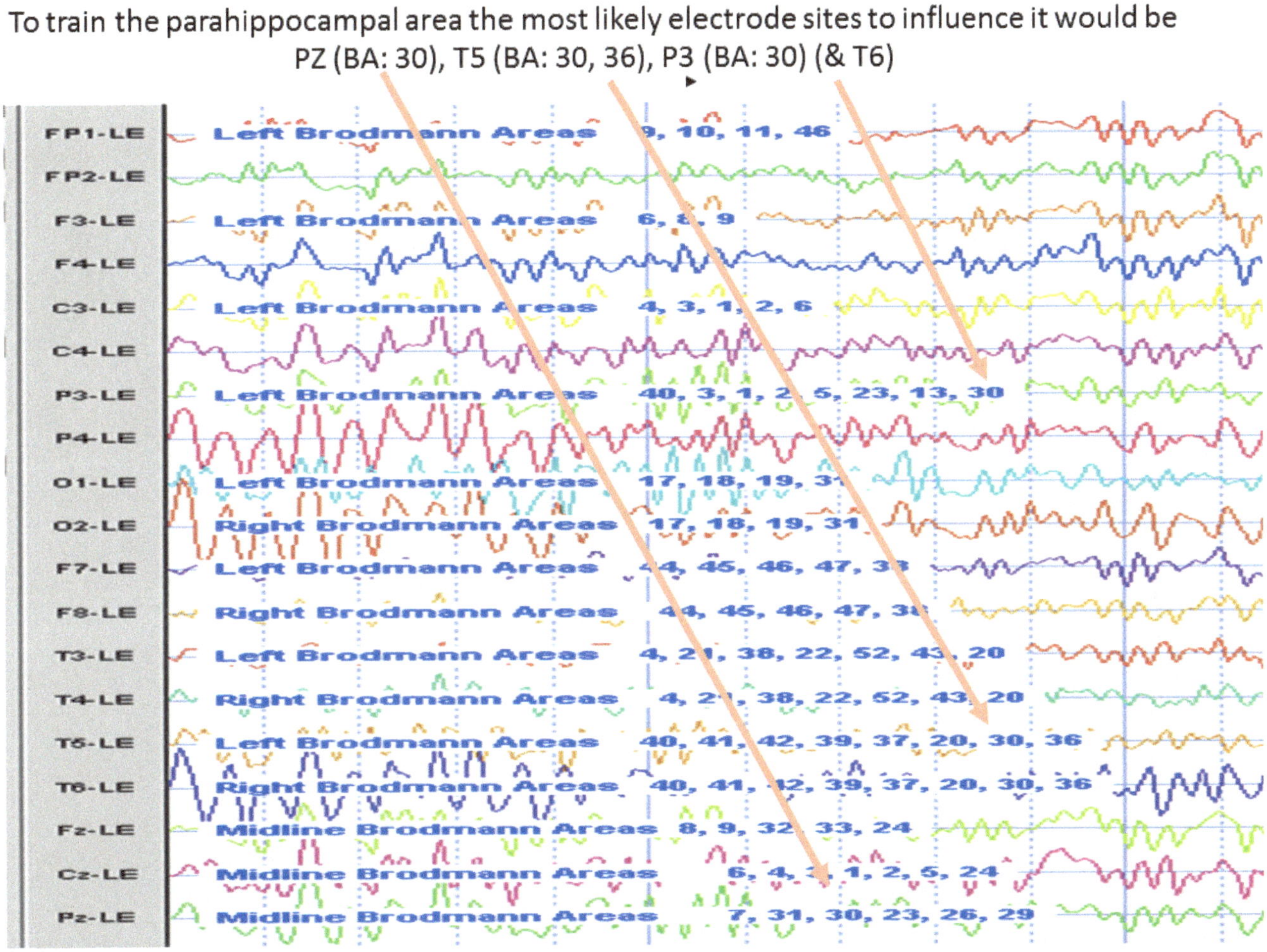

Functions of the area between F7 and T7 and between F8 and T8, and effects of lesions on CMSs that are important for memory.

Temporal Lobe Functions and Epilepsy

The hippocampus and amygdala have the lowest **seizure thresholds** of all brain structures and, when injured, they may develop seizure activity and thus give rise to temporal lobe epilepsy. Automatisms associated with **temporal lobe epilepsy** (TLE) include staring, searching, groping, lip smacking, spitting, laughing, crying, clenching the fist, confused talking, and so on. Common visceral reactions associated with **TLE auras** include feelings of a racing or fluttering heart. Body sensations include numbness, tenseness, pressure, and heaviness. Feelings of strangeness or familiarity are also common and déjà vu occurs in up to 20% of such patients, usually with right cerebral seizures within the temporal lobe. Some claim to have feelings like wanting something but not knowing what. Olfactory hallucinations are not uncommon. There may also be gustatory sensations. Fear is one of the most common feelings, including feelings of panic, or of something horrible about to happen. There may be sexual sensations.

Hence, there is a large range of auras and experiential phenomenon associated with temporal lobe seizures, many of which reflect the possible activation of those structures innervated by the amygdala. Indeed, many of these same feelings and behaviors can be triggered by direct stimulation of the amygdala. In addition, patients may act out on these emotions and auras. There have been reported instances of patients suddenly lashing out and even attempting to attack those close by while in the midst of a seizure. Some patients exhibit behaviors indicative of extreme fear, or conversely, extreme pleasure, including laughter and mirth.

Depression (lasting from hours to weeks) may occur as an immediate sequela to the seizure. Some patients experience confusion. A depressive aura may also precede a seizure by hours or even days. Some patients complain of emotional blocking, and feelings of emptiness. Patients have also described a sense of dissociation and being out of and looking at their own body (Joseph, 2000). The diverse phenomena associated with TLE are a reflection of the diverse functions of the temporal lobe.

Insula

BA 13
C3-T7; C4-T8

Key areas of the Affect network include the **cingulate gyrus and Brodmann areas 24, 25 and 33, plus the anterior portion of the insula, BA 13.** These areas have connections with the amygdala, septum, medial and orbitofrontal cortex, anterior insula, ventral striatum (nucleus accumbens), periaqueductal grey, and the autonomic brain stem motor nuclei. BA 25 has direct connections with the nucleus of the solitary tract in the medulla, as is discussed in a section on HRV training and the stress response in another part of *The NFB Book.*

BA 13 Insula

The insula is an infolding of the cortex between the inferior frontal cortex and the temporal pole. It is a portion of the cerebral cortex that is folded deep within the lateral sulcus. The lateral sulcus may also be called a fissure. It separates the temporal lobe from the parietal and frontal lobes. Thus it is not visible in the diagrams in this book that show the Brodmann areas. It is therefore outlined in the following illustration.

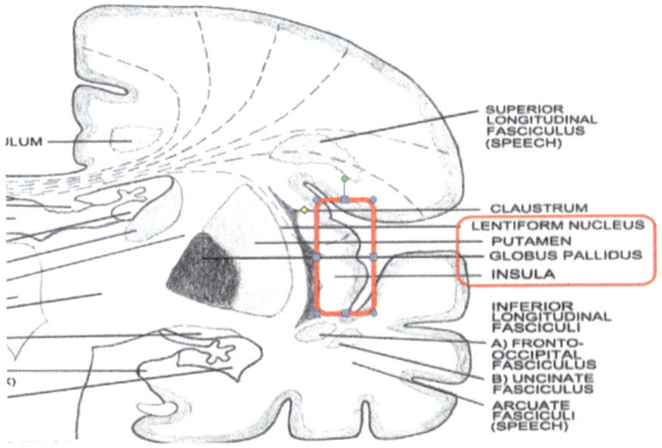

Figure to illustrate the relative position of the insula with respect to the frontal (superior) lobe, temporal (inferior) lobe, and the basal ganglia (medial). In this figure the cingulate cortex is superior/medial with the cingulum (just the label "...LUM" is visible) shown running through its central core. Below the cingulate cortex are dashed lines that indicate the corpus callosum.

Insula (BA 13 and Close to BA 43)

When dissecting the human brain, the insular cortex may be seen by placing your hands on each side of the lateral sulcus and then separating the frontal and temporal lobes and looking between them. The insular cortex is continuous with these two lobes, but it becomes an infolding of the cortex rather than expanding laterally during early development. It may be possible to have an effect on this important area of the cortex using an electrode site between C3 and T7, or C4–T8 on the right. Alternatively, LORETA NFB may have a more direct influence. After 19-channel data collection is done, and before using LORETA NFB, we observe what frequency is (or frequencies are) outside the database norms for BA 13, the insula, using LORETA. If that same frequency is outside database norms near a site between C3 and T7, then we may first try surface NFB to normalize it while we do tasks related to the patient's symptoms.

Due to the importance of the insula for normal balance between the sympathetic nervous system (right insula) and the parasympathetic nervous system (left insula), we always combine NFB with HRV training. Since we cannot specifically target the small area of neurons responsible for a specific network, we use cognitive strategies and tasks to try to have the person's brain activate particular networks while our NFB encourages appropriate EEG activation. Symptoms targeted for improvement would include those symptoms that might be expected to be related to an important aspect of the functioning of the insula and networks connected to the insula. Training to help a client where the insulae are affected, as they might be after a TBI, is a complicated endeavor. These patients will show a decrease in heart rate variability (HRV) measurements so it makes sense to combine NFB with HRV training.

The insula is of import in the **Affect network** and is a key component in some executive functions. It may also be involved in the Default network. The two insulae play a role in diverse functions linked to **emotion** and the regulation of the body's **homeostasis**. These include higher level emotions such as love, joyfulness, appreciating humor, expressing fear or disgust, and evaluating sexual arousal. It has some role in conscious sensing of heat, touch, vibration, taste, and olfaction. Its activity is increased, along with that of the amygdala and anterior cingulate cortices, in emotion-related tasks.

These areas have been shown to be linked to heart rate responses and to the presentation of emotional facial expressions (Yang, 2007).

The insula is involved in **Executive networks and in perception and motor** control. It is activated in networks for comprehension, understanding word meanings, and verbal memory. It has a role in cognitive functions including categorization, action planning, being aware of errors, and verbal memory. It is linked to networks that involve perception and motor control. It is important in **self-awareness.** One can immediately see that the insula (possibly different areas in the insula) is thus important in **Affect, Executive, Salience, and Default networks.** As part of the Salience network, it has a role in turning the Default mode off and on (Gotman, 2005). The right insula is a key in switching between central Executive and Default modes during attentional tasks (Sridharan, 2008).

The insulae are important in **autonomic** nervous system control and **affect**. As is noted above, the left insula influences the parasympathetic system and the right insula influences the sympathetic system. The right insula is involved in conscious emotional and physical self-awareness. With the amygdala, the **right insula activity decreases when** there is increased activity of prefrontal regions that regulate responses to negative emotional stimuli. That is, cognitive reappraisal of negative emotional stimuli can down-regulate the insula and amygdala (Lutz et al., 2009). **In contrast, the right insular cortex is activated** with feelings of disgust, which elicits avoidance behavior. You may recall that due to Davidson's work (1990), we tend to associate avoidance with right frontal activation, as contrasted to approach behavior, which is more associated with left frontal activation. Activation of the insula may also occur with fear.

The insular cortex plays a role in the experience of **bodily self-awareness**. There are mirror neuron-like links between external and internal experience that are related to the functioning of the insula. It plays a role in the affect component of pain, depression, anxiety, and feelings of hopelessness (Sheline et al., 2009). The insula is believed to process convergent information in order to produce an **emotionally relevant context for sensory experience**. The insulae send output to a number of other limbic-related structures, such as the amygdala, the ventral striatum, the nucleus accumbens, and the orbitofrontal cortex, as well as to motor cortices. The insular cortex has been suggested to have a role in **anxiety** disorders, and emotion dysregulation. While the amygdala may be more involved in social anxiety, activation of the insula may be more related to trait anxiety and the processing of threat assessment (Shah et al., 2009).

Anatomical Connections

The insula is an important area because of its multiple connections. The insula has major connections to the hippocampus and the hypothalamus. Connections to the hypothalamus influence the autonomic nervous system, as has been described previously. The **right insula** affects the **sympathetic** and the **left** affects the **parasympathetic** nervous system, in part through connections to the nucleus accumbens, which balances the sympathetic and parasympathetic systems (Nagai et al., 2010). Nagai states, "The insular cortex has **reciprocal connections** with the anterior cingulate gyrus, amygdala, entorhinal cortex, medial and orbitofrontal cortex, and temporal pole, and has afferent connections with hippocampus formation."

Additionally, the insular cortex has dense reciprocal connections **with subcortical autonomic** core centers including the lateral hypothalamic area, nucleus tractus solitarius, and parabrachial nucleus, and these centers are also reciprocally connected to each other.

Importance in HRV Training

Of particular importance to the biofeedback practitioner who uses HRV training is the influence of these structures on **vagal efferent** output. These connections, and thus the whole affect network, may be influenced by both NFB and BFB, and thus we suggest that practitioners consider combining NFB with BFB interventions. Changes in heart rate can correlate with activity in the right middle insula because the right insula influences the sympathetic nervous system.

The heart and the **baroreflex** system have direct **vagal afferent** connections to the nucleus of the **solitary tract (NST)**. This was discussed earlier with an illustration under the Frontal Lobes, "Importance of Heart Rate Variability (HRV) Training – Connections to NST in Brain Stem." The NST, in turn, connects to the parabrachial nucleus (respiratory control), the locus coeruleus (norepinephrine production and a key in understanding the stress response), the thalamus, hypothalamus (control of the autonomic nervous system and pituitary outputs), the amygdala, and the cingulate cortex.

These connections mean that this network has roles not only in **mood modulation** but **also** in related physiological **regulation of the autonomic nervous system and of endocrine** functions. In addition, this Affect network is also important in conditioned emotional learning, vocalizations expressing internal (emotional) state, assessing motivational content, and in assigning **emotional valence** to internal and external stimuli. However, the major function of this network is to modulate autonomic activity and internal emotional responses. If one had to pick one key structure that could regulate the whole network, it would most likely be the anterior cingulate cortex (Devinsky et al., 1995).

BAs 14, 15 and 16 are found in monkeys but not in humans, so they are not discussed in this text.

Cingulate Gyrus

Fz, Cz, Pz
Anterior FCz: Executive BA 32; Affect BAs 24, 25, 33
Central Cz: Affect BA 24
Posterior Pz: Affect – Executive – Default BAs 23, 31; 29, 30, 26

Important connections exist to the insula for all of these areas.

BA 32

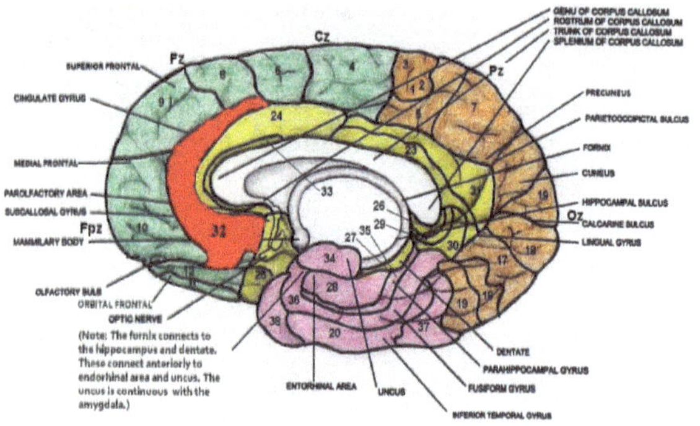

BA 24

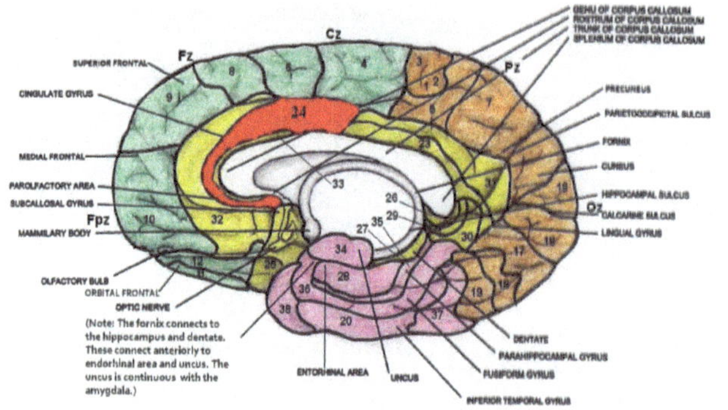

BA 25

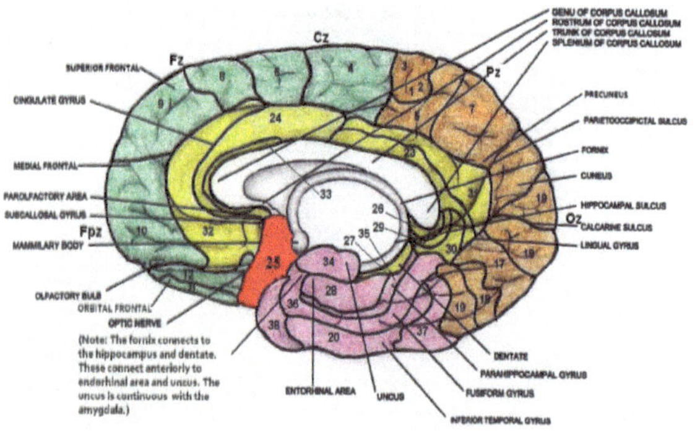

BA 33

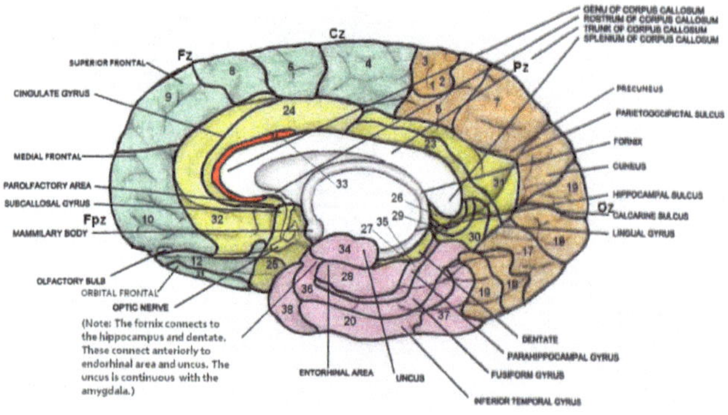

Introduction to the Cingulate Gyrus

BAs 24, 25, 33

FCz

Anterior Cingulate Cortex

Many functions are influenced by the anterior cingulate cortex (ACC). The ACC contains a very high density of opioid receptors. It is involved in the emotional experience of **pain**. It is important in possible gating functions for pain between cortical and subcortical structures. It is part of neural networks involved in the identification and the conscious perception of pain. It is involved in **sexual** arousal. It is important in **attention** networks, both auditory and visuospatial.

It may be involved in more complex functions such as having a sense of **balance** and even timekeeping. It is important in **monitoring** stimuli and in response selection. The ACC may detect the need for executive control, and may signal the prefrontal cortex to provide that control. (This latter function is poor in patients who have ADHD.) It is an important component in **reward** networks that involve both Executive networks (the DLPC) and Affect networks (limbic system including medial, orbital, and insular cortices and the nucleus accumbens, amygdala, and the ventral tegmental area). These same areas, plus the left temporal-occipital junction, are involved in networks related to the **appreciation of humor** (Moran et al., 2004).

As noted at the beginning of this section, the ACC has close connections with the insula. **Negative stimuli** will activate the insula and amygdala. Both fear and disgust will activate the insula. Disgust is a powerful emotion that results in avoidance behavior, which we previously noted may involve the non-dominant hemisphere (NDH). Disgust activates the right insular cortex plus the right medial and orbital prefrontal cortex, the hippocampus and amygdala. We have also noted previously that all of these areas are involved in Affect networks.

However, the **prefrontal cortex does exert control over insula and amygdala** activity. It can down-regulate these areas during reappraisal of negative stimuli. There may be problems with this regulation in certain psychiatric syndromes, such as in **borderline personality disorder** (Donegan et al., 2003). The anterior cingulate cortex has direct connections to all of these areas, and it thus influences all of these control mechanisms.

Of interest to the NFB practitioner is evidence from other fields of research, such as **protein analysis**, which shows that the ACC is structurally damaged in major psychiatric disorders. **Disease-specific protein changes within the ACC** have been found in psychiatric disorders such as depression, bipolar disorder, and schizophrenia. This includes cytoskeletal and mitochondrial dysfunction. Thus, protein changes in the ACC have been shown to be important components of the neuropathology of major psychiatric disorders (Beasley et al., 2006). This evidence concerning the wide-ranging involvement of the ACC gives further support to our **emphasis during initial NFB sessions on normalizing** the QEEG abnormalities associated with the ACC. It also helps explain the positive effects that have been observed in hundreds of patients treated with single-channel neurofeedback at Cz and FCz.

The **ventral portion of the Affect network** also involves other structures such as the amygdala and hippocampus. Like the ACC, damage to the **hippocampal formation (BAs 27, 34, 35, 36)** has been implicated in a number of **psychiatric disorders** including depression, bipolar disorder, schizophrenia, and addictive disorders. The Internet or Rex Canon's summary (Cannon, 2012, p163) offer specific references. There is decreased hippocampal volume in persons who have executive dysfunction with depression (Frodl et al., 2006).

When reading about these structures, the reader may encounter the term **'piriform lobe.'** The piriform lobe or piriform complex is a three-layered cortex that consists of the cortical amygdala, uncus, anterior parahippocampal gyrus (Brodmann area 27), entorhinal cortex, lateral olfactory gyrus, and the cingulate cortex just above the corpus callosum. The 'piriform lobe' is considered to be a part of the **paralimbic** system. It is quite clearly involved in the Affect network. Certain parts of this system may be influenced by NFB training on surface sites over the temporal lobe and at Cz, as well as by LORETA z-score NFB. In addition, the network as a whole may be influenced in a positive manner using HRV training, as might be expected due to the afferent connections of the vagus to the nucleus of the solitary tract in the medulla and the previously outlined connections of this nucleus to important structures that are involved in the Affect network.

BAs 8, 9, 32, 33, 24

Fz:

Fz placement is posited to influence the following Brodmann areas in the central area of the frontal cortex: BA 9 in the prefrontal cortex, BAs 33, 32, 24, related to the ACC, and BA 8 (ventral). It also may influence the frontal eye fields in terms of **motor control, focus, and action observation.**

Anterior Cingulate Gyrus and Medial Prefrontal Cortex

Functions related to Affect networks in the **medial frontal cortex, BA 32, and anterior cingulate cortex** (ACC) include: emotional inhibition, modulation of emotions (sensitivity) and behavioral responses. As previously noted, it also has a role in motivation and attention. BA 32 is the 'dorsal' ACC, and has an important role in Executive networks.

Functions related to **Executive networks in the medial frontal cortex** executive system include: action monitoring, shifting attention, judgment of events (emotional and cognitive), cognitive flexibility or inflexibility, obsessive thoughts, compulsive behaviors, excessive worrying, argumentativeness, oppositional behavior or 'getting stuck' on certain thoughts or actions. **Monitoring** enables the brain to evaluate errors and the quality of action execution and alerts the executive control mechanisms to allocate resources and take corrective action.

Dysfunction in the rostral anterior cingulate gyrus and the medial frontal lobe, as might be observed in a patient with an obsessive compulsive disorder, may be reflected in evoked potentials at Fz and Cz; namely, low amplitude and a long latency for the P400 component as compared to a database.

Dorsal Central Midline Structures (DCMS)

The dorsomedial prefrontal cortex (DMPFC) and the supragenual anterior cingulate cortex (SACC) are connected with the lateral prefrontal cortex. In a meta-analysis of studies on the **cognitive control of emotion**, the dorsal prefrontal regions were characterized by functions that included reappraisal and evaluation of, and explicit reasoning concerning, emotional stimuli (Ochsner and Gross, 2005). This dorsal CMS could also be involved in reappraisal and evaluation of self-related stimuli. It has a strong **evaluative or judgmental** component. It is involved in tasks involving reading other people (**theory of mind**) (Frith and Frith, 2003). In PET studies, in addition to the dorsal medial prefrontal cortex (DMPC) and the temporal pole, it is **the ventral medial prefrontal** cortex that has been shown to be involved in **self-referenced tasks** and to knowledge about one's self (D'Argembeau et al., 2005).

Patients with lesions in **dorsal CMS** show disturbances in social interactions (Damasio, 2003). Northoff and his colleagues make clear statements as to the importance of CMSs. To paraphrase their conclusions, they note that **self-referential processing** is mediated by cortical midline structures. Since the CMS are densely and reciprocally connected to subcortical midline regions, they posit an integrated cortical–subcortical midline system underlying understanding self and self-in-relation-to-others. They conclude that self-referential processing in CMS constitutes the **core of our sense of self** and is critical for elaborating experiential feelings of self (Northoff et al., 2006). This self-referential processing is one aspect of the Default network. These kinds of findings strongly support the importance of combining either single-channel NFB at CZ (or FCZ) or LORETA z-score NFB with HRV training.

Anterior Cingulate, Other Connections

As previously described under "FCz," the Anterior Cingulate Cortex (ACC) may be thought of as the keystone for both Affect and Executive networks. It is crucial in monitoring errors. As previously stated, the ACC connects with the medial and orbital prefrontal cortex, insula and the entire limbic system. In addition, it receives input from the brain stem that, importantly for work with NFB and BFB, includes vagal afferents from the heart to the nucleus solitarius in the medulla. As previously noted, this nucleus connects to the locus coeruleus (LC) (noradrenaline production) and, both directly and through the LC, it connects to the hypothalamus and to the limbic system including the insula and the ACC. These are important connections for understanding a number of related disorders. Indeed, Porges (2007) has stated that one characteristic of some psychiatric problems, such as anxiety disorders, autism spectrum disorders (ASDs), **reactive attachment** disorder, and even the **hyper-vigilance** seen in people with ADHD, is **an inability to inhibit defensive reaction** responses in what would normally be considered safe environments. The anterior cingulate appears to be a central component in these disorders that involve the Affect network. The **ACC** also has direct links to the hypothalamic-pituitary-adrenal (HPA) axis. These connections play a major role in the human stress response and hence, once again, we stress the importance of treatment that combines HRV training with NFB to control stress (Thompson & Thompson, 2007). Affect can be complex and involves a system of Executive and Affect subnetworks. An example is depression.

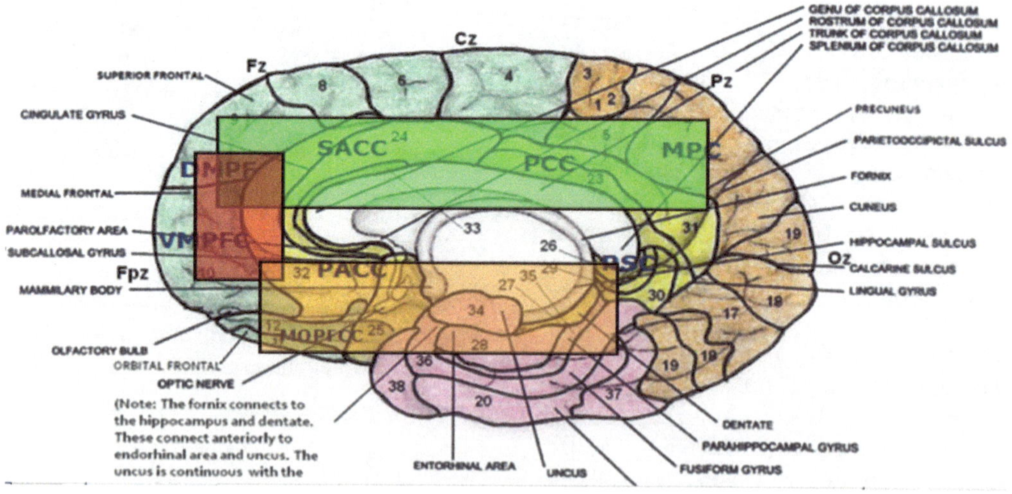

Areas of the Executive and Affect networks involved in depression (adapted after de Ridder, 2010)

- ***Executive/Cognitive*** *Aspects of Network =* ***GREEN*** *(BAs 9 and 46, 23, 24, 31, 32, 40)*
- ***Affect/Vegetative*** *Aspects of Network =* ***ORANGE*** *(BAs 25, 13, anterior insula, hippocampus, hypothalamus)*
- ***Integration and connection*** *of Cognitive and Vegetative =* ***RED*** *(BAs 24, 9, 10, 11) (red box can be extended down to include BA 11).*

In depression, the **vegetative/autonomic Affect** network symptoms involve a ventral compartment (e.g., sleep disturbance, loss of appetite and libido), which includes the hypothalamic-pituitary-adrenal axis, hippocampus, insula (**BA 13**), subgenual (SG) cingulate (**BA 25**), and the brainstem. It should be noted that the solitary nucleus connects to BA 25 and this could be one important factor in understanding how HRV training can have positive effects in depression.

Sleep disturbance is a major factor in depression. Sleep disturbances **will decrease cortisol**, **increase inflammatory responses** (related to **increase in cytokine IL6)** and the risk of infectious disease, and **decrease cellular immunity.** For example, studies have demonstrated that shift workers report more colds than nonshift workers. Some studies give a general overview saying that adults are at risk when they have less than five or more than nine hours of sleep. Others suggest that most adults need eight to nine hours and are at risk of flu when they have less than seven hours. Both stress and sleep deprivation can increase pro-inflammatory cytokines. This will increase the severity of depression, and is usually associated with **poor concentration, anhedonia** symptoms, and social withdrawal (Prather, Rabinovitz, Pollock & Lotrich, 2009; Prather, Marsland, Hall, Neumann, Muldoon & Manuck, 2009; Buysse et al., 2011).

The **executive components** of the Affect network in depression are found in the dorsal compartment, which modulates attentional and sensory-cognitive symptoms (e.g., **apathy, attentional and executive deficits**). This includes the dorsolateral prefrontal cortex (**BAs 9 and 46**), the dorsolateral anterior cingulate (**BA 24'**), posterior cingulate (**BA 23, 31**), the inferior parietal lobe (**BA 40**), and the **striatum**. The dorsal prefrontal components, including the ACC, are also involved in the cognitive control of emotion including reappraisal, evaluation, and explicit reasoning concerning emotional stimuli.

Information **concerning cognition and emotion** from the two compartments (dorsal and ventral) is **integrated** by the rostral anterior cingulate (BA 24), medial frontal cortex (**BAs 9 and 10**), orbital frontal cortex (**BA 11**), and frontopolar areas, as is illustrated in the above figure. **Depressive ruminations** may involve the **Default network** with connections involving the posterior cingulate and the subgenual cingulate areas (Berman et al., 2011).

The **central-midline areas shown for depressive disorders are also important in drug abuse and in bipolar** disorders. Robbins has reviewed substance abuse and its relation to these neuroanatomical structures (Robbins et al., 2009). **Bipolar** disorder is a severe and recurrent illness involving periodic cycling of both manic and depressed states. This disorder can result in significant impairments, including high rates of divorce and suicide, high rates of alcohol and substance abuse, and erratic work performance despite, at times, remarkably productive intervals in the manic phase. Bipolar disorder is often diagnosed late in the course of the illness, or may be initially misdiagnosed as other illnesses, such as unipolar depression (Nusslock et al., 2012). Children may be first be given a diagnosis of ADHD, which is later recognized as being bipolar disorder in their adolescence.

In bipolar disorder, there is **manic state-related increased activity in the left dorsal anterior cingulate,** and left head of the caudate (Blumberg, 2000). In QEEG assessments, it has been our experience that high amplitude spindling beta may be seen with LORETA analysis showing a source in both the ACC and the frontal lobes, particularly the right NDH frontal lobe.

Cingulate Cortex

In the **foregoing section, we dealt with the principle functions** of the first division, the **Affect network components**. Now we will review the **second and third components** of the anterior cingulate cortex, **executive and motor** respectively.

Fz and also Cz; Second Division of the Anterior Cingulate Cortex: Cognition Division (Dorsal)

A second, major division of the anterior cingulate cortex is the executive division. In the previous discussion of the functions of the ACC, the Affect network was emphasized. The executive division includes **Brodmann areas 24'and 32'**. (Note that 24', read as 24 prime, refers to the more dorsal layer of BA 24.) We are not able, using LORETA, to make this fine distinction between areas involved with the Affect network (e.g., BAs 24, 33) and areas mainly said to be involved with the Executive network (BAs

24' and 32'). The executive division also has **connections to the DLPFC** and other areas of the frontal cortex involved in **attention, concentration, planning, evaluating,** and all aspects of executive/cognitive functioning.

Other important functions of the executive components of the ACC include initiation, motivation, and **goal-directed behavior**. **Maintaining attention is a key function** and attention to space is to the contralateral side. However, the reader should recognize that **not all attentional processes** are related to ACC functioning. For example, the left dorsolateral cortex is activated during reading and semantic processing, but the ACC is not activated, even though reading requires attention (Peterson, 1990). The ACC is important in the **retrieval of short-term memory**. It is involved in the assessment of the **motivational content** of internal and external stimuli before movement.

The ACC is important in the **regulation of context-dependent behavior patterns** seen in disorders such as **Anxiety, Panic, Obsessive Compulsive (OCD), Sociopathic Personality, and Asperger's syndrome**. The neuroanatomy of panic disorder has been reviewed by Gorman (Gorman et al., 2000).

Third Division of the Anterior Cingulate (Motor)

A third network of functioning that involves modulation by the anterior cingulate cortex is motor control. The locations for this ACC motor regulation are the motor areas in the **cingulate sulcus and nociceptive cortex** that communicate with the **midline and intralaminar thalamic** nuclei (Peterson, 1990, p280). The motor area has projections to the **spinal cord and to the red nucleus**. It has some control over premotor functions.

The cingulate cortical site includes the **nociceptive area,** which is important in **response selection** and in cognitively demanding information processing. The major function of this cortical area is in response selection associated with skeletomotor activity and responses to noxious stimuli.

Anterior Cingulate
BAs 32, 24, 25, 33
FCz
Affect (and Executive) Networks

BA 32

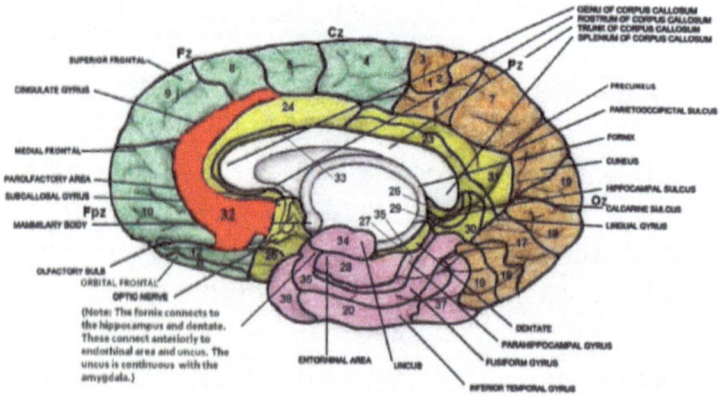

Brodmann area 32 comprises the most anterior (rostral) portion of the anterior cingulate cortex. It is also **called the dorsal anterior cingulate**. It is part of the **Executive network**. It is under Fz and FCz when doing neurofeedback. The dorsal region of anterior cingulate gyrus is associated with rational thought processes and may be seen to be active during the Stroop task. It is also a part of the **Affect** network, and this is involved in regulation of mood and appraising of emotions, including negative emotions, and also rewards. It is an area involved in the anticipation of stimuli and the **detection** of unexpected errors, or when rewards were expected but not received. This area is important in the regulation of mood. It is part of the network involved in **identifying pain**. It is also important in sustaining a response set.

BA 24

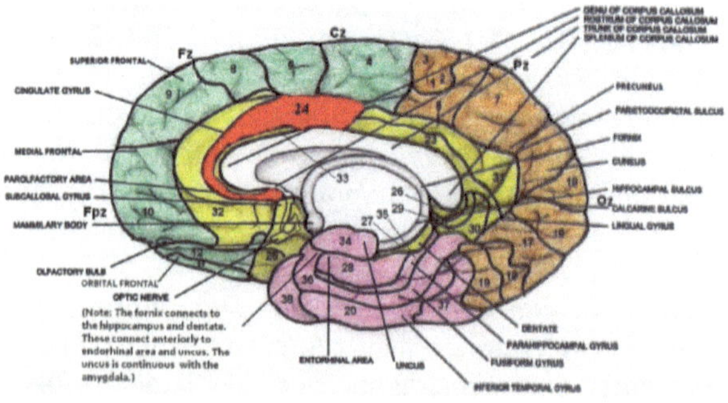

Brodmann area 24 includes a large portion of the anterior cingulate gyrus. The anterior aspect of the cingulate has already been mentioned when discussing the frontal lobes and NFB at FCz. The posterior portion of BA 24 lies under an electrode placed at Cz, which is probably the most frequently used location for single-channel neurofeedback, especially with children. Much of our work with NFB is done to influence the networks associated with the anterior cingulate cortex including BA 24. The anterior cingulate is associated with the Affect, Executive, Salience, and Default networks. It can be described as the **hub of the emotional brain (also called the Affect network or the limbic** system), and we often find that BA 24 is the source location for frequencies that are outside database norms when we do a LORETA analysis of the QEEG in people with anxiety disorders or people with autism spectrum disorders, including Asperger's syndrome.

CZ is a primary site for feedback when we are working with ADHD. In this disorder we are usually decreasing whatever frequency range has excessive slow-wave activity (such as 4–8 Hz or 3–7 Hz in children, 3–10 Hz in some adolescents and adults), enhancing SMR (12–15 Hz or 13–15 Hz), which encourages the client to be calm and relaxed while also focused and concentrating. For part of each session we often change the enhance frequency to 15–18 Hz beta while the client is learning and carrying out cognitive strategies. This can be extraordinarily helpful, as reported in our published case series (Thompson & Thompson, 1998, 2010). The dorsal areas of the ACC are more related to Executive network functions, and the ventral and rostral ACC to the Affect network. Both the rostral-ventral ACC (more under Fz) and the posterior cingulate cortex, BA 31, under Pz, are related to Default network functions.

Brodmann area 24 is also important in a large number of **Executive network** functions, including both inductive and deductive reasoning. It is critical to memory networks, and its functions include aspects of working memory, prospective memory, delayed memory, mental timekeeping, and inhibition. It is important in most aspects of **attention,** including auditory and visual-spatial attention, and divided attention. It is linked to networks responsible for verbal fluency and object naming. It is important in the ability to multitask. It is a key link in Affect network and will influence all aspects of mood and mood swings. It even has some role in such diverse areas as sexual arousal, taste, and pain endurance.

Due to the number of networks that involve the anterior cingulate cortex, when doing NFB, we also use metacognitive training and tasks. We do NFB to normalize frequencies that are outside database norms while the patient is doing tasks related to correcting their symptoms in order to activate particular networks that are relevant to their problems. If working at CZ, the symptoms targeted would be those that might be expected to be related to functioning of the anterior cingulate for a particular patient. In this manner, using metacognitive strategies and related tasks, we postulate we can be a little more specific with respect to involving and constructively optimizing the functions of networks that are important for that person.

BA 25

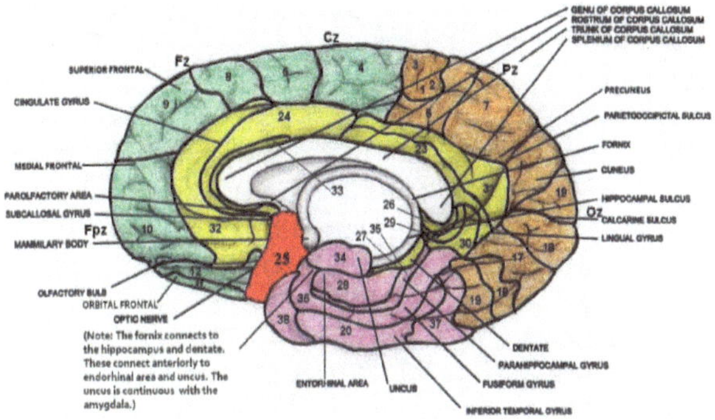

Brodmann area 25 is also called the subgenual area, area subgenualis, or subgenual cingulate because it is "below the knee" of the corpus callosum. It may be influenced by work done with NFB at Fz and Cz by virtue of its involvement in networks that also involve the more superior aspect of the cingulate gyrus under Cz and the medial aspect of the frontal lobe under Fz. It is also involved in moral reasoning.

BA 25 is very deep in the midline cortex. LORETA NFB may have a much more direct effect. This is an area that is very important in the **Affect network.** It is an area that is considered a key to intervention with patients who have an intractable depression. This region is rich in **serotonin** transporters and is considered to influence a vast network. It influences areas such as the hypothalamus and brain stem, which are involved in changes in appetite and sleep; the amygdala and insula, which affect mood and anxiety; the hippocampus, which plays an important role in memory formation; and some parts of the frontal cortex responsible for self-esteem.

A surgical procedure that involves **deep brain stimulation** (DBS) in BA 25 has been used to treat intractable depression (Mayberg et al., 2005). DBS has also been used to treat obsessive compulsive disorder as reviewed by Greenberg et al. (2006). In 2005, Helen S. Mayberg and collaborators described how they successfully treated a number of depressed people — individuals virtually catatonic with depression despite years of talk therapy, drugs, even shock therapy — with pacemaker-like electrodes (deep brain stimulation) in Brodmann area 25 (Mayberg et al., 2005; Kennedy et al., 2011). BA 25 is said to be **metabolically overactive** in treatment-resistant depression, and this appears to correlate with poor therapeutic response to traditional treatments for depression.

However, of importance to the practitioner who uses a combination of NFB and BFB, the **solitary nucleus** has direct connections to BA 25. Thus HRV training will send vagal afferent feedback to the medulla, solitary nucleus, and thus be potentially helpful in influencing BA 25, and thereby, perhaps, the symptoms of depression related to dysfunction in this area of the cortex. Indeed, depressed patients have been shown to be helped by HRV training (Karavidas et al., 2007). In addition, NFB combined with psychotherapy has been shown to affect virtually the same areas as DBS with similar beneficial results and a much less invasive procedure for patients who have depression that does not respond to traditional therapies (Paquette et al., 2009).

BA 33

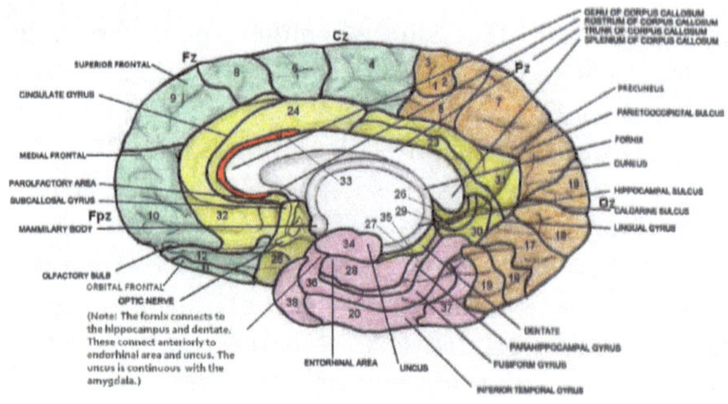

Brodmann area 33 is another part of the rostral anterior cingulate gyrus and thus is a part of the Affect network. It may be particularly important in emotions related to hearing pleasant music. It is important also in networks that involve sexual arousal.

The Caudal Division of the Cingulate Cortex – Posterior Cingulate Cortex

BAs 31, 23
Pz
Posterior Cingulate Gyrus

BA 31

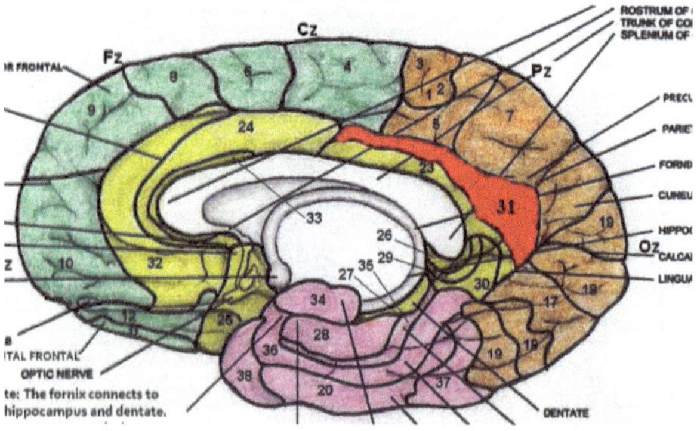

BA 23

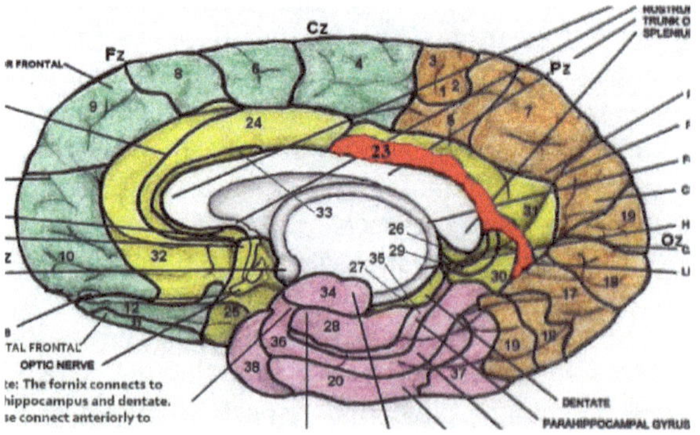

Pz lies above the posterior cingulate gyrus **Brodmann area 31 and below it, Brodmann area 23.**

BA 31

Brodmann area 31 is an association cortex area in the posterior part of the cingulate gyrus. As with other parts of the posterior cingulate, a portion of BA 31 is in the medial parietal lobe. It is a region that is crucial for the **evaluation of stimuli**. It is important in **memory** and has a role in **pain** perception. It is important in **attention, comprehension**, and **visual processing** (Choo et al., 2012; Choo et al., 2009). It has a key role in the **integration and synthesis** of almost all sensory input. In our work with university students whose chief complaint is an inability to **assimilate new information during a lecture**, we are finding hypocoherence (sometimes called disconnects) between Pz (over the posterior cingulate) and central temporal, central, and frontal areas. With NFB training directed at changing this, they have improved and become successful in their learning. Without research, this remains a clinical observation only. BA 31 is also important in evaluative judgment and precautionary reasoning. In keeping with part of this Brodmann area being in the medial parietal lobe, it has functions related to parietal **associational integration of sensory inputs.** The cingulate part of this area is a cortical component of the limbic system. It is a key component of the **Default network** and is important in self-evaluation. It is one area involved in the distinction of **'self' from 'other.'**

The posterior cingulate region is also important in the **recall of episodic information,** and it is one of several brain areas that produce anterograde amnesia when damaged. This occurred with the TBI experienced by the 52-year-old woman whose case is described below. Other functions include visuospatial processing and memory. It is part of networks involved in **identification of pain**. This area of the cingulate has connections to the hippocampus, posterior parietal cortex, posterior parahippocampal gyrus, and to the dorsal striatum.

The cingulate gyrus part of this area is a cortical component of the **limbic system** and is thus a part of the Affect network in addition to its roles in the Executive and Default networks.

BA 23

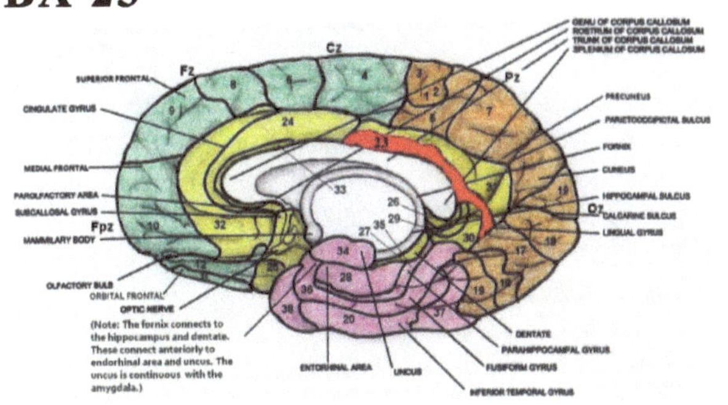

Brodmann area 23 is involved in the **Default network** when the brain is not engaged in active tasks and it is important in aspects of thinking about self versus other(s) and 'self-in-the-world.' Like BA 31, it is also part of the networks for the **synthesis and integration of incoming sensory information**. It is important in learning complex procedures, memory encoding and retrieval, learning complex procedures, visual discrimination, lexical categories, and high order tasks such as **evaluation and judgment**. It is involved in classical **conditioning** and in the conditioning of fear. It is linked to emotions evoked by words. It also has a role in processing temperature.

The following case assessment reveals difficulties that encompass many of the areas described above under the dominant hemisphere temporal – parietal area and cingulate gyrus (described below). Twenty-one years before presenting at our center, a 52 year old woman was hit in the jaw. She fell backwards, striking her head on the hard floor. She was briefly unconscious. When she awoke she was told that she had tried to strangle her girlfriend who found her and was attempting to help her by putting her in a car to transport her to hospital after the assault. She remembers thinking she was outside her own body and that she could see parts of her (forearm, hand) separated from her and floating in space. She had been a brilliant student, perhaps genius level intelligence, able to sort accounting figures and sheets with ease in a part-time job while she was a student. After the injury she had difficulty with even relatively simple accounting, and still cannot order figures in proper columns and rows. Putting numbers and charts together and organizing things — putting all the little pieces together to see the big overall picture — is still, as it has been for the last 21 years since her injury, extremely difficult. There are also major problems with memory. She will pay her phone bill three times, not realizing she already paid it. She will purchase oranges when she goes shopping even though she has far too many already at home. She will sometimes pick up the phone and look at it and say to herself, "What do I do with this?" She has difficulty recalling timelines in terms of what year things happened since the injury. On the other hand, she has an excellent and very detailed and precise memory from long before the injury.

Below are some of the EEG findings for this client that appear to correlate with her symptoms.

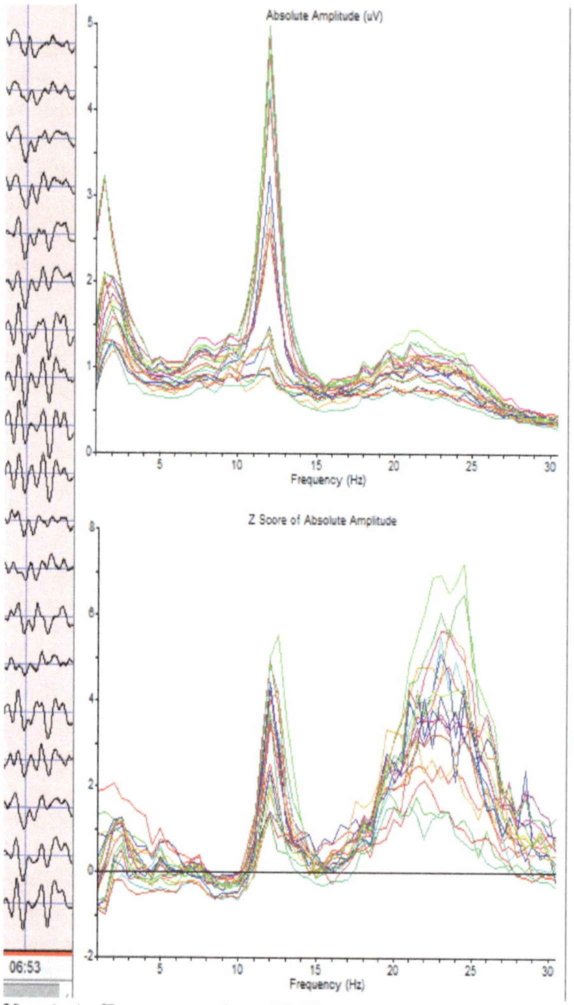

X axis is Frequency 2 to 30 Hz
Y axis is amplitude on the top figure & bottom figure it is standard deviations -2 to +8.

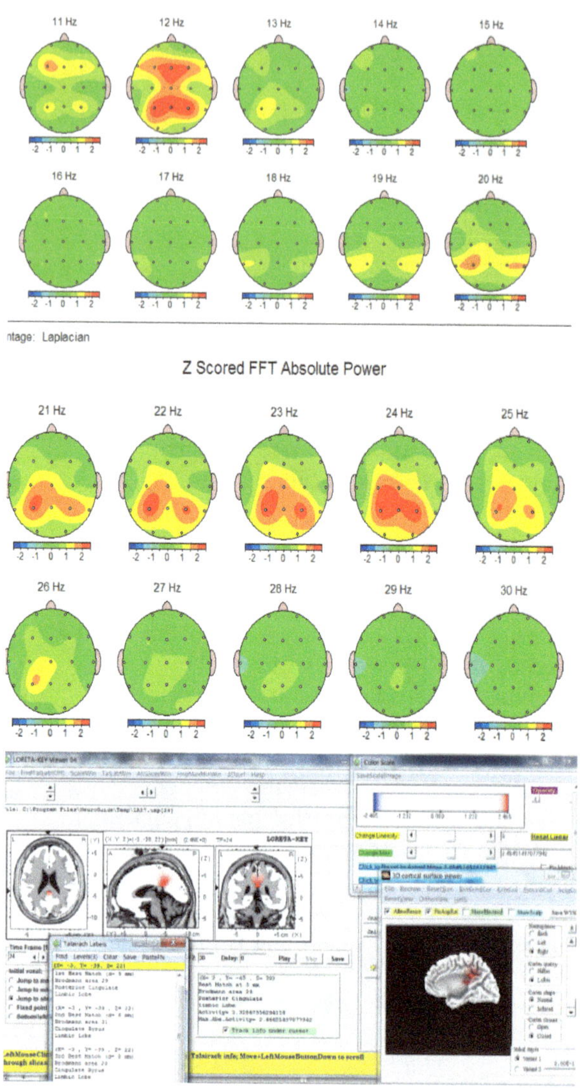

EC 24 Hz 2.5 sd, posterior cingulate BAs 29, 31, 23

LORETA shows high-amplitude spindling beta 24 Hz, which was 2.5 standard deviations above the database mean with a source in the posterior cingulate BAs 29, 31, 23. We postulate that this may contribute to the patient's difficulties with synthesis and integration of new incoming information. She feels this is a key issue. Her particular learning problems with columns and rows of figures could relate to injury to the DH, left, angular gyrus area. Her difficulties with memory may relate to her being well outside database norms in areas that reflect EEG activity influenced by BAs 31, 29, and the left angular gyrus, the supramarginal gyrus, the left entorhinal cortex, parahippocampal area, and the inferior frontal gyrus near and including the rostral ventral cingulate gyrus BA 25. The involvement of BA 25 and the anterior cingulate including BA 24 and right insula may all be related to her easily precipitated extreme anxiety. The spindling beta in the parietal regions may contribute to a major difficulty handling any 'startle' response, whether it be auditory or visual. Despite all these difficulties, she is a very pleasant, hard working individual who has been finding ways to cope with her deficiencies for two decades.

Posterior Cingulate Gyrus and Anterior-Medial Aspects of the Parietal Lobe Overlap

BAs 26, 29, 30, Pz:

BA 26: Medial Parietal Lobe/Posterior Cingulate

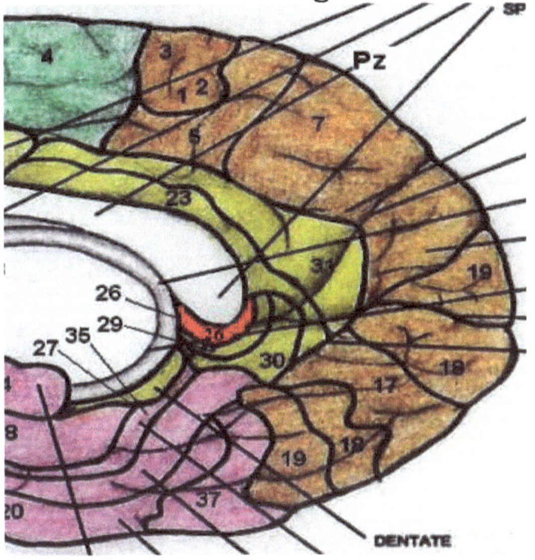

Brodmann area 26 lies in the retrosplenial region of the cerebral cortex. It is a narrow band located in the isthmus of the cingulate gyrus in the medial parietal lobe. It is bounded externally by the granular retrolimbic area, BA 29. It is an area of the association cortex in the transitional region between the posterior cingulate gyrus and the medial temporal lobe; this area is a cortical component of the limbic system.

It has been suggested that in post-traumatic stress disorder (PTSD), triggering traumatic memories may reduce blood flow in this area (as reflected in PET scan data). It is assumed that this represents a decrease in the activation of BA 26. This may correspond to an increase in activity in the motor cortex and represent readying for motor action in response to the stressful stimuli (posted in *Brain* by Dr Justin Marley on April 10, 2012).

BA 29

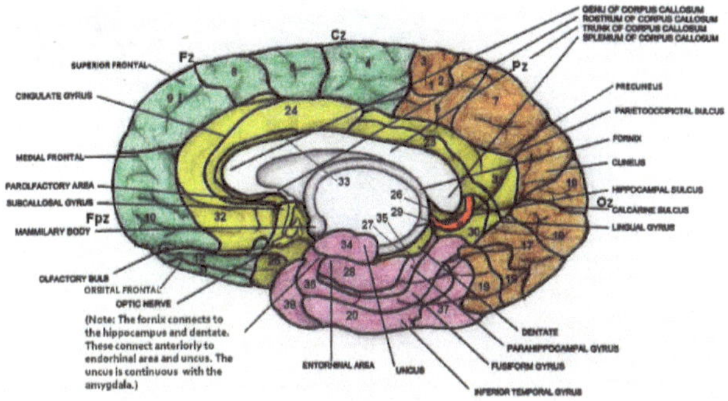

Brodmann area 29 is a medial area of the cortex that may include functions that also relate to the posterior cingulate and the posterior medial aspect of the temporal lobe. It is a part of the **paralimbic cortex**. It may be involved in **semantic associations** (not conscious) and novelty, but its functions are not as well researched as other areas. It lies between the posterior cingulate and the hippocampal area and we posit that it may be an important link between the integration and synthesis of new information in the posterior cingulate area and memory.

BA 30

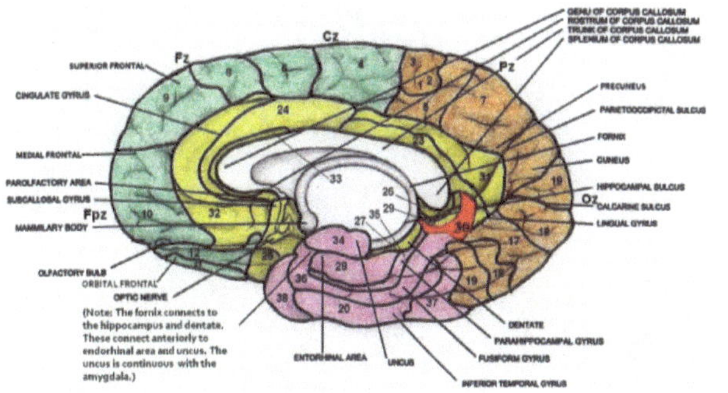

Brodmann area 30 is in the retrosplenial region and is a part of the **cingulate cortex and cuneus**. It is a **transitional area** between the **posterior cingulate cortex and the temporal lobe.** The retrosplenial region includes **Brodmann area 26 and Brodmann area 29,** as well as **Brodmann area 30**. The retrosplenial cortex has dense reciprocal projections with both the anterior thalamic nuclei and the hippocampus. Thus it is likely that it has functions in the **Affect, Memory, and Default networks**. It has a role in attending to speech, listening to sentences and, in particular, to **emotional aspects of words**. It is part of the paralimbic cortex and has direct links to the anterior thalamus and other limbic areas, and thus is important in **mood regulation**. It is in an area that is one of the **central midline structures (CMS)** involved in the **Default** network, and thus has a role in appraisal of one's self (**insight**). All of these functions mean that we are alert to its possible dysfunction in people with Asperger's syndrome.

Parietal Lobes

Introduction

Brodmann areas under Pz that may be influenced by NFB at this site include: BA 7 somatosensory cortex and working memory, BA 31 Posterior Cingulate Gyrus, and BAs 23, 26 and 28, which are medial and can be seen in midsagittal section views of the cerebral hemispheres. Areas 26 and 28 might require LORETA neurofeedback training.

Anatomical Boundaries

The parietal lobe is defined by four anatomical boundaries: the central sulcus (Rolandic fissure) separates the parietal lobe from the frontal lobe; the parieto-occipital sulcus separates the parietal and occipital lobes; the lateral sulcus (Sylvian fissure) is the most lateral boundary separating the parietal lobe from the temporal lobe; and the medial longitudinal fissure divides the two hemispheres, and thus the two halves of the parietal cortex.

Immediately posterior to the central sulcus, the most anterior part of the parietal lobe is the postcentral gyrus (Brodmann area 3), the secondary somatosensory cortical area. Separating this from the posterior parietal cortex is the postcentral sulcus, which can be seen just posterior to the central sulcus in the figure from *Gray's Anatomy*.

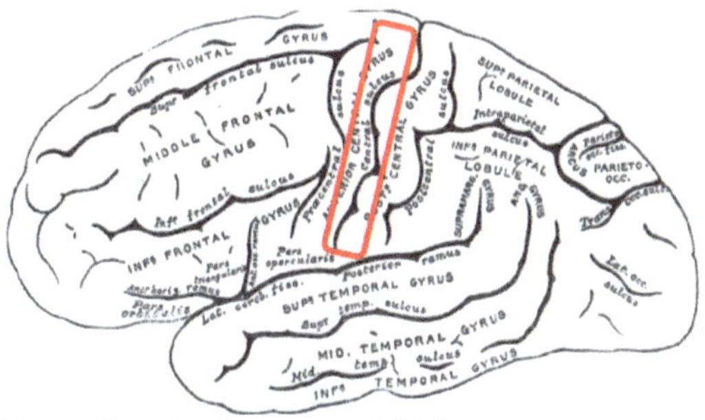

From Gray's Anatomy, 1918.
This drawing shows the Central Sulcus

From Gray's Anatomy *(1918). This drawing shows the Central Sulcus.*

Functions

The parietal lobe plays an important role in **integrating sensory information** from exterior sensory inputs and from various parts of the body. It is important in the **knowledge of numbers** and in seeing relationships between numbers. Particularly on the **NDH right side**, it perceives the **manipulation of objects in space.** Portions of the parietal lobe are involved with visuospatial processing. The parietal association cortex contains areas responsible for **perception of space**, and for localization of **self in relation to objects in space**. These areas can encode the location of objects. Although multisensory in nature, the posterior parietal cortex is referred to as the **dorsal stream for vision** (as opposed to the ventral stream in the temporal lobe). This dorsal stream has been called both the **'where'** stream (as in spatial vision) and the **'how'** stream (as in vision for action). The ventral intraparietal (VIP) area receives input from a number of senses (visual, somatosensory, auditory, and vestibular).

The **medial intraparietal (MIP)** area neurons are part of the central midline structures (CMSs) and dorsally may be more involved in the integration and synthesis of incoming sensory information and in communicating this information to the temporal and frontal cortices.

The **anterior intraparietal** (AIP) area contains neurons responsive to **shape, size and orientation** of objects to be grasped, as well as for manipulation of the hands. It responds both to viewed and remembered stimuli. It has the necessary connections to the frontal lobes and the frontal eye fields so that **goal-related activity can be 'remapped'** when the eyes move. It is also claimed that both the left and right parietal neural systems play a role in self-transcendence, a personality trait that may measure predisposition to spirituality.

The parietal lobe is divided into two hemispheres – left and right. The **left hemisphere** plays a more prominent role for right-handers and is involved in symbolic functions in **language and mathematics**. The **right parietal** lobe plays a more prominent role for true left-handers, and is specialized for images and for the understanding of **maps**. These are functions that require the perception and retention of **spatial relationships**. The parietal association cortex enables individuals to **read, write, and solve mathematical** problems. The sensory inputs from the right side go to the left side of the parietal lobe and vice versa.

Damage to the right parietal lobe can result in the loss of imagery and the ability to visualize spatial relationships. This was one of the problems of the 44-year-old woman who had encephalitis as a young woman in the example given earlier. Extensive damage will result in a neglect of the left side of space and the left side of the body. The person will be unaware of this loss and this is called **anosognosia**. Representing the left side may even be neglected when drawing. A novel treatment for this disorder is to use mirrors to fool the person into thinking that their left is their right so that they will move their left limb.

Damage to the **left parietal** lobe will result in different problems that include problems in mathematics, reading, writing, and understanding symbols. Damage to the left side of the parietal lobe, however, will not result in neglect of the right side of space and body.

Cortical Information Flow

There is considerable evidence that a person's cortex is essentially divided into two functional streams: an occipital-parietal-frontal pathway that processes 'where' information, and an occipital-temporal-frontal pathway that provides the 'what' information to the individual (Ungerleider and Mishkin, 1982, reported in Kim & Robertson, 2001).

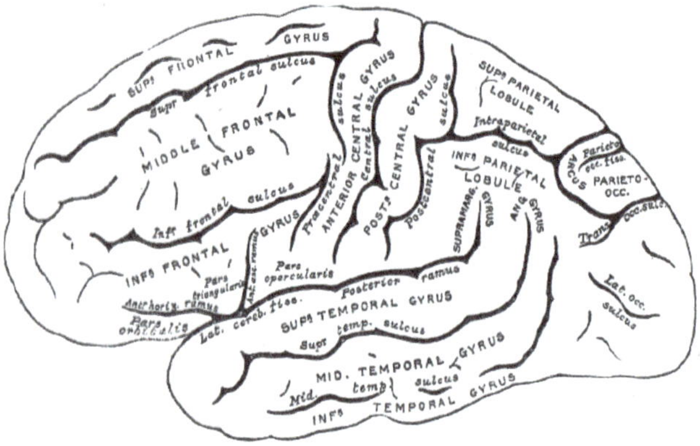

Gray's Anatomy *(1918)*

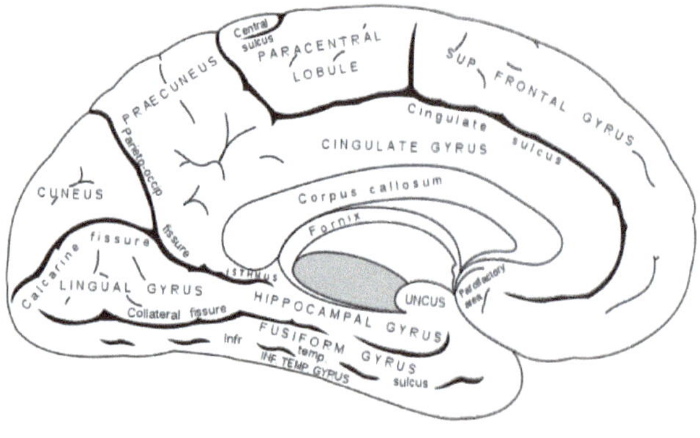

Gray's Anatomy *(1918), midsagittal section*

Parietal Lobes, Dorsal Lateral Aspect

BA 7; BA 7:
Pz:
Somatosensory Association Cortex

BA 7

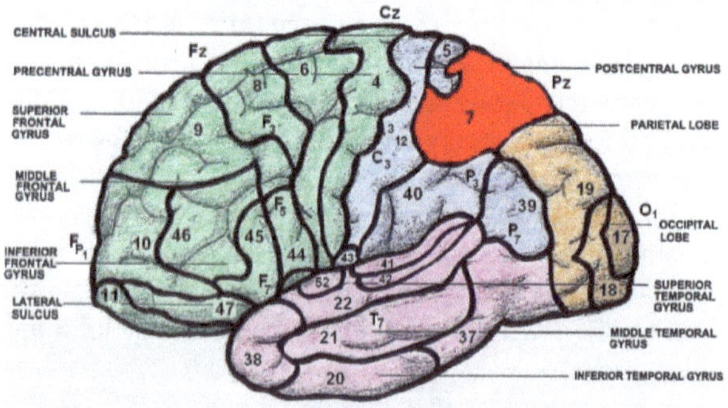

BA 7

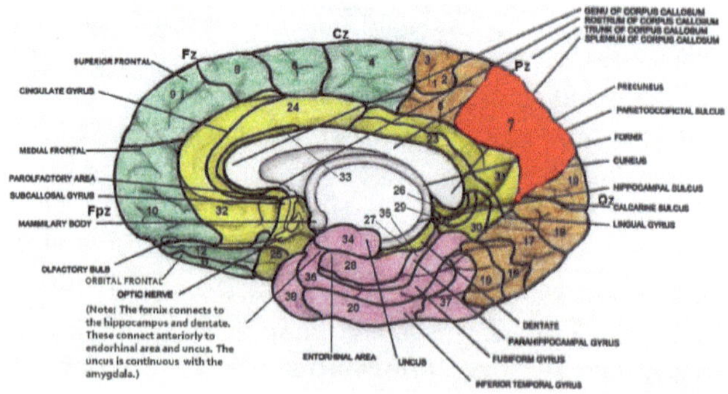

Dorsal and Lateral Aspects of BA 7

This somatosensory association cortex is one key area in the **Default** network, and it has motor, memory, attention, and cognitive and emotional understanding functions. It is involved in the perception of pain. In the **nondominant hemisphere** it is important in the **conscious awareness of visuospatial** events and in **understanding emotions**. It is important in **working memory** and comprehension. It is involved in visuomotor coordination (reaching to grasp an object) and bimanual manipulation.

In the **dominant** (left hemisphere) this area includes various networks that are involved in such functions as: **verbal comprehension**, episode recall, hand-writing and spelling, language, imaging, shifting attention, and the use of tools.

In the **nondominant** (right hemisphere) this area participates in understanding emotions, gestures, nuance, and innuendo. It is critical to **visual-spatial comprehension** including attention, mental rotation, stereopsis, and judgments or estimates that involve visual and spatial aspects of drawings and of the environment. This area is also part of the networks that are involved in a perception of personal space. It is important in visuospatial memory.

In both hemispheres, the **superior** parietal lobe is involved in rhythm detection, semantic categorization, temporal context recognition, and tactile localization, while the **inferior** parietal lobe is involved more in tactile recognition. In both hemispheres mirroring functions are present, which are important in learning manipulation of objects and tools. **Lesions** may result in **ideomotor apraxia** (inability to perform skilled purposeful movements unrelated to weakness, paralysis, lack of coordination or sensory loss). Lesions can result in **astereognosis**. This is a form of tactile agnosia where the subject is unable to identify common objects by feeling them if there is a barrier that prevents them from seeing the object. As with so many areas of the brain already discussed, it is one part of the working memory networks for motor, verbal, visual, auditory, and even emotional functions and is involved in the **conscious recollection of previous experiences**. It is also part of the networks (that include the anterior cingulate cortex) for the perception of **pain**.

Important for all of our work with NFB, this area in the nondominant hemisphere, in conjunction with frontal areas, is involved in a **sustained attention network,** particularly with respect to **visual-motor attention.**

Syndromes Associated with Parietal Lobe Functions

The following syndromes are briefly described in this book for the sole purpose of helping the practitioner understand some of the functions that may be affected when NFB is carried out over parietal lobe sites. Many are very rare syndromes so it is not necessary to learn them, just note how the symptoms relate to a particular area of cortical damage.

BAs 40 and 39 DH: Gerstmann's Syndrome

Gerstmann's syndrome is associated with lesions in the dominant (usually left) parietal lobe. This syndrome is characterized by four primary symptoms:

- Dysgraphia/agraphia: deficiency in the ability to write
- Dyscalculia/acalculia: difficulty in learning or comprehending mathematics
- Finger agnosia: inability to distinguish the fingers on the hand
- Left-right disorientation

The lesions causing one or more of these symptoms are attributable to dysfunction in the **angular and supramarginal gyri** near the temporal and parietal lobe junction. Such dysfunction may occur after a stroke or a TBI. In addition to exhibiting the above symptoms, many adults also experience **aphasia**, which is a difficulty in expressing oneself when speaking, and in understanding speech and written communications. Often both reading and writing are also affected.

In children the symptoms that have been associated with this syndrome may be developmental, but most cases are not identified until the child reaches school age and must learn to read and do math. As would be expected, these children exhibit poor handwriting and spelling skills, and difficulty with math functions, including adding, subtracting, multiplying, and dividing. They have an inability to differentiate right from left. They may even have difficulty discriminating among individual fingers. In addition to the four symptoms listed that are part of this syndrome, many children also suffer from constructional apraxia, an inability to copy simple drawings. Frequently, there is also an impairment in reading. Children with a high level of intellectual functioning, as well as those with brain damage, may be affected with the symptoms associated with this syndrome.

BA 7, Lateral Aspect

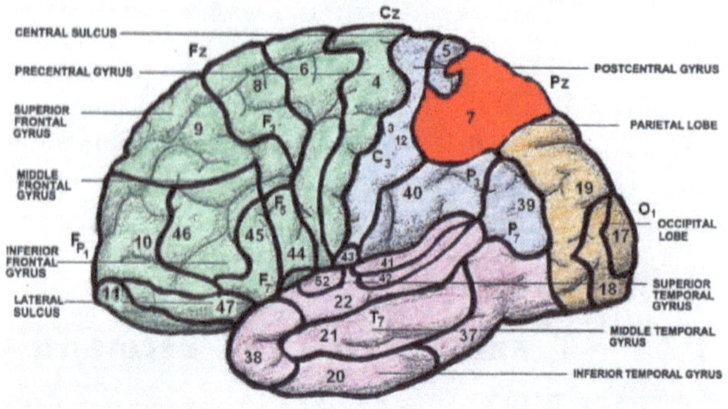

Bálint's Syndrome

Bálint's syndrome was named in 1909 for the Austro-Hungarian neurologist Rezső Bálint. It is associated with bilateral parietal – occipital lesions (Ropper, Allan, Brown, Robert, 2005). People who suffer from this syndrome have an inability to perceive the visual field as a whole (**simultanagnosia**), difficulty in fixating the eyes (**ocular apraxia**), and inability to move the hand to a specific object by using vision (**optic ataxia**). Optic ataxia is associated with difficulties reaching toward objects in the visual field opposite to the side of the parietal damage.

Since simultanagnosia is the inability to perceive simultaneous events or objects in one's visual field, people with Bálint's syndrome perceive the world erratically, as a series of single objects, rather than seeing the wholeness or Gestalt of a scene. It is a specific deficit of attention. Recovery in simultanagnosia may be related to finding meaning to the total scene and thus expanding their very restricted attentional window. Simultanagnosia is a profound visual deficit. It impairs the ability to perceive multiple items in a visual display, while **preserving the ability to recognize single** objects. It may be difficult for the person to disengage from an object once it has been selected and move to other objects or to retain a sense of that first object while viewing a second object. The patient sees their world in a patchy, spotty manner.

Ocular apraxia is exemplified by the inability to carry out familiar movements when asked to do so. As previously described, persons with apraxia understand commands and are willing to carry them out; however, they are physically unable to perform the task. In optic apraxia there is an inability to voluntarily guide eye movements and change to a new location of visual fixation. The most frequent and disabling deficit is the symptom of unilateral spatial neglect. This neglect manifests as a bias of spatial representation and attention on the same side as the lesion, while ignoring the opposite side. This was described above under dysfunction of the right parietal lobe. In addition, there are disturbances of space representation after traumatic damage to the right hemisphere's parietal lobe.

Optic ataxia is the inability to guide the hand toward an object using visual information where the inability cannot be explained by motor, somatosensory, visual field deficits, or acuity deficits. Optic ataxia is seen in Bálint's syndrome, where it is characterized by an impaired visual control of the direction of arm-reaching to a visual target, accompanied by defective hand orientation and grip formation. It is considered a specific visuomotor disorder, independent of visual space misperception. Optic ataxia is also known as misreaching or dysmetria and it refers to a lack of coordination of movement, typified by undershoot or overshoot of intended position with the hand, arm, leg, or eye. It is sometimes described as an **inability to judge distance** or scale. Bálint described a patient who, while cutting a slice of meat that he held with a fork in his left hand, would search for it outside the plate with the knife in his right hand. The ability to grasp an object is also impaired.

Anatomical Lesions Causing Symptoms in Bálint's Syndrome

The visual difficulties in Bálint's syndrome are usually due to damage to the top part of the temporal-occipital lobes on both sides of the brain. The temporal-occipital area refers to the lateral and posterior portions of the brain. In Bálint's syndrome, the superior or dorsal part of the parietal lobes on both sides of the brain may also be affected. The parietal lobes are the middle portion of the dorsal aspect of the brain. There is usually bilateral damage to the posterior parietal cortex. The damage and the syndrome can originate from single or multiple strokes, Alzheimer's disease, intracranial tumor, or brain injury; in short, anything causing damage to the posterior superior areas of the parietal lobe (BA 7).

Parietal Lobes, Medial Dorsal Aspect

BA 7
Pz:

BA 7: Cuneus, Precuneus

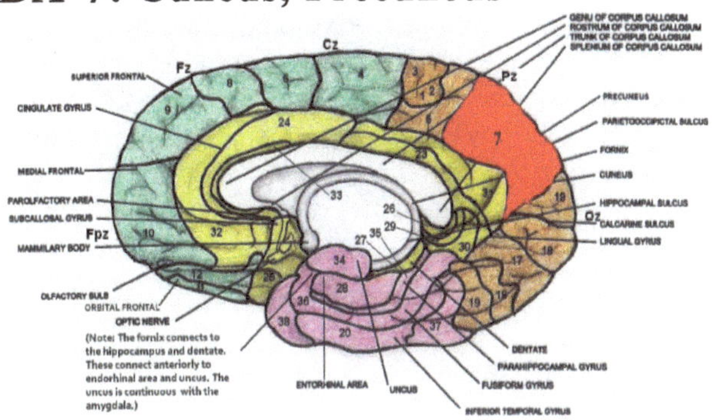

The medial superior areas of the parietal lobe are called the cuneus and precuneus. These areas are responsible for the **organization, integration, and synthesis** of auditory, visual and kinesthetic inputs and for orientation in space. They are some of the last areas to become myelinated. It is important in high-level functions including attention, self-referential and self-recognition tasks, theory of mind, working memory, and many other cognitive processes. The **precuneus** has a role in visual-spatial imagery, episodic memory retrieval, and taking a perspective on 'self.' These posterior medial areas have a very high metabolic rate. There is a decrease in this Default mode activity during non-self-referential, goal-directed tasks. Thus a patient might not feel anxiety when they are absorbed in a cognitive task.

These areas have extensive connections to other medial and lateral parietal areas, the superior temporal cortices, both the medial and dorsolateral frontal cortices, the orbital surfaces of the frontal lobes, and the anterior cingulate (Cavanna, 2006). In other words, they are an important part of the Default network.

BA 5 (Previously discussed in 'Central Region)

The posterior portion of **BA 5** is important in the perception of tactile objects, the body, and in orienting in extrapersonal space. As previously mentioned, damage to these areas may contribute to agnosia and apraxia.

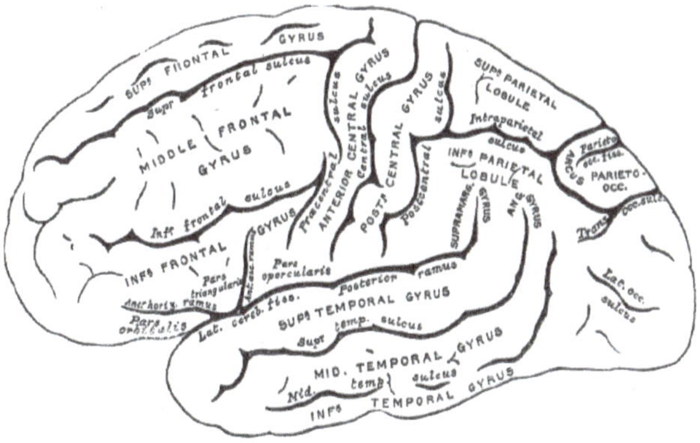

Gray's Anatomy *(1918)*

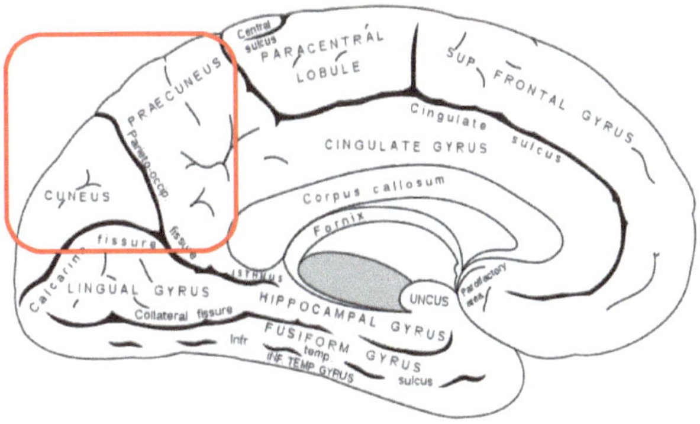

Gray's Anatomy *(1918), midsagittal section to view medial aspects of parietal lobe*

The precuneus, cuneus, and the posterior cingulate may be more active at rest and activation will be attenuated during a motor or cognitive task. These areas subserve core consciousness and represent **self in relationship to the world**. They are involved in monitoring the outside world and are important for psychologically assessing and evaluating 'self-in-the-world.' This is a form of visual and emotional response analysis and involves making decisions about another person as compared to oneself (Seger, Stone & Keenan, 2004). Perhaps importantly, it has direct connections to the inferior right parietal lobe (between P4 and T6/P8), which is part of the **right parietal to frontal Mirror Neuron** network for imitating. Such imitation involves interpreting innuendo and understanding the meaning of communications by others in order to be able to imitate others. Difficulties with all of these functions are observed in patients who have Asperger's or an autism spectrum disorder.

A seven-year-old autistic girl developed an apparent excess of high frequency beta in the P4 area during NFB training. This occurred at the same time as she improved in her social functions and became almost indistinguishable in her behavior from her bright, socially competent, non-autistic, twin sister. Even her mother immediately saw the correlation and said, "Don't train down that high beta. Everything is going so well!" This increase in activation at P4 appeared to represent a compensatory change. We use this case as one of our examples when we warn professionals to be careful when using z-score training and to not use one-size-fits-all protocols and normalize everything, but rather to carefully assess the patient before determining which frequencies and sites are appropriate for that individual's NFB training regimen.

The precuneus appears to be involved in self-related mental representations during rest—in other words, **self-consciousness**. In our assessments of patients who exhibit high levels of **anxiety**, we may note high amplitude of high-frequency beta in this posterior medial area. We also sometimes see spindling beta more than 2 SD above the database means between P4 and P8 (T6) in the general area of the right angular gyrus. We have postulated that this type of finding might correlate with the observed hyper-vigilant state in these patients and thus relate to their anxiety. This is observed in some **hypervigilant** patients who have **difficulties falling asleep** and going back to sleep when they awaken during the night.

Temporal-Parietal Junction, Lateral Aspect

(As it relates to learning, dominant hemisphere language comprehension, nondominant hemisphere prosody functions)

BAs 39, 40
T7-P3 x C3-P7;

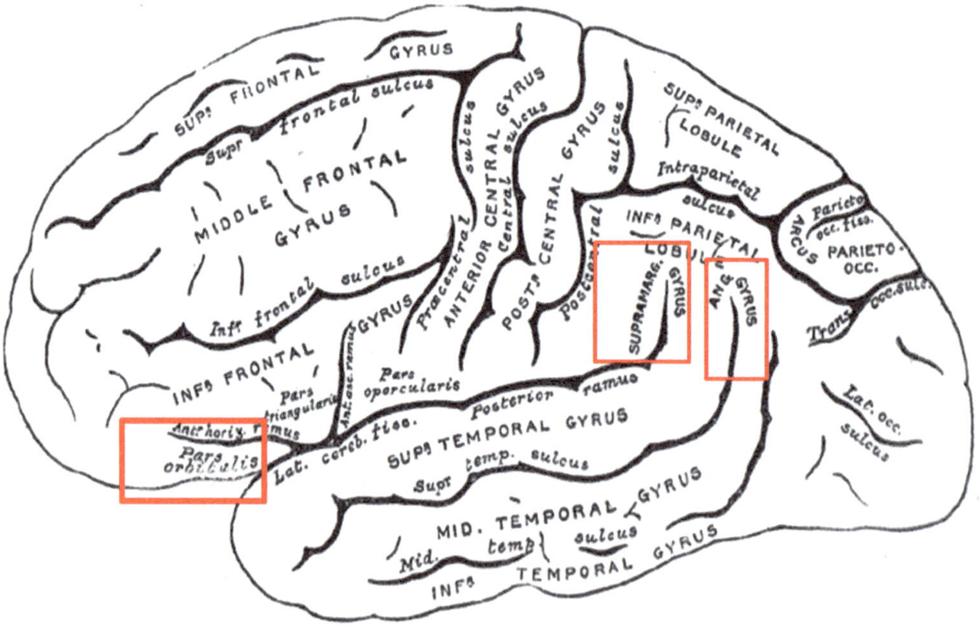

Figure to show the temporal-parietal junction. Adapted from Gray's Anatomy *to show the angular and supramarginal gyri. Also identified is the pars orbitalis*

Introduction

In the **dominant hemisphere** the temporal-parietal junction comprises Wernicke's area. This area encompasses part of BAs 39 and 40 in the supramarginal and angular gyrus areas, and extends inferior into the posterior superior aspect of the temporal lobe, taking a small posterior portion of BAs 41, 42 and 22. Functions of this area and the homologous area in the nondominant hemisphere differ. For the most part, dominant hemisphere, left-sided lesions interfere with verbal comprehension and memory processes, whereas **nondominant** (right-sided) lesions interfere with visuospatial (nonverbal) processes and the interpretation and comprehension of emotional aspects of language and gestures and nuance and innuendo in communications.

The left frontal operculum area (F5, or Broca's area) is the key area for speech articulation. However, the temporal lobe (BAs 21 and 22) and the supramarginal gyrus, angular gyrus, and insula are involved in auditory and verbal representation. These areas (see figure below) and their connections, such as via the **arcuate fasciculus**, are all involved in **letter and word perception and recognition.** These areas with their connections to the frontal lobe have been described in other sections of this monograph. They are important in the **comprehension** of abstract verbal forms, object naming, word recall (involving the hippocampus for auditory information on the left and visual information on the right), and perception of complex verbal relationships.

Patients with frontal lobe lesions have difficulty in the temporal organization of information, such as lists of words. A name can pass through Wernicke's area and then, via the angular gyrus, arouse associations in other areas of the cortex. In this manner the **angular gyrus is a connecting link** between sensory input and speech production areas. It is an important association cortex that **combines auditory and visual** information that are both necessary for reading and writing. It is involved in the steps between reading and speaking. Damage to the angular gyrus can result in **alexia** (inability to read) with **agraphia** (inability to write). The patient is unable to match spoken letter sounds to written letters. They can only spell the very simplest words.

Right hemisphere lesions in the parietal-temporal-occipital cortex can result in an inability to understand temporal relationships (future planning), visual-spatial defects, and problems in retaining a visual image. A study directed at investigating the neuroanatomical correlates of difficulties with the clock drawing test (CDT), which is usually considered to be a parietal lobe test, indicated that impaired performance on the CDT most strongly correlated with damage to right parietal cortices (supramarginal gyrus) and to left inferior frontal-parietal opercular cortices. In the CDT, the person is asked to draw a clock and to set the time to twenty minutes 'til four. Time setting errors were predominant in people with left hemisphere lesions, perhaps because of the interpretation of language involved in the setting of the hands to "twenty minutes 'til four." Visual spatial errors predominated in patients with right hemisphere damage; for example, leaving out numbers from the left side of the clock or bunching up all the numbers on the right side (Tranel, Rudrauf, Vianna & Damasio, 2008).

Left hemisphere lesions in these general areas result in **aphasia**, inability to evoke a visual image in response to a word, inability to organize sequentially, and the inability to draw proper angles and copy designs.

Introduction to Lateral Aspect, Dominant Lobe, Temporal-Parietal Junction, Approximately at the Center of an 'X' drawn between T7-P3 and C3-P7

Wernicke's Area

At approximately the center of an 'X' drawn between T7-P3 and C3-P7 is a site that lies roughly over the angular gyrus and the supramarginal gyrus, which is usually referred to as Wernicke's area. Carl Wernicke (1848 – 1905) was a German psychiatrist and anatomist who identified this area as being related to language comprehension.

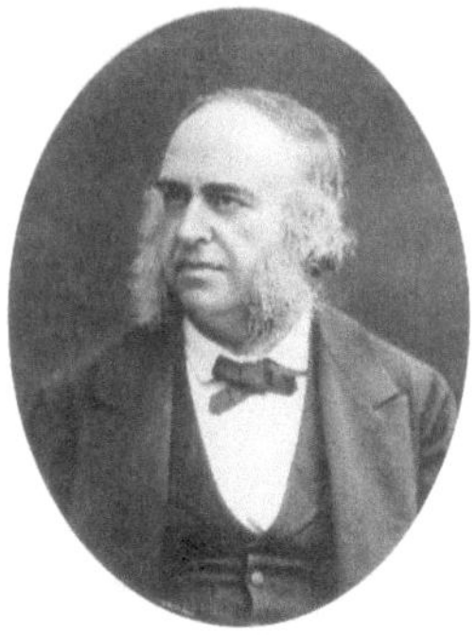

Carl Wernicke (1848 – 1905)

Wernicke's area lies mainly in the posterior, superior temporal gyrus, and spans the region between temporal and parietal lobes. It plays a key role (in tandem with Broca's area in the frontal lobe) in language. Both Wernicke's aphasia and Broca's aphasia have been described elsewhere in this text and, for ease of reading, a portion of this is copied below. The functions of the left temporal lobe are not limited to simple perception of what one hears but extend to comprehension, naming, verbal memory, and other language functions.

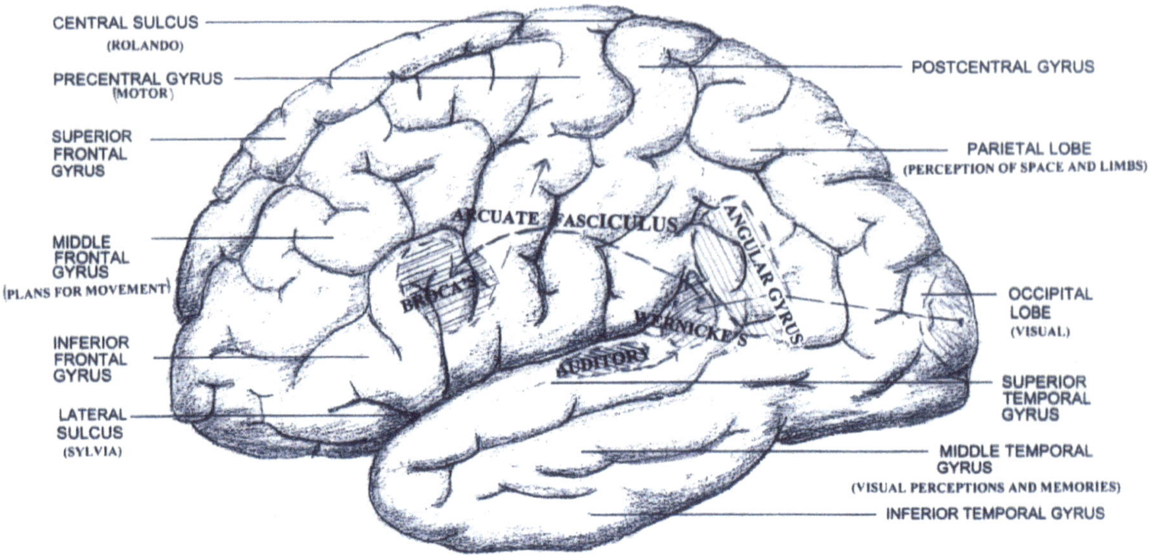

Lateral View of the Left Cerebral Hemisphere to show Broca's and Wernicke's Areas *(Amanda Reeves after Smith, 1962; Carlson, 1986). The left frontal operculum area (F5, or Broca's area; BAs 44 and 45), is the key area for speech articulation. However, the temporal lobe (BAs 21 and 22) and the supramarginal gyrus, angular gyrus, and insula are involved in auditory and verbal representation. These areas and their connections, such as via the* ***arcuate fasciculus*** *between Wernicke's and Broca's areas, are all involved in* ***letter and word perception and recognition.*** *These areas with their connections to the frontal lobe are important in the* ***comprehension*** *of abstract verbal forms, object naming, word recall (involving the hippocampus for auditory information on the left and visual information on the right), and perception of complex verbal relationships. The proximity of Wernicke's area to the auditory cortex is important for all of these functions.*

Wernicke's area is known to be important for **understanding** speech. Understanding involves the inferior parietal lobe and the auditory association area of the superior temporal gyrus. If there is damage to this area, speech will still be fluent and grammar will be good, but the person will **speak nonsense.** They speak a kind of jargon in which (without understanding what they are saying) they substitute inappropriate words or the wrong words to the extent that they are unable to understand their own speech. These people have similar difficulties with understanding when reading and expressing themselves when writing.

A **lesion near Wernicke's** area in the posterior section of the left temporal lobe leaves the individual with an inability to analyze word meanings.

Damage to the **connections between the auditory cortex** and **Wernicke's area results in** the person being able to hear sounds but they are **word deaf.** They cannot understand the meaning of spoken words, yet they are able to read, write, and speak normally.

Damage to **connections between Wernicke's** and **Broca's** areas leave the individual unable to repeat what is said to them if it is more complex than a single word or phrase, particularly if the sounds are unfamiliar. That is, unless the words have meaning that can be recognized in some other way.

Communication between Wernicke's and Broca's areas involves the superior longitudinal fasciculus and a portion of it called the arcuate fasciculus, a band of very long association fibers running anterior to posterior in each cerebral hemisphere. These fibers run from the frontal lobe through the parietal lobe above and below the insula and around the end of the lateral sulcus. It has branches to the temporal lobe, and branches that run all the way posterior to the occipital lobe. Clearly, in the left hemisphere, this communication link is essential for speech. There are two pathways, direct and indirect, between

Wernicke's and Broca's areas (Catani & Jones, 2005). Damage to the direct pathway may produce conduction aphasia, whereas damage to the indirect pathway spares the ability to repeat speech but impairs comprehension. The symptoms of conduction aphasia suggest that the connection between posterior temporal cortex and frontal cortex plays a vital role in short-term memory of words and speech sounds that are new or have just been heard. The arcuate fasciculus connects these two regions and circulates information back and forth, possibly contributing to short-term memory.

In the majority of people with tone deafness, the superior arcuate fasciculus in the right hemisphere is not functioning properly. This suggests a disconnection between the posterior superior temporal gyrus and the posterior inferior frontal gyrus. The posterior superior temporal gyrus may be the origin of the disorder.

Comprehension in these individuals can be improved if they can visualize what is being talked about. They are not, however, able to repeat even a short series of unrelated words. They may, on the other hand, understand what is said, be able to speak well, and intelligently answer a question.

In contrast, in some individuals, the opposite problem can occur. An overactive connection between **Wernicke's** and **Broca's** areas may result in the involuntary repeating of words or phrases (**echolalia**).

Broca's Area (BAs 44, 45)

As previously described in the frontal lobe section, damage to **Broca's area** interferes with the individual's ability to instruct the motor cortex and results in defects in the articulation of speech. Damage to Broca's area and its **association areas** may result in a condition where the person is able to understand what has been said to him and be conscious of what he wants to say, but not be able to say it. This person may substitute staccato nouns and verbs so that the flow of his speech is lost and it sounds like a telegram without connecting words such as 'if,' 'and,' or 'but.' Ungrammatical speech and writing errors may be observed. In some instances these persons may also fail to understand spoken or written grammar. There is difficulty with prepositions. Broca's aphasia is usually accompanied by motor symptoms with right hemiparesis and right central facial paresis.

Damage to the **connections to speech areas** from their **surrounding cortex** may result in the person being unable to **understand speech.** However, they can repeat words or finish well-known phrases (e.g., "roses are red...").

BA 39: Angular Gyrus, Introduction

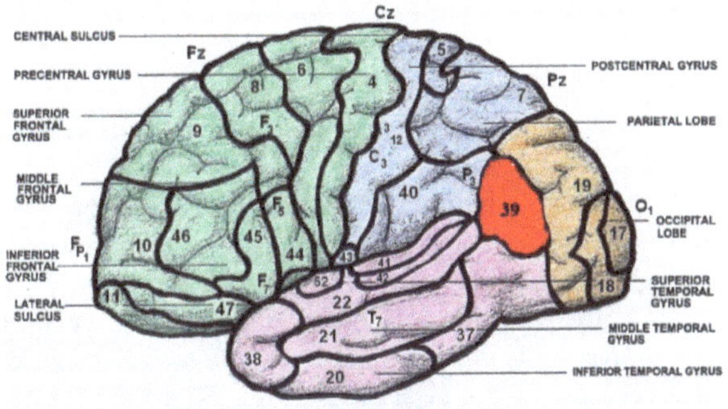

Brodmann area 39 is the region of the parietal lobe that sits at the occipital-parietal-temporal junction behind (posterior to) the lateral fissure. It is immediately posterior to the supramarginal gyrus. It involves visual-spatial-language skills and therefore **visual word recognition.** The left hemisphere angular gyrus is required for reading. Damage to this area can result in **alexia** (inability to read) and in **agraphia** (inability to write). It is important in the dominant hemisphere for generating sentences and verbal creativity. It is involved in networks for higher executive functions such as inferential reasoning. It is necessary for arithmetic calculations and numerical facts. (Note that BA 44 is also important for doing arithmetic.)

Learning Difficulties

Dysfunction of this area can result in a number of other learning difficulties, too. These may include difficulties with calculations (also intraparietal sulcus area), **left-right discrimination,** and technical competence. These persons may show symptoms of **agraphia** including reversing letters, reversing order of letters, crossing lines and difficulties copying material. They may also have **apraxia** (inability to execute a learned movement on demand) and dysphasia, including difficulties with meanings of words (a type of **semantic aphasia**), labeling objects, or interpretation of pictures such as cartoons. Identification of shape, size, and texture may be difficult. In more general terms, some individuals may not have major deficits but merely be clumsy, have a poor sense of direction, poor ability to draw, and they may be poor at spelling. All of these learning problems, though frequently said to stem from the dominant hemisphere, may also involve the nondominant hemisphere. Damage in this area and also in BA 40 is related to **Gerstmann's syndrome,** a condition that was originally described as including problems in four areas: writing (agraphia or dysgraphia), math calculations (dyscalculia), recognizing fingers (finger agnosia), and left-right discrimination. However, more often patients will exhibit only one or two or three but not all four of these symptoms. (For more details see: Mayer, Martory, Pegna, Landis, Delavelle & Annoni, 1999).

Of interest with respect to the autism spectrum disorders, this area is important for functions related to **Theory of Mind,** that is, the ability to theorize about what is in another person's mind and appreciate their point of view. Its functions also include spatial focusing, **action sequences**, and situational context. **Action authorship** – one's judgment concerning whether an action was done by them or by someone else – is also a function of this area. Sight reading of music is another function (particularly in the non-dominant hemisphere). It is even involved in reflective self-awareness and seeing things differently from others, which may be functions of the Default network.

When there is a **disconnect between the left angular gyrus and the left visual cortex**, words cannot be recognized in the normal fashion. However, an intact right visual cortex can still recognize letters and convey that information via the corpus callosum to the left hemisphere speech and language areas. The letters may, therefore, be named. As the patient says the sequence of letters out loud the word can be recognized through the auditory input from his/her own voice. Subvocalizing can also work. Although the individual cannot read silently, he may be able to read slowly out loud and understand what he is reading. He can also write sentences or copy words from a page.

BA 40: Supramarginal Gyrus, Introduction

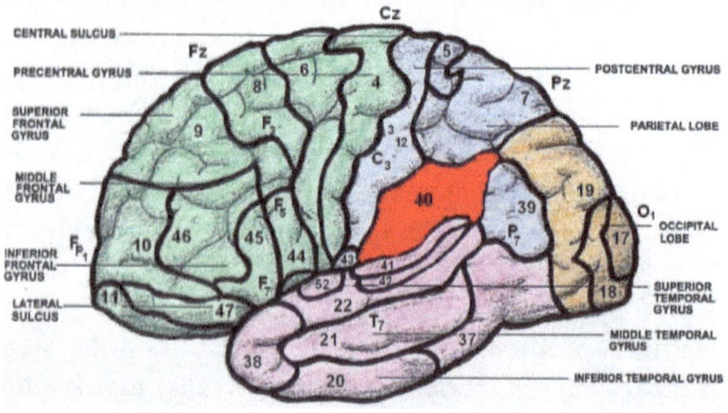

Brodmann area 40 is in the inferior parietal lobe and contains the supramarginal gyrus. In the **dominant** hemisphere it is important in attending to phonemes, verbal creativity, formation of sentences, categorization, and semantic processing. It is crucial for arithmetic calculations with integers. The left (dominant hemisphere) supramarginal gyrus is a general nodal point for **short-term auditory working memory** that is involved in both **music and linguistic** processing. It is important for the short-term memory of linguistic phonology and short-term pitch memory. It is an area that links kinesthetic memories with auditory commands. It may be part of networks for the conscious recollection of previously experienced events.

In **both hemispheres** this area is important in **deductive reasoning** and the ability to sustain attention. These areas are also important in other cognitive activities, such as distinguishing same and different, conflict detection, and for emotional working memory.

Lesions can result in so-called **ideomotor apraxia**, associated with deficits in the ability to plan or complete motor actions that rely on semantic memory. The patient can perform an action automatically, such as tying shoelaces, but the action cannot be performed on request. When there are lesions in BA 40 in the **dominant** hemisphere, the patient will exhibit errors in writing, spelling, word choice, and syntax. Right–left disorientation is common, as is **acalculia** (difficulty with simple arithmetic including addition, subtraction, multiplication and division).

Nondominant Supramarginal Gyrus

In the nondominant hemisphere, the supramarginal gyrus is important for visual grasping, **gesture** imitation, visual-motor planning, **music** performance, and in empathy. Deficits can result in **constructional apraxia,** which involves such problems as an inability to copy designs, difficulty with block construction tasks, inability to locate places on a map.

Mainly in the **nondominant** hemisphere, BA 40 is also important for imitation of movements and same or different discrimination. **Astereognosis** may occur. In this disorder, the patient cannot identify common objects by touch. In the nondominant hemisphere, the supramarginal gyrus is one of the areas near the temporal-parietal junction involved in prosody, which refers to **speech intonation, rhythm**, and emphasis. Thus dysfunction can result in **sensory aprosodia,** which involves difficulties with understanding the emotional content in communication, that is, reading tone of voice, **nuance**, and innuendo, as well as reading body language. Impairments in empathy and understanding the intentions of others may also be observed.

Lateral Aspect, Nondominant Lobe Temporal-Parietal Junction; Approximately at the Center of an 'X' Drawn Between T8-P4 and C4-P8

This is a site that lies approximately over the angular gyrus and the supramarginal gyrus in the non-dominant hemisphere. In most people this is near the temporal-parietal junction in the right hemisphere over **BAs 40, 39 and 22.** It is the homologous site to Wernicke's area in the dominant hemisphere. The functions of this area were noted above under BA 39 and 40. They include: **spatial-emotional-contextual** perception, symbol recognition, ability to understand emotional tones, and the comprehension of **innuendo**, nuance, and the emotional aspects of both gesture and verbal communications (Ross, 1981). It can also be important in nonverbal memory. Low activity in this area, as indicated by high amplitude slow waves (theta or alpha), in our experience, is often seen in patients who have Asperger's syndrome. The same symptoms of sensory aprosodia can be present after a stroke affecting this area, as reported by Ross (1981).

Parietal Lobes – Lateral and Inferior

P3 and P4; P7 and P8; BAs 40, 39, 37

BA 40

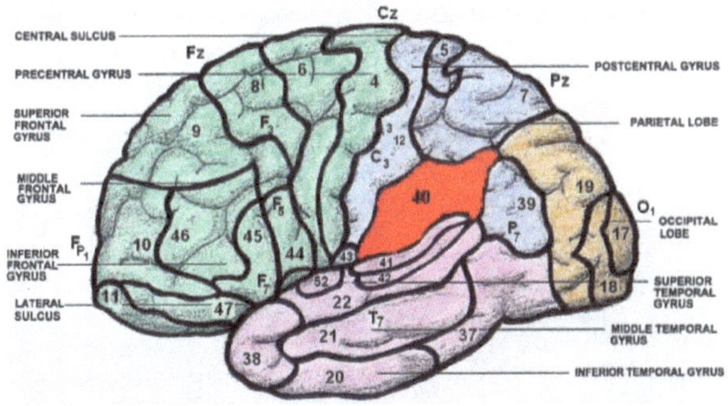

Brodmann area 40 is part of the parietal cortex in the human brain. The functions of the supramarginal gyrus and the angular gyrus as they are involved in language comprehension and learning were covered above in the temporal – parietal junction discussion ,of Wernicke's area. This will not be repeated here. The **inferior part of BA 40** is in the area of the supramarginal gyrus, which lies at the posterior end of the lateral fissure, in the inferior lateral part of the parietal lobe. This location may underlie its involvement in the **integration of tactile and proprioceptive** information and in somatosensory spatial discrimination. **Same and different** differentiation involves this area in conjunction with the ACC and the prefrontal cortex. It is part of the networks for memory.

The **supramarginal gyrus** part of Brodmann area 40 is the region in the inferior parietal lobe that is involved in reading, both in regards to meaning and phonology. It is important in the network for **deductive** reasoning, as was previously discussed. It has **mirror neuron** functions. In the nondominant hemisphere in particular, it is involved in visual-motor activity including the imitation of gestures.

Dysfunction in this area can have effects on all of the learning functions described above under the angular gyrus. BA 40 lies just superior to Brodmann area 41 and the auditory cortex and lesions in this region of the temporal lobe may affect auditory comprehension as described above under the heading: Temporal Lobe and Frontal Lobe – A Functional Unit. This area is also important, particularly in the non-dominant hemisphere, in a network for sustained attention.

P4; BA 40 – Right Hemisphere

An electrode placed over or near P4 may influence activity emanating from BA 40 and also other Brodmann areas including: 3, 1, 2, 5, 23, 13 and 30. In general terms, the functions of these areas include spatial position, visualization of spatial organization, context, left-side body awareness. As previously mentioned, damage to this area results in anosognosia for left body and space. These and other functions are described above under the nondominant parietal lobe functions.

When this area is overactive, which may correlate with increased beta activity, it may relate to the person being hypervigilant with a **'busy brain.'** As previously mentioned, hyperactivity in this area may correlate with **hypervigilance** and can make it difficult for that individual to fall asleep. Some people may be anxious (even exhibit panic attacks) but at the same time be bright intellectually.

P3; BA 40 – Left Hemisphere

An electrode placed over or near P3 may influence activity emanating from BA 40 and also other Brodmann areas including: 3, 1, 2, 5, 23, 13 and 30. NFB at this site can influence activity in the supramarginal gyrus that may include cognitive reasoning, attention, spelling and verbal short-term memory, imagination (BAs 40, 24, 10). It may also influence activity in the angular gyrus (BA 39) and functions such as the recall of a series of numbers (digit span), with dysfunction resulting in a syndrome called acalculia. These and other functions have been described above under the dominant parietal lobe functions.

Note: Overactivity in the parietal lobe may be accompanied by **parietal spindling beta**. In the parietal region, however, this spindling beta may reflect sensory hypersensitivity or sensory defensiveness (auditory, visual, kinesthetic). It is important for the NFB practitioner to be aware of this because using NFB to decrease the spindling beta can be helpful for some patients.

The supra marginal gyrus and the angular gyrus are shown in the adjacent figure. One can see that they are approximately in Brodmann areas 40 and 39. They lie roughly at the center of an X with lines drawn between C3 - P7 and P3 - T7.

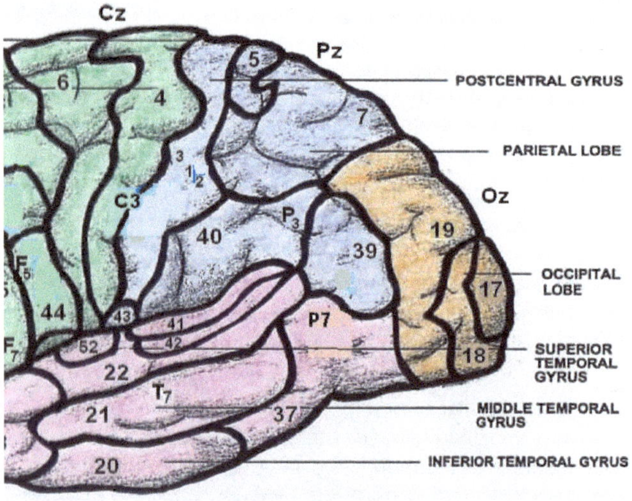

Note the supramarginal gyrus and, just posterior to it, the angular gyrus. They lie just posterior to the lateral cerebral fissure and above the posterior end of the superior temporal gyrus.

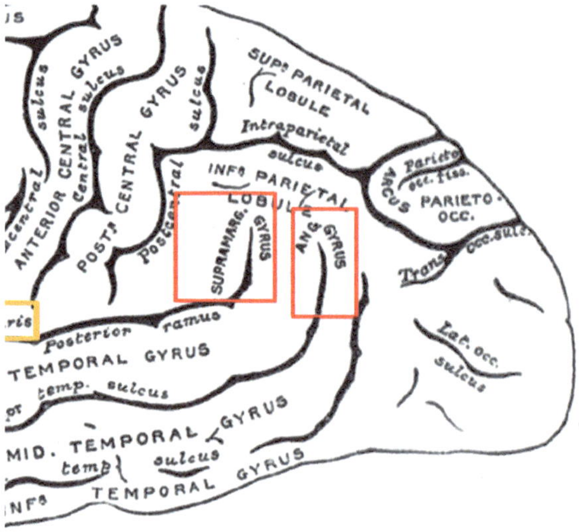

P7; BAs 39, 37

BA 37 (Described under Tempral Lobe)

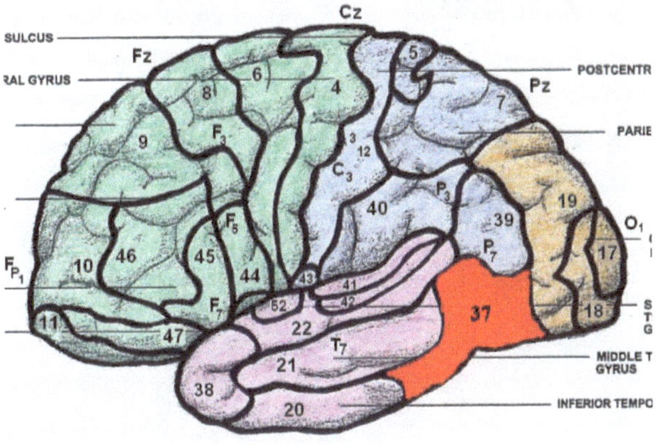

BA 39

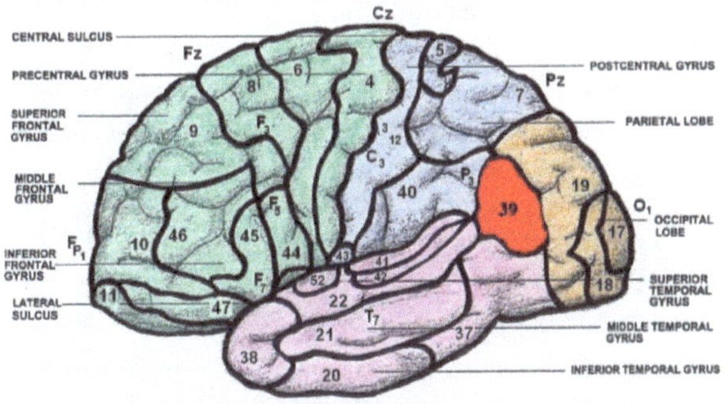

These areas functionally overlap with BA 40 and the posterior portion of BA 22. As described above, BAs 40 and 39 include the supramarginal gyrus and the angular gyrus. In the dominant hemisphere this would include the posterior portion of Wernicke's area and connections to temporal areas. **Sentence generation** and verbal creativity, in addition to right-side **body awareness,** are functions associated with BAs 39 and 37. BA 37 was previously discussed under the medial aspect of the temporal lobes.

Functions include **semantic categorization**, word retrieval, word generation, **face-name** association, attention to semantic relations and associating words with visual percepts. It is important in sign language. It is involved in reading and in making **orthography-phonology links**. Note that orthography refers to a standardized system for using a particular writing system (script) for a language. Children develop links between the sounds of speech (phonology) and how the language is written. BA 37 is involved in this process. It is also part of the networks for deductive reasoning as was described under the introduction to the frontal lobes. NFB carried out over P7 may also influence aspects of other Brodmann areas such as: BAs 40, 41, 42, 20, 30, 36, and possibly BA 21.

P8

In the **nondominant hemisphere, P8** lies over BAs 39 and the posterior superior portion of BA 37. BA 37 is important for drawing. Other functions of these areas include left-side body awareness and fear. As previously described, damage to this area results in **anosognosia** for the left side of the body and space. NFB carried out over P8 may also influence aspects of other Brodmann areas in addition to BA 39 and BA 37, such as BAs 40, 41, 42, 20, 30, 36, and possibly 21.

In the **dominant hemisphere, P7** lies over BAs 39 and the posterior superior portion of BA 37. Apart from reading, functions of these areas include calculations, verbal construction, and meaning. For many areas of the parietal lobes under both P3 and P4, P7 and P8, **focusing and refocusing attention** is another function. Attention, however, also involves large networks of activity that connect the occipital and parietal regions to central midline structures, as well as many areas in the temporal and frontal lobes. We postulate that one way to have appropriate effects on focusing, and concentrating aspects of attention, is to have the client use mental strategies and carry out specific tasks while doing the NFB training. In this manner we posit that the appropriate Attention networks will be activated and trained.

We did **not** show an area for attention in the networks, because, like memory, Attention networks involve such a large number of cortical areas. Frontal, central and parietal ares are all involved. **Focusing and refocusing attention** is one key to efficient cognitive functioning. For visual stimuli, the **frontal eye fields** (approximately between F3 and C3) connect to the superior colliculus in order to turn the eyes towards an object of interest. These areas are **reciprocally connected to the lateral inferior parietal** areas. Lateral inferior parietal (LIP) neuronal activity is necessary in order to disengage attention from a current stimulus in order for focus to change to a different stimulus. Related to this function, lateral intraparietal area (LIP) **salience mapping** is a function that is important in order to pay attention and to rank items in a visual field for locus of attention (Bisley et al., 2006). LIP areas connect to: frontal eye field (FEF), superior colliculus, pulvinar, inferior temporal BA 20 (visual pattern recognition). It determines the relative significance of incoming information, and transfers this salience data to other appropriate cortical areas. However, decisions as to how this salience information is used depend on the function and needs of areas that receive these projections from LIP and are not made in the parietal cortex.

Vestibular Connections to Inferior Parietal-Temporal BA 22, Posterior Insula

Symptoms of **nausea and vertigo** and even choking may be associated with inferior parietal lobe and BA 22 dysfunction. Nausea may also be associated with the posterior area of the insula. On the other hand, persons who suffer from Meniere's disease, a disorder of the inner ear, experience episodes of vertigo, nausea, vomiting, diminished hearing, and tinnitus and may demonstrate pathology in BA 25, 38, and 10. They may be treated with restriction of salt/caffeine/tobacco and may be prescribed diuretics, meclizine, and benzodiazepines (reference, Neurology on the web from the University of Kansas Medical Center).

Further posterior, the parieto-occipital cortex is important in **procedural memory**. This, again, is just an initial link in one aspect of the memory network systems that have been discussed under the cingulate gyrus, medial aspects of the temporal lobes, the Papez circuit, and the Executive areas of the frontal lobes.

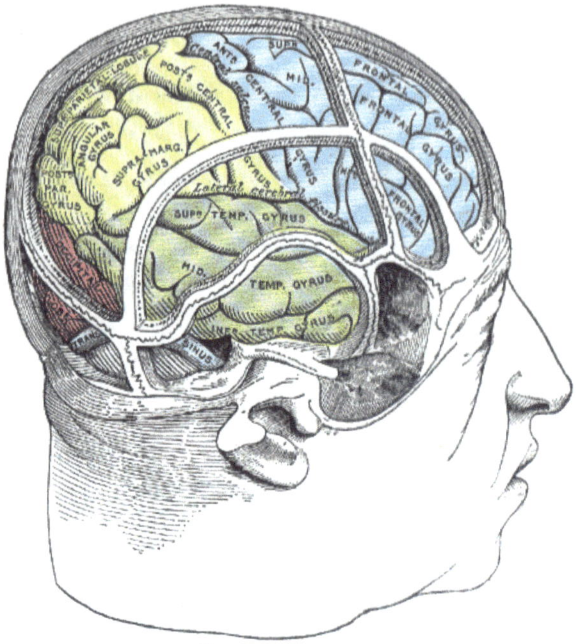

Gray's Anatomy 20th edition *(1918) (public domain)*

This figure from Gray's Anatomy *is included to assist the reader in visualizing the relationship of the angular gyrus and the supramarginal gyrus to the scalp. One can see that these areas would be in a region covered in part by P8 (T6) and P4 on the right and P7 (T5) and P3 on the left.*

Occipital Regions: O1, O2

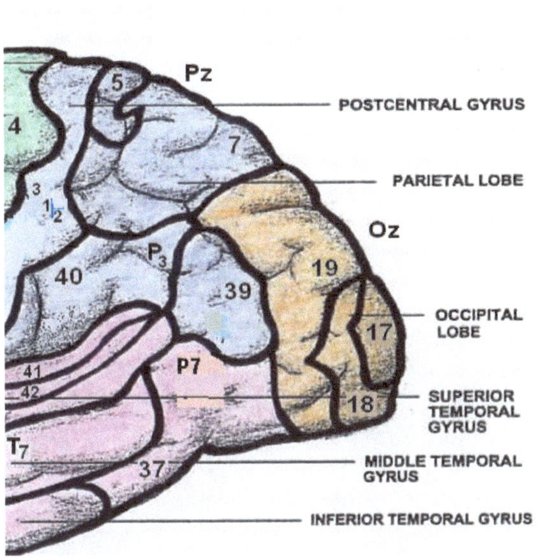

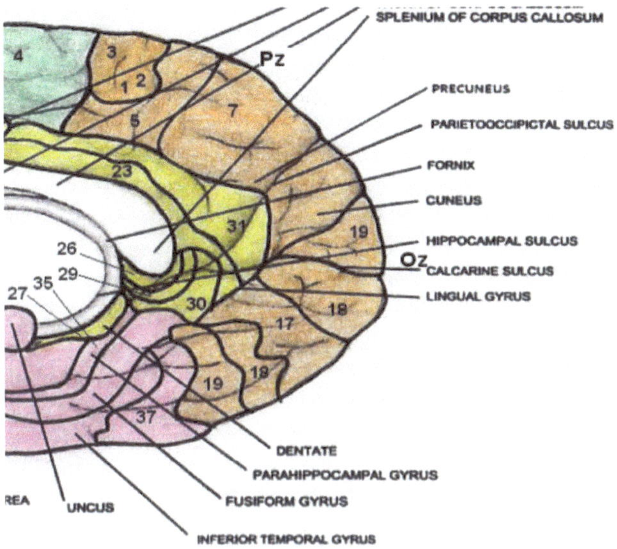

BAs 17

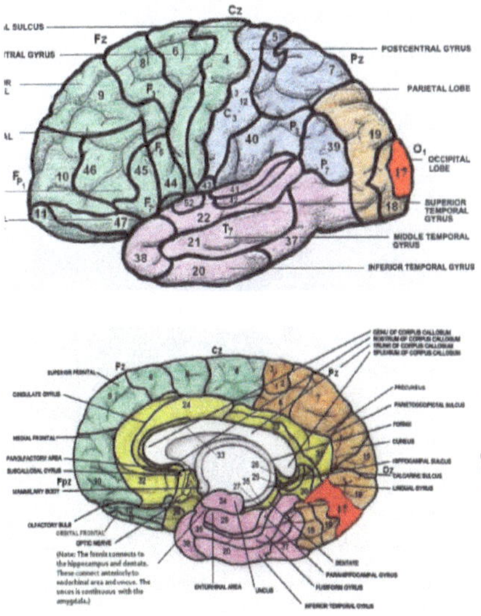

BA 18

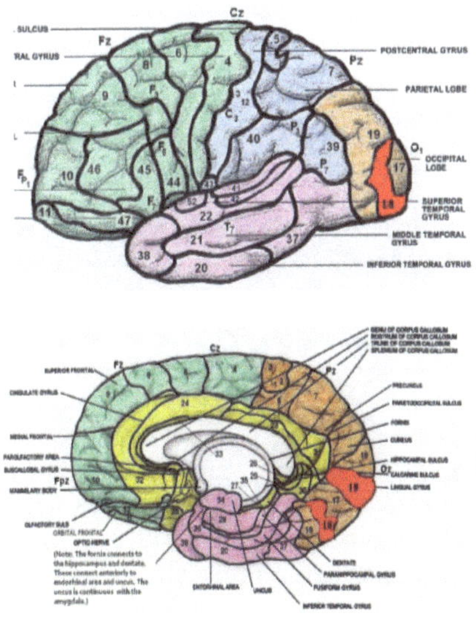

BA 19

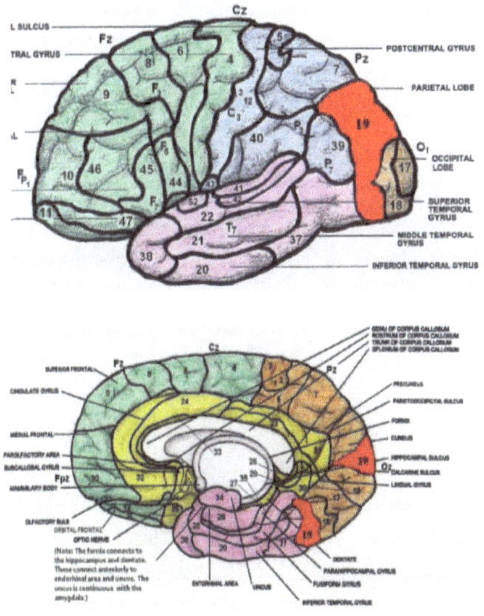

Neurofeedback in the occipital area may have effects on: BAs 17, 18, the visual cortex; BA 19, the visual association cortex; and BA 31, the posterior cingulate gyrus. The area below the calcarine sulcus responds to the upper half of the visual field while above the calcarine suclus responds to the lower half of the visual field. The primary visual cortex (V1) corresponds precisely to the visual field. Complete bilateral lesions of the occipital lobes can result in **Anton's Syndrome**, a condition in which there is cortical blindness with denial of being blind. BA 17 detects intensity of light and recognizes color, contours and patterns. **More complex functions**, such as face encoding, **require networks**. For faces this may include BAs 17, 18, 19 (occipital); 44, 45 (frontal); 37 (fusiform); and the right hippocampal formation.

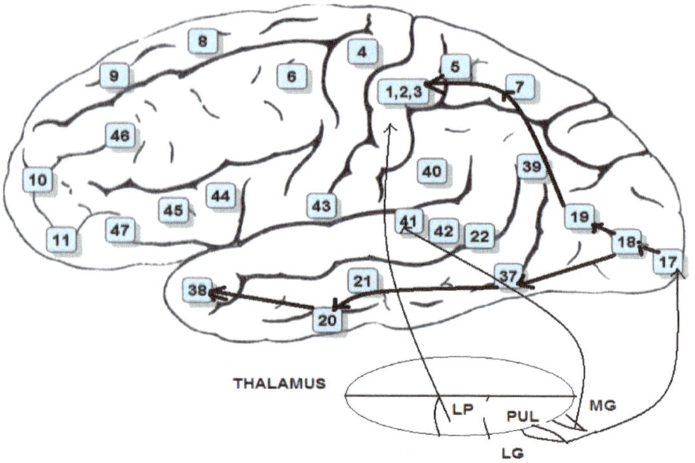

Reference: Adapted from Quantitative EEG, Event-Related Potentials and Neurotherapy. *Juri D. Kropotov, Academic Press, Elsevier: San Diego CA, 2009. Drawing after* Gray's Anatomy.

LG = Lateral geniculate
MG = Medial geniculate
PUL = Pulvinar
Visual stimuli from the lateral geniculate go to Brodmann area 17 of the visual cortex. Auditory stimuli from the medial geniculate go to Brodmann area 41 of the auditory cortex.
LP = Lateral posterior thalalmic nucleus (to BAs 1, 2, 3 of the somatosensory cortex)
In this diagram the medial and lateral geniculate (MG and LG) are illustrated as loops attached to the posterior portion of the thalamus. Diagram below shows location.

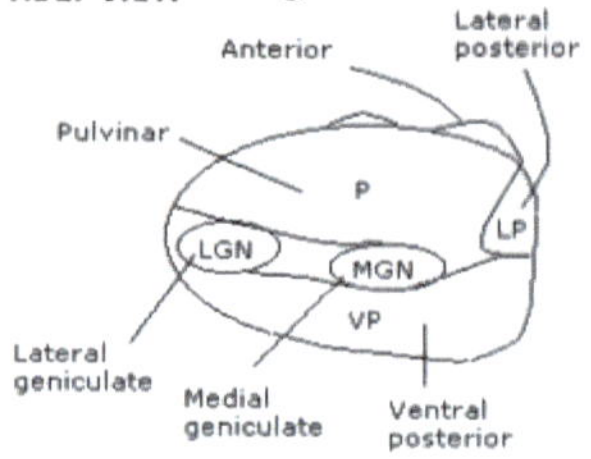

BA 17

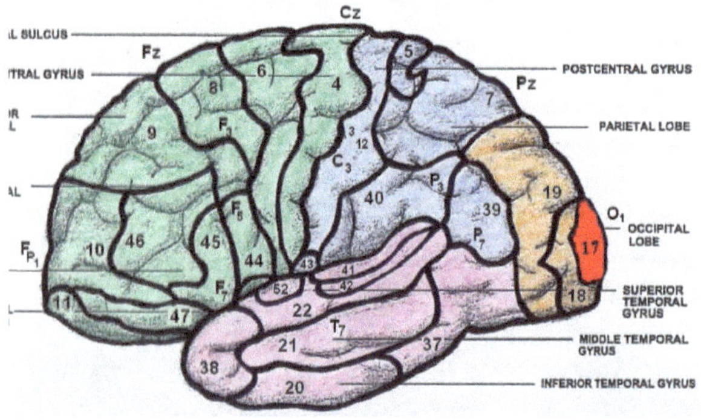

BA 17

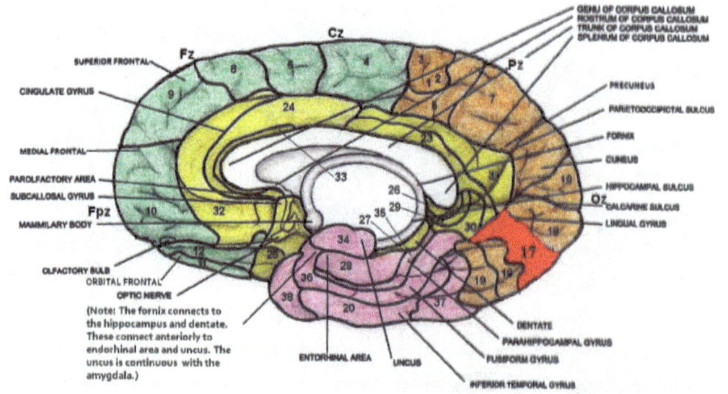

The **primary visual cortex is BA 17.** It is sensory cortex located in and around the calcarine fissure (calcarine 'sulcus' in figure above) in the occipital lobe. BA 17 receives information directly from its ipsilateral lateral geniculate nucleus in the thalamus. It is an area that is important in perception of light intensity, distinguishing visual patterns, contours, colors, and motion. It is also involved in perception of spatial orientation. BA 17 transmits information to two primary pathways, called the dorsal stream and the ventral stream, as noted by Kropotov (2009). The dorsal stream goes to the dorsomedial area and then to the posterior parietal cortex. The **dorsal stream** is referred to as the **'Where Pathway'** or the 'How Pathway.' It is associated with motion, representation of object locations, and control of the eyes and arms, especially when visual information is used to guide reaching or saccades. **Saccades** are a mechanism for fixation. They are rapid intermittent eye movements, as occurs when the eyes fix on one point after another in the visual field. Saccades are quick, simultaneous movements of both eyes in the same direction and are initiated cortically by the frontal eye fields (FEF), or subcortically by the superior colliculus.

The **ventral stream** goes to the inferior and middle temporal cortex and to the entorhinal cortex. The ventral stream is referred to as the **'What Pathway.'** It is associated with form recognition and object representation. It is also associated with storage of long-term memory. The ventral stream is associated with discrimination of shapes, textures, objects, and faces.

BA 18

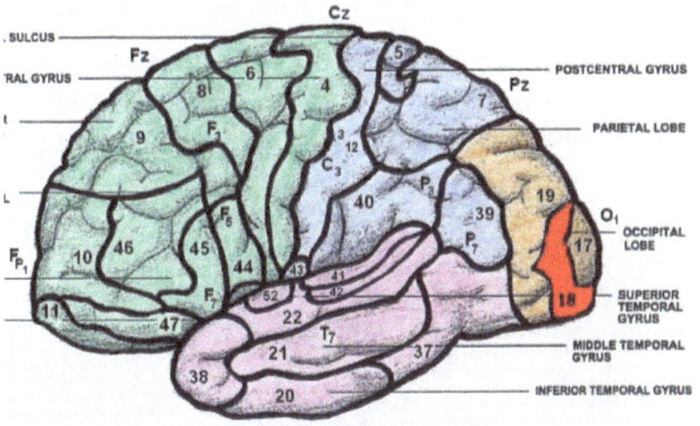

BA 18

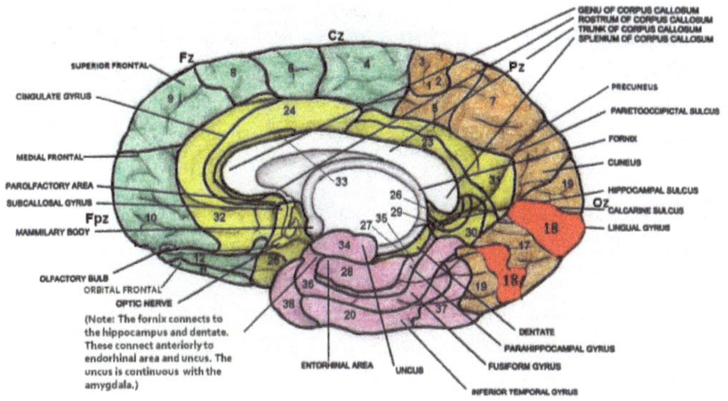

Brodmann area 18 is in the secondary visual cortex (V2), which is also called the **prestriate** cortex. It is a visual association area. BA 18 is important in the **perception** of light intensity, motion, and in monitoring **color, shape**, and visual **patterns**. It is also involved in distinguishing whether a stimulus is part of the **figure or the ground**. Object recognition memory is a function of this part of the cortex, as is converting short term object memory to long-term memory. **Face-name association** and word and face encoding are related to this area. However, this and most other functions noted here also involve BA 19.

Lesions can result in **visual agnosia,** a condition in which the patient is unable to recognize patterns, objects, faces, colors. Oliver Sacks' book *The Man Who Mistook His Wife for a Hat* describes a neurological patient with a lesion in this area. In the dominant hemisphere damage/dysfunction may result in an inability to read (alexia). Topographical agnosia may occur. The patient may be unable to track visual motion patterns and discriminate finger gestures. **Orientation and selective attention** may be compromised.

BA 19

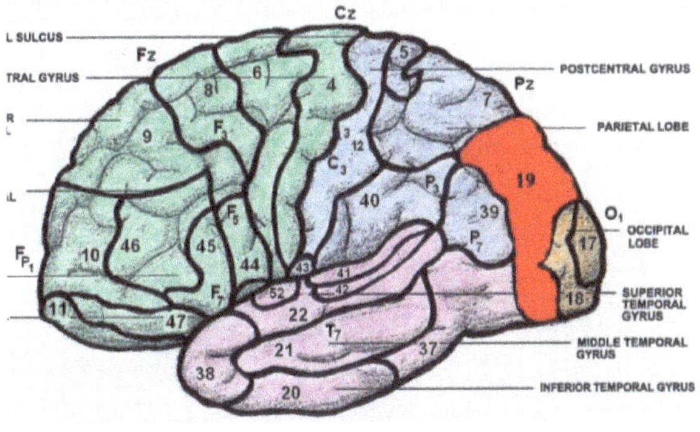

BA 19

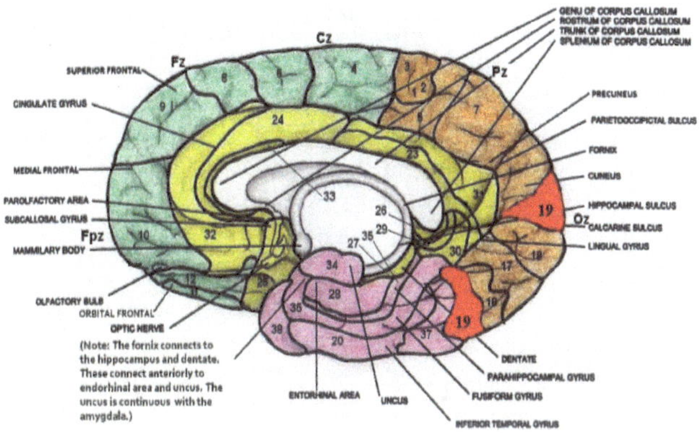

Brodmann area 19 is the associative visual area (V3). It overlaps in functions such as **light intensity** and **pattern detection** with BA 18. Brodmann area 19 refers to a region in the occipital cortex that borders the parietal and temporal lobes. It comprises parts of the lingual gyrus, the cuneus, the middle occipital gyrus, and the superior occipital gyrus of the occipital lobe. It is bounded anteriorly by the parieto-occipital sulcus and rostrally by Brodmann areas 39 (parietal lobe) and 37 (temporal lobe), and posteriorly by BA 18 (occipital lobe). BA 19 along with BA 18 comprise the **extrastriate** (or peristriate) cortex.

Brodmann area 17 is the **striate** cortex. It is the primary visual cortex. In normally sighted humans, **Brodmann areas 18 and 19 are** the **extrastriate cortex. The extrastriate cortex is a visual association** area, with feature-extracting, **shape and pattern** recognition, attentional, and multimodal integrating functions. It is one of the areas that can detect **light intensity**. Although functions of BA 18 and 19 overlap, only area 19 is important in the **spatial orientation of a stimulus (i.e., "Where is it?")**. It is also one of the areas along with the fusiform gyrus for processing **phonological**

properties of written words. Brodmann area 19 has been noted to receive inputs from the retina via the superior colliculus and pulvinar nucleus of the thalamus, and may contribute to **focusing attention**. It is involved in visual-spatial orientation and in sustained attention. It is possible it also contributes to the phenomenon of blindsight.

Blindsight refers to being cortically blind due to a lesion in the striate cortex. These persons can respond to visual stimuli that they do not consciously see. If such a patient is asked to detect and localize a visual stimulus or to discriminate amongst visual stimuli on their blind side they may be accurate as to location or type of movement. This is known as Type 1 blindsight.

Type 2 blindsight is when a patient states that there has been a change, such as a movement, within their blind area. Blindsight is said to challenge the common belief that perceptions must be conscious in order to affect our behavior. Blindsight suggests that it may be possible that that human behavior can be guided by sensory information of which the person is not consciously aware. It is **the converse of** the previously mentioned form of anosognosia (**Anton's agnosia). Anton's agnosia is also called** Anton-Babinski syndrome where there is complete cortical blindness and denial of that blindness. This denial may include confabulation concerning a supposed visual experience.

In patients blind from a young age, this area has been found to be activated by somatosensory stimuli. (For more detail and a clinical example, see Doidge, 2010.) Because of these findings, it is thought that area 19 is the differentiation point of the two visual streams, of the 'what' and 'where' visual pathways. The **dorsal** region may contain motion-sensitive neurons, and **ventral** areas may be specialized for object recognition. It discriminates according to light intensity and patterns. It monitors color and shape. It is a key area for visual attention, orientation, selection, and is part of the working memory network for visual and spatial inputs. It is a part of networks for visual imagery, and inferential reasoning. It is an area that may also be involved in theory of mind and in memory tasks.

As previously discussed with respect to the inferior temporal cortex, Kropotov (2009) has demonstrated that one can follow the time sequence after a visual stimulus using evoked potentials. This is shown in the heavy black lines in the above figure. Visual stimuli travel from the lateral geniculate (LG) to the occipital lobe and auditory stimuli go from the medial geniculate (MG) to BA 41 in the auditory cortex.

From front to back, frontal cortex to occipital lobes, the pathways in our brains are finely tuned and organized with awe-inspiring complexity. As we try to influence particular areas and functions, we must always respect these intricate interconnections and forever strive to understand them better.

Appendices

Table of Networks and Brodmann Areas

The lists become too long if one tries to be specific; therefore only highlights are given.

FUNCTION of NETWORK	**Brodmann areas** **(Major sites only)**	**Comment** (Only a few areas noted; networks for attention and for memory, for example, involve many other areas.)
Executive	**6, 8, 9, 10, 44, 45, 46, 47 (24, 32, 33), 39, 40**	Dorsolateral frontal Cingulate, Parietal (supramarginal, angular)
Memory	**34, 35, 36, 37, 31, 29, 20, 21, 28, 35, + 9, 10, 6**	Ventral central midline + frontal for working memory and spatial memory + temporal for visual, auditory memory and memories of past events . Other areas for some aspects: 8, 9, 10, 45, 46, 47
Attention	**7, 39, 31, 24, (+ right frontal: 10, 6, ...)**	Sustained attention nondominant frontal-parietal area. Visual: 17, 18, 37; For speech: 38, 47, 22, 23, 24.
Learning and Language	**39, 40, 35, 22 posterior, 44, 45, 46, (37, 39, 47)**	Mainly dominant hemisphere for language and many other areas are also involved; e.g., 6, 8, 9, 10, 24, 31, 32, 33, 38, 40 , 5, 7, even 20, 21, 22)
Affect	**23, 24, 32, 33, 25, 34, 13, 9, 10, 11, 12, 38, 47, 34, 35, 36**	Central midline structures/cingulate, medial frontal and orbital frontal
Default	31, 23; 29, 30 39, 40; (21) 24, 32, 10, 9 24, 10, 32, (11, 25) 28, 35, (27, 48)	Posterior Cingulate & Retrosplenial cortex Inferior Parietal Lobe (& Temporal) Dorsal Medial Prefrontal Cortex Ventral Medial & (in brackets) functionally related areas: Inferior Prefrontal & Subgenual Cingulate Hippocampal Region (Medial Temporal)
Integration of Information	**31, 23, 29, 26, 30**	Posterior cingulate, midline cuneus and precuuneus
Somatosensory	**1,2,3, 5, 40, (7, 40, 31)**	Sensorimotor strip
Motor	**4, 6, 8, (planning 6, 13, 40, 32, 33)**	Sensorimotor strip – It is now known that there is overlap between traditional primary sensory and motor areas.
Visual	**17, 18, 19, (integration 20)**	Occipital and inferior temporal
Auditory	**41, 42, 22, (21, 38)**	Temporal (frontal lobes then become involved)
Gustatory	**43**	
Olfactory	**34, 11**	

The phrase 'preferential recruitment' may be used. It can refer to functionally related BAs becoming activated when any one of the corresponding group are activated. In work using NFB it is an important concept because it implies that when the practitioner encourages activity at a specific site, that other areas will be influenced if they are linked by networks to that site.

Table of Regions of Interest, Lobules, Brodmann Areas

TABLE II	LOBULES			
REGIONS of INTEREST	Frontal-Brodmann Areas	Temporal-Brodmann Areas	Parietal-Brodmann Areas	Occipital-Brodmann Areas
Anterior Cingulate	25,24,32,33,10			
Extra-Nuclear - 1	13,47			
Inferior Frontal Gyrus - 1	9,10,11,44,45,46,47			
Medial Frontal Gyrus - 2	6,8,9,10,11,25,46,47			
Middle Frontal Gyrus	6,8,9,10,11,46,47			
Orbital Gyrus	11,47			
Paracentral Lobule - 3	5,6,31,4			
Precentral Gyrus - 3	4,6,43,44			
Rectal Gyrus	11,			
Subcallosal Gyrus - 2	25,34,13,			
Superior Frontal Gyrus	6,8,9,10,11			
Fusiform Gyrus		20,36,37		
Inferior Temporal Gyrus		20,21,37		
Insula		13,		
Middle Temporal Gyrus - 1		21,20,38,37,22,39		
Parahippocampal Gyrus		28,30,35,36,34		
Sub-Gyral - 1		20,21,37,40,6		
Superior Temporal Gyrus		13,21,22,38,39,41,42,		
Transverse Temporal Gyrus		41,42,		
Uncus		20,28,36		
Angular Gyrus -1			39,	
Cingulate Gyrus			23,24,31,32	
Inferior Parietal Lobule			7,39,40	
Postcentral Gyrus			1,2,3,5,7,40,43	
Posterior Cingulate			23,29,30,31	
Precuneus			7,19,31,39	
Superior Parietal Lobule - 1			7,	
Supramarginal Gyrus -1			40,	
Cuneus				7,17,18,19,30
Inferior Occipital Gyrus - 1				17,18,19
Lingual Gyrus				17,18,19
Middle Occipital Gyrus - 1				18,19,37,

Groupings of Brodmann areas according to regions of interest and lobes of the brain.
From Neuroguide.com. Reprinted with permission.

Order of Description of Functions

Lobes, Networks, Brodmann Areas, 10-20 Sites

Lobes or Cortical Areas	Associated Networks	Principle Brodmann Areas	10-20 Sites
Frontal (Lateral & Medial)	Executive Networks Medial: Executive and Affect Networks Medial (BA 9, 10): Default Network	8, 9, 10, 46, 45, 44, 6 47 Lateral and Medial discussed together for each BA --Inferior prefrontal 9, 10, 11, 46, 47	Fz F3, F4 F7, F8 FP1, FP2
Frontal Orbital - Ventral/medial	Affect network – Social (Default network)	11, 12	F9, F10 FPz
Central	Somatosensory Cortex Sensory Network Motor Network	BAs 4, 6, & 1, 2, 3, 5 BAs 1 , 2, 3 Primary (+ 43) Somatosensory Cortex BA 5 Somatosensory Association Cortex BA 4 Primary Motor Cortex BA 6 Motor Association Cortex	Cz C3, C4 Cz C3, C4
Temporal			
- Lateral Aspect	Executive – Auditory	41, 42, 22; 21, (52)	T7 & T8
- Temporal Pole	Executive, Semantic – also Affect Networks	38	T7 & T8 (F7, F8)
Temporal - Medial Aspect - (+ *Amygdala*)	Executive Network – Memory Affect network (+Default)	26, 27, 28 36, 37, (48) 35, 34	(Pz) (P7, P8)
Temporal - Inferior	Object identification; part of the 'what' pathway.	20, 37	T9 & T10
Insula	Affect & Executive	13	C3-T7
Cingulate			
Anterior (ACC)	Affect - Executive - Default	Affect: 24 (also Executive & Default & Salience networks) Affect: 33, 25 Executive: 32 (also Affect & Default)	Cz FCz Fz
Posterior (PCC)	Default Executive – Sensory	23, 31, 26, 29, (30)	Pz
Parietal	Executive, Sensory, Attention, (& Default) Networks; Spatial Awareness, part of the 'where' pathway.	5, 7	PCz, Pz
Temporal – Parietal - Lateral Aspect	Executive Network (& Default) Comprehension/Language Learning Gesture, Emotion, Nuance	39, 40 DH: 39, 40 NDH: 39, 40	P3 & P4
Inferior-Parietal Lateral	Attention & Salience	37	P7 & P8
Parietal Lobes - Medial Dorsal Aspect	Somatosensory Association	7	Pz
Occipital	Visual	17, 18, 19	O1, 02

Important: *The electrodes used for surface EEG NFB may reflect the activity from a number of Brodmann areas. The functions of Brodmann areas overlap with other Brodmann areas. Thus it is inevitable that under each principle BA being discussed, other BAs will be mentioned.*

Summary of Locations of Brodmann Areas

(Remember that BAs can overlap more than one gyrus and a gyrus can have more than one BA associated with it.)

- Areas 1, 2 & 3 – Primary Somatosensory Cortex (frequently referred to as Areas 3, 1, 2)
- Area 4 – Primary motor cortex
- Area 5 – Somatosensory association cortex
- Area 6 – Premotor cortex and supplementary motor cortex (also called secondary motor cortex or supplementary motor area)
- Area 7 – Somatosensory association cortex
- Area 8 – Includes frontal eye fields
- Area 9 – Dorsolateral prefrontal cortex
- Area 10 – Anterior prefrontal cortex (most rostral part of superior and middle frontal gyri)
- Area 11 – Orbitofrontal area (orbital and rectus gyri, plus part of the rostral part of the superior frontal gyrus)
- Area 12 – Orbitofrontal area (used to be part of BA11, refers to the area between the superior frontal gyrus and the inferior rostral sulcus)
- Area 13 (& 14) – Insular cortex
- *Areas 14, 15 (anterior temporal lobe) & 16 – Not found in humans*
- Area 17 – Primary visual cortex (V1)
- Area 18 – Secondary visual cortex (V2)
- Area 19 – Associative visual cortex (V3)
- Area 20 – Inferior temporal gyrus
- Area 21 – Middle temporal gyrus
- Area 22 – Superior temporal gyrus, memory comparison area of auditory cortex, the posterior part is considered to contain a portion of Wernicke's area in the Dominant Hemisphere
- Area 23 – Ventral posterior cingulate cortex
- Area 24 – Ventral anterior cingulate cortex
- Area 25 – Subgenual cortex (part of the ventromedial prefrontal cortex)
- Area 26 – Ectosplenial portion of the retrosplenial region of the cerebral cortex
- Area 27 – Part of piriform cortex
- Area 28 – Posterior entorhinal cortex
- Area 29 – Retrosplenial cingulate cortex
- Area 30 – Part of cingulate cortex
- Area 31 – Dorsal posterior cingulate cortex
- Area 32 – Dorsal anterior cingulate cortex
- Area 33 – Part of anterior cingulate cortex
- Area 34 – Anterior entorhinal cortex (on the parahippocampal gyrus)
- Area 35 – Perirhinal cortex (on the parahippocampal gyrus)
- Area 36 – Parahippocampal cortex (on the parahippocampal gyrus); fusiform gyrus
- Area 37 – Fusiform gyrus, occipitotemporal gyrus
- Area 38 – Temporopolar area (most rostral part of the superior and middle temporal gyri)
- Area 39 – Angular gyrus (part of Wernicke's area in Dominant Hemisphere)
- Area 40 – Supramarginal gyrus (part of Wernicke's area in Dominant Hemisphere)
- Areas 41 & 42 – Primary and Auditory Association Cortex
- Area 43 – Primary gustatory cortex
- Area 44 – Pars opercularis. Contains mirror neurons and is part of Broca's area in Dominant Hemisphere
- Area 45 – Pars triangularis. Broca's area in Dominant Hemisphere
- Area 46 – Dorsolateral prefrontal cortex
- Area 47 – Inferior prefrontal gyrus
- Area 48 – Retrosubicular area (a small part of the medial surface of the temporal lobe)
- *Area 49 – Parasubiculum area in a rodent*
- *Areas 50 & 51 – Found in monkeys*
- Area 52 – Parainsular area (at the junction of the temporal lobe and the insula)

Multiple Choice Questions

Choose the answer that is *most correct.* Sometimes, more than one answer may be partially correct. Questions are designed as a teaching aid only.

Section 1: Brodmann Areas and Networks

1. A Brodmann Area (BA) delineates a particular cortical area that has a specific function that differs from other Brodmann areas.
   T True
   F False
2. Inhibition of cortical areas and networks is extremely important. One inhibitory mechanism that is available involves links from the frontal cortex to subcortical structures that are broadly labelled the 'basal ganglia.' These connections can focus action while simultaneously inhibiting areas that are not necessary for a particular task. This mechanism is often described as a sequence in the following order:
   a. Cortex, putamen, thalamus, globus pallidus, cortex
   b. Cortex, locus coeruleus, solitary nucleus, cortex
   c. Cortex, putamen, globus pallidus, thalamus, cortex
   d. Cortex, caudate, nucleus ambiguous, thalamus, cortex
3. The lentiform nucleus comprises:
   a. The globus pallidus laterally, the innominate and anterior perforated area superiorly, and the subthalamus medially
   b. The putamen laterally, globus pallidus medially and the innominate substance, which contains the anterior perforated area, inferiorly
   c. The nucleus accumbens laterally, the putamen medially, the thalamus inferiorly, and the solitary nucleus posterior
   d. The thalamus medial, the nucleus accumbens lateral, the innominate, which contains the anterior perforated area, inferiorly.
4. The relationship between the putamen, globus pallidus, and thalamus is:
   a. The putamen activates the globus pallidus.
   b. The putamen activates the globus pallidus, which can inhibit the thalamus.
   c. The putamen inhibits the globus pallidus. The globus pallidus inhibits the thalamus.
   d. The putamen inhibits the globus pallidus. The globus pallidus activates the thalamus.
5. The dominant hemisphere is:
   a. The right hemisphere in left-handed persons
   b. The left hemisphere only in right-handed persons
   c. The left hemisphere in right handed and many left-handed persons
   d. The right hemisphere in all left-handed persons and some right-handed persons
6. The anterior cingulate cortex is a major component of the following networks:
   a. The Affect network but not the Executive or Salience networks
   b. The Executive but not the Salience or Affect networks
   c. The Salience and Executive networks but not the Affect network
   d. The Affect, Executive and Salience networks
7. The lobes of the brain that are usually considered crucial for all executive functions, including the voluntary control of attention, the inhibition of inappropriate and/or unwanted behavior, the planning of actions and executive decision making are:
   a. The temporal lobes
   b. The frontal lobes
   c. The parietal lobes
   d. The occipital lobes
8. The following areas most involved in handwriting are:
   a. Broca's area
   b. Wernicke's area
   c. Gurstman's area
   d. Exner's area
9. Tactile apperceptive agnosia refers to an inability to:
   a. Visually identify items in their immediate environment
   b. Recognize objects based on feeling their shape
   c. Recognize faces
   d. Execute a learned action with the hands
10. Constructional apraxia refers to an inability to:
   a. Name an object even though the person can recognize it
   b. Move a limb voluntarily
   c. Construct or even draw an object
   d. Have in mind the concept of an object

11. Frontal lobe damage that affects the ability to perceive a 'pattern' (such as knowing that you are looking at a car and not a tree or a plane) is called:
    a. Constructional apraxia
    b. Anomia
    c. Aphasia
    d. Associative agnosia
12. After a stroke, a person may have nonfluent speech but good comprehension. This may be called:
    a. Broca's aphasia
    b. Anomia
    c. Wernicke's aphasia
    d. Apraxia
13. The following are true concerning the term 'mirroring' as it is used today in psychology and medicine:
    a. Infants learn by mirroring their mothers
    b. Mirroring was discovered in monkeys near the International 10-20 System site F5
    c. Mirroring functions are a characteristic of an area near the temporal-parietal junction.
    d. All of the above
14. Sensory aprosodia is a term that is used to describe:
    a. Nonfluent speech but good comprehension
    b. Fluent speech, poor repetition, poor comprehension of both written and spoken propositional language.
    c. Inability to plan movement related to an object because the patient has lost the perception of the object's purpose.
    d. Unable to detect the meaning of nuance, innuendo, and tone of voice that reflects emotions.
15. Deductive arguments are:
    a. Arguments that can be evaluated for validity where the premises provide absolute grounds for accepting the conclusion
    b. Arguments that must be evaluated for plausibility or reasonableness
    c. Never valid but entirely reliable
    d. Primarily a function of the right prefrontal areas
16. Nondominant (usually right) hemisphere dominance is thought of as being characterized by:
    a. Stimulus seeking behavior, seeking novelty and change, extroverted
    b. Excellent verbal comprehension
    c. Inability to easily comprehend novelty
    d. Relying on stable patterns and routines
17. The dominant neurotransmitter in:
    a. The dominant left frontal lobe is noradrenaline
    b. The dominant left frontal lobe is dopamine
    c. The nondominant right frontal lobe is dopamine
    d. Both frontal lobes is serotonin
18. The major functions usually attributed to the dominant (usually left) hemisphere include:
    a. Sensing the Gestalt
    b. Attention to spatial relationships
    c. Letter and word perception and recognition
    d. Synthesis and integration of sensory inputs
19. One major connecting link between neurons in the entorhinal area with the orbital surface of the frontal lobe is called the:
    a. Cingulum
    b. Uncinate fasciculus
    c. Superior longitudinal fasciculus
    d. Arcuate fasciculus
20. Overactivity of the right prefrontal area is often thought to be related to:
    a. Difficulties with expressive language
    b. Inability to interpret nuance and innuendo
    c. Irritability, impulsivity, tactless, and even manic behavior
    d. Approach behavior and positive thoughts
21. The Nucleus Basalis of Meynert (NB) is a diffuse grouping of neurons within the basal forebrain that projects to widespread areas of the neocortex and represents the main source of:
    a. Noradrenaline
    b. Serotonin
    c. Neocortical acetylcholine (Ach)
    d. Dopamine
22. The Nucleus Basalis of Meynert and the cholinergic enervations to the hippocampus and temporal lobes are the first to be affected by:
    a. Pick's disease
    b. Alzheimer's disease
    c. Huntington's
    d. Asperger's
23. The ventromedial prefrontal cortex is an important area for:
    a. Regulating auditory memory
    b. Shifting attention from interpreting gestures to comprehending emotional tone of speech
    c. Solving arithmetic problems
    d. Tonic inhibition of the amygdala (also reactivating past emotional associations and events, therefore essentially mediating pathogenesis of PTSD)

24. The right insula can:
    a. Decease heart rate
    b. Influence the parasympathetic side of the autonomic nervous system
    c. Influence the sympathetic side of the autonomic nervous system
    d. Decrease peristalsis
25. The anterior cingulate cortex Brodmann area 24 is:
    a. Of primary importance in the default and affect network.
    b. A key structure involved in speech production.
    c. Important for clear handwriting.
    d. Has motor control of the hands.
26. In depression the **vegetative/autonomic Affect** network symptoms involve:
    a. A ventral compartment (e.g., sleep disturbance, loss of appetite and libido), which includes the hypothalamic-pituitary-adrenal axis, hippocampus, insula (BA 13), subgenual cingulate (BA 25) and the brainstem.
    b. A dorsal compartment, which modulates attentional and sensory-cognitive symptoms (e.g., apathy, attentional and executive deficits). This includes the dorsolateral prefrontal cortex (BAs 9 and 46), the dorsolateral anterior cingulate (area 24'), posterior cingulate (BA 31), the inferior parietal lobe (BA 40), and the striatum.
    c. The left, dominant, dorsolateral prefrontal cortex
    d. The right parietal temporal junction and the right supramarginal gyrus (BA 40) and angular gyrus
27. The left frontal operculum (F5) (Broca's area) is the key area for:
    a. Verbal comprehension
    b. Speech articulation
    c. Understanding innuendo
    d. Spatial perception
28. Encoding of visuospatial patterns activates:
    a. The left inferior prefrontal cortex and the left medial temporal lobe
    b. The right inferior prefrontal cortex and the right medial-temporal lobe
    c. The right superior temporal lobe (BA 41)
    d. The left superior temporal lobe (BA 41)
29. The integration of auditory, visual, perceptual and memory inputs that can assist reading can include: phonemic (letter to sound), lexical (sight words), and semantic (meaning) inputs to:
    a. Areas near the right temporal parietal junction
    b. Areas near the left prefrontal cortex
    c. Areas near the right prefrontal cortex
    d. Areas near the left temporal parietal junction
30. The auditory association area can include:
    a. BA 20 and BA 38 of the temporal lobe
    b. BA 41, BA 42 and BA 22 of the superior temporal gyrus
    c. BA 1, BA 2, BA 3 of the sensory cortex
    d. BA 44, BA 45 of the frontal cortex
31. A person whose speech is fluent with good grammar, but whose speech doesn't seem to make sense, a person who speaks without understanding what he or she is saying and substitutes inappropriate or the wrong words in his or her sentences in a jargon that is just nonsense, will most likely suffer from dysfunction in Wernicke's area, which is found in:
    a. The right dorsolateral prefrontal cortex
    b. The inferior parietal lobe and the auditory association area of the superior temporal gyrus in the nondominant hemisphere
    c. The inferior parietal lobe and the auditory association area of the superior temporal gyrus in the dominant hemisphere
    d. The precuneus and posterior cingulate (BA 31) of the dominant hemisphere
32. A region of the brain that is involved in visual-spatial-language skills and visual word recognition, and can be involved in learning disabilities including alexia (inability to read), agraphia (inability to write), difficulties with calculations, left-right discrimination, and technical competence is the:
    a. Angular gyrus in the dominant hemisphere
    b. Ventral rostral cingulate gyrus
    c. Parahippocampal gyrus in the dominant hemisphere
    d. Hypothalamus

33. A region of the brain that is involved in spatial-emotional-contextual perception, symbol recognition, ability to copy emotional tones, and the comprehension of innuendo, nuance, and the emotional aspects of both gesture and verbal communications is the:
    a. Angular gyrus and the supramarginal gyrus in the dominant hemisphere
    b. Angular gyrus the supramarginal gyrus in the nondominant hemisphere
    c. Parahippocampal gyrus and the fusiform gyrus in the dominant hemisphere
    d. Parahippocampal gyrus and the fusiform gyrus in the nondominant hemisphere
34. An area of the cortex that plays an important role in autobiographical memories and, in particular, spatial memories is the:
    a. Dominant hemisphere, entorhinal cortex (EC) BAs 34 and 28 – hippocampus system
    b. Nondominant hemisphere, entorhinal cortex (EC) BAs 34 and 28 – hippocampus system
    c. Dominant hemisphere, left frontal operculum (F5) (close to Broca's area BAs 44, 45)
    d. Nondominant prefrontal area BA 9, BA 10, BA 46
35. The most important areas for encoding and consolidation of long-term memories lie in:
    a. The dominant hemisphere parahippocampal gyrus
    b. The septal area of the frontal lobe
    c. The hippocampus
    d. The structures in the entire Papez circuit
36. Extensive damage to which area of the cortex will result in anosognosia, a neglect of the contralateral (opposite side) of space and the body and a lack of awareness of the loss:
    a. The left/dominant temporal cortex
    b. The right/nondominant temporal cortex
    c. The left/dominant parietal cortex
    d. The right/nondominant parietal cortex
37. One or more of the following symptoms – dysgraphia, dyscalculia, finger agnosia, left-right disorientation – are most likely related to dysfunction in the:
    a. The left/dominant temporal cortex
    b. The right/nondominant temporal cortex
    c. The left/dominant parietal cortex
    d. The right/nondominant parietal cortex
38. Persons who demonstrate an inability to perceive the visual field as a whole (simultanagnosia), have difficulty in fixating the eyes (ocular apraxia), and show an inability to move the hand to a specific object by using vision (optic ataxia) have Bálint's syndrome. These difficulties are most often related to lesions in:
    a. Both temporal lobes
    b. The dominant prefrontal cortex
    c. The right parietal lobe
    d. Parietal-occipital area bilaterally
39. A person's cortex may have a cortical stream for information flow related to the 'what' of information (in contrast to the 'where' of information) that goes along:
    a. occipital-temporal-frontal pathway
    b. occipital-parietal-frontal pathway
    c. dominant temporal- nondominant frontal pathway
    d. nondominant parietal- dominant temporal-frontal pathway
40. The cuneus and precuneus are found in:
    a. The superior temporal cortex
    b. The medial superior portion of the parietal lobe
    c. The inferior lateral aspect of the parietal lobe
    d. The anterior portion of the occipital lobe
41. The cuneus and precuneus, along with the posterior cingulate gyrus, are areas that are responsible for the:
    a. Comprehension of verbally presented material including phonemic (letter to sound), lexical (sight words), and semantic (meaning)
    b. Organization, integration and synthesis of auditory, visual and kinesthetic inputs and for orientation in space
    c. Spatial-emotional-contextual perception, symbol recognition, ability to copy emotional tones, and the comprehension of innuendo, nuance, and the emotional aspects of both gesture and verbal communications
    d. The inhibition of cortical networks
42. Nondominant parietal lobe functions include:
    a. Spatial position, opposite side body awareness, visualization of spatial organization, context
    b. Cognitive reasoning, attention, spelling, verbal short-term memory, imagination
    c. Comprehension of verbally presented material including phonemic (letter to sound), lexical (sight words), and semantic (meaning)
    d. Appreciation of fine art, such as paintings and sculptures

43. Lateral inferior parietal (LIP) neuronal activity is necessary for which of the following:
    a. The organization, integration and synthesis of auditory, visual and kinesthetic inputs
    b. Disengage attention from a current stimulus in order for focus to change to a different stimulus
    c. Interpretation of metaphors
    d. Pattern recognition
44. Visual information comes to the occipital lobes from the:
    a. Medial geniculate of thalamus
    b. Lateral geniculate of thalamus
    c. Lateral posterior nucleus of the thalamus
    d. Pulvinar
45. Brodmann area 24 is located in:
    a. The temporal cortex
    b. The parietal cortex
    c. The anterior cingulate gyrus
    d. The posterior cingulate gyrus
46. Long-term potentiation is a process wherein:
    a. A post-synaptic cell is enhanced so that it can depolarize more readily in response to a neurotransmitter
    b. A presynaptic membrane is encouraged to inject more neurotransmitter into the synaptic space
    c. The presynaptic axon develops more receptors
    d. The postsynaptic dendrite increases its capacity to transmit Mg^{++} ions
47. In the membrane of the postsynaptic receptor site:
    a. Ca^{++} blocks the NMDA (N-methyl-D-aspartate) receptor sites
    b. Na^{++} blocks the NMDA receptor sites
    c. Mg^{++} blocks the NMDA receptor sites
    d. Mg^{++} blocks the APMA (alpha-amino-3-hydroxy-5-methyl-4- isoxazole-propionic acid) receptor sites
48. A unique property of the NMDA (N-methyl-D-aspartate) receptor is its voltage-dependent activation. This means that, when glutamate causes an influx of sodium into the AMPA (alpha-amino-3-hydroxy-5-methyl-4- isoxazole-propionic acid) post-synaptic terminal, an electrical voltage depolarization change takes place that allows the:
    a. Mg^{2+} block of the NMDA receptor site to be released
    b. Ca^{2+} block of the NMDA receptor site to be released
    c. Ca^{2+} to pass through the receptor site, which then allows the Mg^{2+} block of other AMPA receptor sites to be released
    d. Na^{+} to pass through the receptor site, which then allows the Ca^{2+} block of other AMPA receptor sites to be released

END OF BRODMANN AREA MONOGRAPH QUESTIONS

Answers

References: Some of the questions involve more than just neuroanatomy, so an author's name may be given in order to facilitate finding a reference in the reference list.

1. [F]
2. [c]
3. [b]
4. [c]
5. [c]
6. [d]
7. [b]
8. [d]
9. [b]
10. [c]
11. [d]
12. [a]
13. [d]
14. [d] (Ross, 1981)
15. [a]
16. [a]
17. [b]
18. [c]
19. [b]
20. [c]
21. [c] (Divac, 1975; Mesulam and Van Hoesen, 1976)
22. [b]
23. [d] (Thayer et al., 2012)
24. [c] (Oppenheimer, S. 2001)
25. [a]
26. [a] (Paquette et al., 2009)
27. [b]
28. [b] (Kichhoff et al., 2000)
29. [d]
30. [b]
31. [c]
32. [a]
33. [b]
34. [b] (Damasio, 2003)
35. [d]
36. [d]
37. [c]
38. [d] (Roper, A. & Brown, R. et al.)
39. [a] (Ungerleider & Mishkin, 1982)
40. [b] (Smith, C.G. 1962, *Basic Neuroanatomy,* University of Toronto Press)
41. [b]
42. [a] (Thatchern 2012)
43. [b] (Bisley, J., Goldberg, M.E., 2006, *J. Neurophysiol.* 95 1696–1717)
44. [b] (Smith, C.G. 1962)
45. [c] (Thompson et al., 2007)
46. [a] (Cooke & Bliss, 2006)
47. [c] (Cooke & Bliss, 2006)
48. [a] (Malenka & Bear, 2004; Cooke & Bliss, 2006)

References

Primary Reference:

Dan Lloyd (dan.lloyd@trincoll.edu); Brownell Professor of Philosophy
Trinity College; 300 Summit Street, Hartford, CT 06106; Personal Communications, 2007.

Secondary References:

Achard, S., Salvador, R., Whitcher, B., Suckling, J. & Bullmore, E. (2006). A resilient, low-frequency, small-world human brain functional network with highly connected association cortical hubs. *J Neurosci, 26*(1), 63–72.

Alexander, G.E., DeLong, M.R. & Strick, P.L. (1986). Parallel organization of functionally segregated circuits linking basal ganglia and cortex. *Annual Review of Neuroscience*, *9*, 357–81.

Amodio, D.M. & Frith, C.D. (2006). Meeting of minds: the medial frontal cortex and social cognition. *Nature Reviews Neuroscience, 7*, 268–277.

Aron, A.R., Robbins, T.W. & Poldrack, R.A. (2004). Inhibition and the right inferior frontal cortex. *Trends in Cognitive Sciences*, *8*(4), 170–177.

Astur, R.S. & Constable, R.T. (2004). Hippocampal dampening during a relational memory task. *Behav Neurosci, 118*, 667–675.

Astur, R.S., St. Germain, S.A., Baker, E.K., Calhoun, V., Pearlson G.D. & Constable, R.T. (2005). FMRI hippocampal activity during a virtual radial arm maze. *Appl Psychophysiol Biofeedback, 30,* 307–317.

Augustine, J.R. (2008). *Human Neuroanatomy: An Introduction.* San Diego, California, Academic Press.

Baehr, E., Rosenfeld, J.P., Baehr, R. & Earnst, C. (1999). Clinical use of an alpha asymmetry neurofeedback protocol in the treatment of mood disorders. In J.R. Evans & A. Abarbanel (Eds.) *Introduction to Quantitative EEG and Neurofeedback.* San Diego: Academic Press.

Baguley, I.J., Heriseanu, R.E., Felmingham, K.L. & Cameron, I.D. (2006). Dysautonomia and heart rate variability following severe traumatic brain injury. *Brain Injury*, *20*(4), 437–444.

Baker, L.D., Frank, L.L., Foster-Schubert, K., Green, P.S., Wilkinson, C.W., McTiernan, A., Plymate, S.R., Fishel, M.A., Watson, G.S., Cholerton, B.A., Duncan, G.E., Mehta, P.D. & Craft, S. (2010). Effects of aerobic exercise on mild cognitive impairment: a controlled trial. *Arch Neurol, 67*(1), 71–79.

Bear, D.M. & Fedio, P. (1977). Quantitative analysis of interictal behavior in temporal lobe epilepsy. *Arch Neurol, 34*(8), 454–67.

Beasley, C.L., Pennington, K., Behan, A., Wait, R., Dunn, M.J. & Cotter, D. (2006). Proteomic analysis of the anterior cingulate cortex in the major psychiatric disorders: Evidence for disease-associated changes. *Proteomics, 6*(11), 3414–3425.

Beauregard, M., & Paquette, V. (2006). Neural correlates of a mystical experience in Carmelite nuns. *Neuroscience Letters*, *405,* 186–190.

Beauregard, M. & Levesque, J. (2006). Functional magnetic resonance imaging investigation of the effects of neurofeedback training on the neural bases of selective attention and response inhibition in children with attention-deficit/hyperactivity disorder. *Applied Psychophysiology and Biofeedback, 31*(1), 3–20.

Berman, M.G., Peltier, S., Nee, E.D., Kross, E., Deldin, P.J. & Jonides, J. (2011). Depression, rumination and the default network. *SCAN, 6*, 548–555.

Bisley, J.W. & Goldberg, M.E. (2006). Neural correlates of attention and distractibility in the lateral intraparietal area. *J Neurophysiol, 95*(3), 1696–1717.

Blumberg, H.P. (2000). Increased anterior cingulate and caudate activity in bipolar mania. *Biol Psychiatry*, *48,* 1045–1052.

Blumer, D. (1975) Temporal lobe epilepsy and its psychiatric significance. In: D.F. Benson, & D. Blumer, editors. *Psychiatric Aspects of Neurological Disease*. Grune and Stratton, New York: pp. 171–198.

Blumer, D. & Benson, D.F. (1982). Psychiatric manifestations of epilepsy. In D.F. Benson, & D. Blumer, eds., *Psychiatric Aspects of Neurological Disease, Volume II,* New York, Grune & Stratton.

Blumer, D. & Walker, A. (1967). Sexual behaviour in temporal lobe epilepsy. *Arch Neurol, 16,* 31–43.

Bogacz, R. Wagenmakers, E.J., Forstmann, B.U. & Nieuwenhuis, S. (2010). The neural basis of the speed-accuracy tradeoff. *Trends in Neurosciences*, *33*(1), 10–6.

Bonelli, R.M. & Cummings, J.L. (2007). Frontal-subcortical circuitry and behavior. *Dialogues in Clinical Neuroscience*, *9*(2), 141.

Bottini, G., Corcoran, R., Sterzi, R., Paulesu, E., Schenone, P., Scarpa, P., Frackowiak, R.S.J. & Frith, D. (1994). The role of the right hemisphere in the interpretation of figurative aspects of language: A positron emission tomography activation study. *Oxford Journals, Medicine, Brain, 117*(6), 1241–1253.

Boulay, C.B., Sarnacki, W.A., Wolpaw, J.R. & McFarland, D.J. (2011). Trained modulation of sensorimotor rhythms can affect reaction time. *Clinical Neurophysiology: Official Journal of the International Federation of Clinical Neurophysiology*, *122*(9), 1820–6.

Brodmann, K. (1909). *Localisation in the Cerebral Cortex.* Translated and Edited by Laurence J. Garey, 1994, London, Smith-Gordon.

Brown, J.W., & Braver, T.S. (2005). Learned predictions of error likelihood in the anterior cingulate cortex. *Science (New York)*, *307*(5712), 1118–21.

Brown, J.W., Bullock, D. & Grossberg, S. (2004). How laminar frontal cortex and basal ganglia circuits interact to control planned and reactive saccades. *Neural Networks: The Official Journal of the International Neural Network Society*, *17*(4), 471–510.

Brunoni, A.R., Valiengo, L., Baccaro, A., Zana, Tamires A., de Oliveira, J.F., Goulart, A., Boggio, P.S., Lotufo, P.A., Bensen, I.M. & Fregni, F. (2013). The sertraline vs electrical current therapy for treating depression clinical study results from a factorial, randomized, controlled trial. *JAMA Psychiatry Published Online,* Feb. 6, 2013.

Buchanan, T.W., Tranel, D. & Adolphs, R. (2009). In P.J. Whalen & E.A. Phelps (Eds.) *The Human Amygdala,* 289–318. New York, Guilford.

Buckner, R.L., Andrews-Hanna, J.R. & Schacter, D.L. (2008). The brain's default network: Anatomy, function, and relevance to disease. *Ann NY Acad Sci, 1124,* 1–38.

Bullmore, E. & Sporns, O. (2012). The economy of brain network organization. *Nature Reviews Neuroscience, 13*, 336–349.

Bullock, D., Tan, C.O. & John, Y.J. (2009). Computational perspectives on forebrain microcircuits implicated in reinforcement learning, action selection, and cognitive control. *Neural Networks : The Official Journal of the International Neural Network Society*, *22*(5–6), 757–65.

Buysse, D.J., Germain, A., Moul, D.E., Franzen, P.L., Brar, L.K., Fletcher, M.E., Begley, A., Houck, P.R., Mazumdar, S., Reynolds, III, C.F. & Monk, T.H. (2011). Efficacy of brief behavioral treatment for chronic insomnia in older adults. *Arch Intern Med, 171*(10), 887–895.

Buzsaki, G. (2006). *Rhythms of the Brain.* New York, Oxford University Press.

Cannon, R., & Lubar, J.F. (2007). EEG spectral power and coherence: Differentiating effects of spatial-specific neuro-operant Learning (SSNOL) utilizing LORETA neurofeedback training in the anterior cingulate and bilateral dorsolateral prefrontal cortices. *Journal of Neurotherapy, 11* (3), 25–44.

Cannon, R., Congedo, M., Lubar, J. & Hutchens, T. (2009). Differentiating a network of executive attention: LORETA neurofeedback in anterior cingulate and dorsolateral prefrontal cortices: Mapping a network of executive attention. *International Journal of Neuroscience, 119* (3), 401–441.

Cannon, R.L. (2012). *Low Resolution Electromagnetic Tomography (LORETA): Basic Concepts and Clinical Applications.* Corpus Christi, Texas, 78411, DMED Press, p160.

Carlson, N.R. (1986). *Physiology of Behavior – Third Edition.* Toronto: Allyn and Bacon Inc.

Cavanna, A.E. & Trimble, M.R. (2006). The precuneus: a review of its functional anatomy and behavioural correlates. *Brain, 129* (Pt 3), 564–583.

Chauhan, N.B., Siegel, G.J., & Lee, J.M. (2001). Depletion of glial cell line-derived neurotrophic factor in substantia nigra neurons of Parkinson's disease brain. *Journal of Chemical Neuroanatomy*, *21*(4), 277–288.

Chiesa, V., Gardella, E., Tassi, L., Canger, R & Lo Russo, G. (2007). Age-related gender differences in reporting ictal fear: Analysis of case histories and review of the literature. *Epilepsia*, *48*(12), 2361–2364.

Choo, I.H., Lee, D.Y., Oh, J.S., Lee, J.S., Lee, D.S., Song, I.C., Youn, J.C., Kim, S.G., Kim, K.W., Jhoo, J.H. & Woo, J.I. (2010). Posterior cingulate cortex atrophy and regional cingulum disruption in mild cognitive impairment and Alzheimer's disease. *Neurobiol. Aging, 31*, 772–779.

Choo, I.H., Lee, D.Y., Lee, J.H., Kim, K.W., Jhoo, J.H., Ju, Y.-S., Yoon., J.C., Kim, S.G., Ha, J. & Woo, J.I. (2009). The prevalence of cognitive impairment with no dementia in older people: The Seoul study. *International Journal of Geriatric Psychiatry, 24*(3), 306–312.

Christopoulos, G.I., Tobler, P.N., Bossaerts, P., Dolan, R.J. & Schultz, W. (2009). Neural correlates of value, risk, and risk aversion contributing to decision making under risk. *J Neurosci, 26* (24), 6469–6472.

Civier, O., Bullock, D., Max, L. & Guenther, F.H. (2013). Computational modeling of stuttering caused by impairments in a basal ganglia thalamo-cortical circuit involved in syllable selection and initiation. *Brain and Language, 126*(3), 263–78.

Cooke, S.F. & Bliss, T.V. (2006). Plasticity in the human central nervous system. *Brain, 129* (Pt 7), 1659–1673.

Coull, J.T. & Nobre, A.C. (1998). Where and when to pay attention: The neural systems for directing attention to spatial locations and to time intervals as revealed by both PET and fMRI. *The Journal of Neuroscience, 18*(18), 7426–7435.

D'Argembeau, A., Collette, F.,,Van der Linden, M., Laureys, S., Del Fiore, G., Degueldre, C., Luxen, A & Salmon, E (2005). Self-referential reflective activity and its relationship with rest: A PET study. *NeuroImage, 25,* 616– 624.

Damasio, A. (2003b). Mental self: the person within. *Nature, 423* (6937), 227. doi:10.1038/423227a

Damasio, A. (2003). Feelings of emotion and the self. *Annals of the New York Academy of Sciences, 1001,* 253–261.

Davidson, R.J. (1995). Cerebral asymmetry, emotion and affective style. In R. J. Davidson & K. Hugdahl (Eds.) *Brain Asymmetry*, Cambridge, Mass: MIT Press, 369–388.

Davidson, R.J. (1998). Anterior electro-physiological asymmetries, emotion, and depression: Conceptual and methodological conundrums. *Psychophysiology, 35*, 607–614.

Davidson, R.J. (2000). Cognitive neuroscience needs affective neuroscience (and vice versa). *Brain Cogn, 42*, 89–92.

Davidson, R.J. (2002). Anxiety and affective style: Role of prefrontal cortex and amygdala. *Biolog Psychiat, 51* (1), 68–80

Davidson, R.J., Abercrombie, H., Nitschke, J.B. & Putnam, K. (1999). *Current Opinion in Neurobiology, 9*, 228–234.

Davidson. R.J., Pizzagalli, D., Nitshke, J.B. & Putnam, K. (2002). Depression: Perspectives from affective neuroscience. *Annual Rev Psychol, 5*(3), 545–574.

De Ridder, D., Van Laere, K., Dupont, P., Menovsky, T. & Van de Heyning, P. (2007). Visualizing out-of-body experience in the brain. *N Engl J Med, 357*, 1829–1833.

De Ridder, D. (2009). An evolutionary approach to brain rhythms and its clinical implications for brain modulation. *Journal of Neurotherapy, (13)*1, 69–70.

De Ridder, D. (2010). Alcohol addiction: A clinical pathophysiological approach. *Proceedings of the ISNR 18th Annual Conference,* Denver, Colorado.

De Ridder, D. (2011). Limbic dysrhythmia and delta pathologies. ISNR Presentation, 2011.

deBeus, R. (2005). Efficacy of attention training for children with ADHD: A randomized double-blind placebo-controlled study. Presented at: The Annual Meeting of the International Society for Neurofeedback and Research. Atlanta, Ga., USA, 7–10 Sept. 2006.

Dedovic, K., Renwick, R., Mahani, N.K., Engert, V., Lupien, S.J. & Pruessner, J.C. (2005). The Montreal imaging stress task using functional imaging to assess the effects of perceiving and processing psychosocial stress in the human brain. *J Psychiatry Neuroscience, 30*(5), 319–325.

Dedovic, K., Duchesne, A., Andrews, J., Engert, V., & Pruessner J.C. (2009). The brain and the stress axis: The neural correlates of cortisol regulation in response to stress. *Neuroimage*, 47(3), 864–871.

Dehaene, S., Le Clec'H, G., Poline, J.-B., LeBihan, D. & Cohen, L. (2002). The visual word form area. A prelexical representation of visual words in the fusiform gyrus. *NeuroReport, 13*, 321–325.

Devinsky, O., Morrell, M. & Vogt, B. (1995). Contributions of anterior cingulate cortex to behavior, *Brain, 118*, 279–306.

Ding, J.B., Guzman, J.N., Peterson, J.D., Goldberg, J.A. & Surmeier, D.J. (2010). Thalamic gating of corticostriatal signaling by cholinergic interneurons. *Neuron, 67*(2), 294–307.

Dobbs, D. (2006). Turning off depression. *Scientific American Mind, 17*(4), 26–31.

Doidge, N. (2007). *The Brain That Changes Itself.* New York, Viking Press.

Donegan, N.H., Sanislow, C.A., Blumberg, H.P., Fulbright, R.K., Lacadie, C., Skudlarski, P., Gore, J.C., Olson, I.R., McGlashan, T.H. & Wexler, B.E. (2003). Amygdala hyperreactivity in borderline personality disorder: implications for emotional dysregulation. *Biological Psychiatry, 54*(11), 1284–1293.

Dranias, M.R., Grossberg, S. & Bullock, D. (2008). Dopaminergic and non-dopaminergic value systems in conditioning and outcome-specific revaluation. *Brain Research, 1238*, 239–87.

Farwell, L. & Donchin, E. (2000).The truth will out. *Academic Press, Psychophysiology, 28*, 531–547.

Fox, M.D., Snyder, A.Z., Vincent, J.L., Corbetta, M., Van Essen, D.C. & Raichle, M.E. (2005).The human brain is intrinsically organized into dynamic, anticorrelated functional networks. *Proceedings National Academy of Science, USA, 102*(27), 9673–9678.

Frank, M.J. (2006). Hold your horses: A dynamic computational role for the subthalamic nucleus in decision making. *Neural Networks : The Official Journal of the International Neural Network Society*, *19*(8), 1120–36.

Fried, I., Wilson, C., MacDonald, K. & Behnke E. (1998). Electric current stimulates laughter. *Nature, 391*(6668), 650

Frith, U. & Frith, C.D. (2003). Development and neurophysiology of mentalizing. *Phil Trans R Soc Lond B, 358*(1431), 459–473.

Frodl, T., Shaub, A., Banac, S., Charypar, M., Jäger, M., Kümmler, P., Bottlender, R., Zetzsche, T., Born, C., Leinsinger, G., Reiser, M., Möller, H.-J. & Meisenzahl, E.M. (2006). Reduced hippocampal volume correlates with executive dysfunctioning in major depression. *J Psychiatry Neurosci, 31*(5), 316–323.

Gevins, A., Smith, M.E., McEvoy, L. & Yu, D. (1997). High-resolution EEG mapping of cortical activation related to working memory: Effects of task difficulty, type of processing, and practice. *Cereb Cortex, 7,* 374 –385.

Glascher, J. & Adolphs, R. (2003). Processing of the arousal of subliminal and supraliminal emotional stimuli by the human amygdala. *Journal of Neuroscience*, *23*, 10274–10282.

Gloor, P., Pellegrini, A. & Kostopoulos, G.K. (1979). Effects of changes in cortical excitability upon the epileptic bursts in generalized penicillin epilepsy of the cat. *Electroencephalogr Clin Neurophysiol*, *46*(3), 274–289.

Gloor, P., Olivier, A., Quesney, L.F., Andermann, F. & Horowitz, S. (1982). The role of the limbic system in experiential phenomena of temporal lobe epilepsy. *Ann Neurol, 12,* 129–144.

Goela, V. & Dolana, R.J. (2004). Differential involvement of left prefrontal cortex in inductive and deductive reasoning. *Cognition, 93*(3), 109–121.

Golby, A.J., Poldrack, R.A., Brewer, J.R., Desmond, J.E., Aron, A.P. & Gabrieli, J.D.E. (2001). Material-specific lateralization in the medial temporal lobe and prefrontal cortex during memory encoding. *Brain, 124*(9), 1841–1854.

Goldapple, K., Segal, Z., Garson, C., Lau, M., Bieling, P., Kennedy, S. & Mayberg, H. (2004). Modulation of cortical-limbic pathways in major depression: Treatment specific effects of cognitive behavioural therapy. *Arch Gen Psychiatry, 61*, 34–41.

Goldberg, E. (2001). *The Executive Brain: Frontal Lobes and the Civilized Mind.* New York: Oxford University Press (paperback 2002).

Goldberg, I., Harel, M. & Malach, R. (2006). When the brain loses its self: prefrontal inactivation during sensorimotor processing, *Neuron, 50*(2), 329–339.

Gorman, J.M., Kent, J.M., Sullivan, G.M. & Coplan J.D. (2000). Neuroanatomical hypothesis of panic disorder revised. *Amer J Psychiatry, 157*(4), 493–505.

Gotman, J., Grova, C., Bagshaw, A., Kobayashi, E., Aghakhani, Y. & Dubeau, F. (2005). Generalized epileptic discharges show thalamocortical activation and suspension of the default state of the brain. *Proc Natl Acad Sci USA, 102*(42), 15236–15240.

Grafman, J. (2002). The structured event complex and the human prefrontal cortex. In D.T. Stuss & R.T. Knight (Eds.), *The Frontal Lobes* (pp. 292–310). New York: Oxford University Press.

Gray, H. (1918). *Anatomy of the Human Body.* Philadelphia, Lea & Febiger.

Gray, L. (2013). The University of Texas Medical School at Houston, FreeScience – Books – Neuroscience Online, Chapter 10, Vestiblar System: Structure and Function. Also, *NeuroScience 2nd edition*, Chapter 11: Vestibular System: Pathways and Reflexes.

Greenberg, B.D., Malone, D.A., Friehs, V., Gerhard M., Rezai, A.R., Kubu, C.S., Malloy, P.F., Salloway, S.P., Okun, M.S., Goodman, W.K. and Rasmussen, S.A. (2006). Three-year outcomes in deep brain stimulation for highly resistant obsessive–compulsive disorder. *Neuropsychopharmacology*, *31*, 2384–2393.

Hagmann, P., Cammoun, L., Gigandet, X., Meuli, R., Honey, C.J., Wedeen, V.J. & Sporns, O. (2008). Mapping the structural core of human cerebral cortex. *PLoS Biology, 6(7*), 1479–1493.

Hamer, M. & Chida, Y. (2009). Physical activity and risk of neurodegenerative disease: A systematic review of prospective evidence. *Psychol Med, 39,* 3–11.

Hampson, M., Driesen, N.R., Skudlarski, P., Gore, J.C. & Constable, R.T. (2006). Brain Connectivity Related to Working Memory Performance *The Journal of Neuroscience, 26(*51), 13338–13343.

Harmon-Jones, E. & Allen, J.J.B. (1998). Anger and frontal brain activity: EEG asymmetry consistent with approach motivation despite negative affective valence. *Journal of Personality and Social Psychology*, *74*(5), 1310–1316.

Hickok, G. (2001). Functional anatomy of speech perception and speech production: psycholinguistic implication. *Journal of Psycholinguistic Research, 30(*3), 225–235.

Holmes, T.H. & Rahe, R.H. (1967). The social readjustment rating scale. *J Psychosom Res, 11*(2): 213–8.333

Holtzheimer, P.E. & Mayberg, H.S. (2011). Stuck in a rut: Rethinking depression and its treatment. *Trends in Neurosciences, 34*(1), 1–9.

Iacoboni, M. & Dapretto, M. (2006). The mirror neuron system and the consequences of its dysfunction. *Nature Reviews and Neuroscience, 7*(12), 942–951.

Iacoboni, M. (2006). Understanding emotions in others: Mirror neuron dysfunction in children with autism spectrum disorders. *Nature Neuroscience, 9*(1), 28–30.

Jacobs, J., Kahana, M.J., Ekstrom, A.D., Mollison, M.V. & Fried, I. (2010). A sense of direction in human entorhinal cortex. *Proc Natl Acad Sci USA, 107*(14), 6487–6492).

Joseph, R. (2000). Neuropsychiatry, neuropsychology, BA 34, uncus, temporal lobe, *Clinical Neuroscience* 3rd Ed. (2000). New York: Academic Press.

Karavidas, M.K., Lehrer, P. M., Vaschillo, E., Vaschillo, B., Marin, H., Buyske, S., Malinovsky, I., Radvansky, D. & Hassett, A. (2007). Preliminary results of an open-label study of heart rate variability biofeedback for the treatment of major depression. *Applied Psychophysiology and Biofeedback, 32*(1), 19–30.

Kennedy, S.H., Giacobbe P., Rizvi, S.J., Placenza, F.M., Yasunori, N.Y., Mayberg, H.S. & Lozano, A.M. (2011). Deep brain stimulation for treatment-resistant depression: Follow-up after 3 to 6 years. *Am J Psychiatry, 168*(5), 502–510.

Kim, M.J., Gee, D.G., Davis, F.C. Loucks, R.A. & Whalen, P.J. (2011). Anxiety dissociates dorsal and ventral medial prefrontal cortex functional connectivity with the amygdala at rest. *Cerebral Cortex, 7*, 1667–1673.

Kim, M.J., Loucks, R.A., Palmer, A.L., Brown, A.C., Solomon, K.M., Marchante, A.N. & Whalen, P.J. (2011). The structural and functional connectivity of the amygdala: from normal emotion to pathological anxiety. *Behavioral Brain Research, 223*, 403–410.

Kirchhoff, B.A., Wagner, A.D., Maril, A. & Stern, C. E. (2000). Prefrontal-temporal circuitry for episodic encoding and subsequent memory. *The Journal of Neuroscience, 20*(16), 6173–6180.

Knezevic, B., Thompson, L. & Thompson, M. (2010). Pilot project to ascertain the utility of Tower of London Test to assess outcomes of neurofeedback in clients with Asperger's Syndrome. *Journal of Neurotherapy, 14*(3), 3–19.

Knoch, D., Gianotti, L.R.R., Pascual-Leone, A., Treyer. V., Regard, M., Hohmann, M. & Brugger, P. (2006). Disruption of right prefrontal cortex by low-frequency repetitive transcranial magnetic stimulation induces risk-taking behavior. *Journal of Neuroscience, 26*(24), 6469–6472.

Konishi, S., Chikazoe, J., Jimura, K., Asari, T. & Miyashita, Y. (2005). Neural mechanism in anterior prefrontal cortex for inhibition of prolonged set interference. *Proc Natl Acad Sci USA, 102*(35), 12584–12588.

Kringelbach, M. & Rolls, E.T. (2005). The human orbitofrontal cortex: Linking reward to hedonic experience. *Nature Reviews Neuroscience, 6*(9), 691–702

Kropotov, J. D. (2009). *Quantitative EEG, Event-Related Potentials and Neurotherapy.* San Diego, CA: Academic Press, Elsevier, 292–309.

Kropotov, J. D., Grin-Yatsenko,V. A., Ponomarev,V. A., Chutko, L. S.,Yakovenko, E. A. & Nikishena, I. S. (2005). ERPs correlates of EEG relative beta training in ADHD children. *International Journal of Psychophysiology, 55,* 23–34.

Kurova, N.S. & Cheremushkin, E.A. (2007). Spectral EEG characteristics during increases in the complexity of the context of cognitive activity. *Neurosci Behav Physiol, 37*(4), 379–385

Kwak, Y.S., Um, S.Y., Son ,T.G. et al. (2008). Effect of regular exercise on senile dementia patients. *Int J Sports Med, 29*(6), 471–474.

La Rovere, M.T., Pinna, G.D. & Raczak, G. (2008). Baroreflex sensitivity: Measurement and clinical implications. *Annals of Noninvasive Electrocardiology, 13*(2), 191–207.

Laird, A.R., Fox, P.M., Eickoff, S.B., Turner, J.A., Ray, K.L., McKay, D.R., et al. (2011). Behavioral Interpretations of Intrinsic Connectivity Networks. *Journal of Cognitive Neuroscience*, 23(12), 4022-4037.

Lévesque, J., Beauregard, M. & Mensour, B. (2006). Effect of neurofeedback training on the neural substrates of selective attention in children with attention-deficit/hyperactivity disorder: A functional magnetic resonance imaging study. *Neuroscience Letters, 394*(3), 216–21.

Levine B., Black S.E., Cabeza R., Sinden M., Mcintosh A.R., Toth J.P., Tulving E. & Stuss D.T. (1998). Episodic memory and the self in a case of isolated retrograde amnesia. *Brain, 121*(Pt 10), 1951–1973.

Li, C-s.R., Huang, C., Constable, R.T., & Sinha, R. (2006). Imaging response inhibition in a stop-signal task: Neural correlates independent of signal onitoring and post-response processing.*The Journal of Neuroscience, 26*(1), 186–192.

Linden, M., Habib, T. & Radojevic, V. (1996). A controlled study of the effects of EEG biofeedback on cognition and behavior of children with attention deficit disorder and learning disabilities. *Biofeedback and Self Regulation, 21*(1), 106–111.

Lisanby S.H., Luber B., Perera T. & Sackeim H.A. (2000). Transcortical magnetic stimulation: applications in basic neuroscience and neurpsychopharmacology. *Int J Neuropsychopharmacol, 3*, 259–273.

Lopez, C., Blanke, O. & Mast, F.W. (2012). The human vestibular cortex revealed by coordinate-based activation likelihood estimation meta-analysis. *Neuroscience, 212*(14), 159–179.

Lubar, J.F. (1995). Neurofeedback for the management of attention-deficit/hyperactivity disorders. In Mark S. Schwartz and Associates, *Biofeedback: A Practitioner's Guide – Second Edition.* New York: Guilford Press, 493–522.

Lundstrom, B.N., Ingvar, M. & Petersson, K.M. (2005). The role of precuneus and left inferior frontal cortex during source memory episodic retrieval. *NeuroImage, 27*, 824–834.

Lutz, A., Greischar, L.L., Periman, D. & Davidson, R.L. (2009). BOLD signal in insula is differentially related to cardiac function during compassion meditation in experts vs. novices. *Neuroimage, 47*, 1038–1046.

Mabbott, D.J., Rovet, J., Noseworthy, M.D., Smith, M.L. & Rockel, C. (2009). The relations between white matter and declarative memory in older children and adolescents. *Brain Research, 1294*, 80–90.

MacLeod, A.K., Buckner, R.L.,Miezin, F.M., Petersen, S.E. & Raichle, M.E. (1998). Right anterior prefrontal cortex activation during semantic monitoring and working memory. *Neuroimage, 7*, 41–48.

Malenka, R. & Bear, M. (2004). LTP and LTD: An embarrassment of riches. *Neuron, 44* (1): 5–21.

Matthews, S.C., Paulus, M. P., Simmons, A. N., Nelesen, R. A. & Dimsdale, J. E. (2004). Functional subdivisions within anterior cingulate cortex and their relationship to autonomic nervous system function. *Neuroimage, 22,* 1151–1156.

Mayberg, H.S. (2003). Modulating dysfunctional limbic-cortical circuits in depression: Towards development of brain-based algorithms for diagnosis and optimised treatment. *British Medical Bulletin, 65,* 193–207.

Mayberg, H.S., Brannan, S.K., Tekell, J.L., Silva, J.A., Mahurin, R.K., McGinnis, S. & Jerabek, P.A. (2000). Regional metabolic effects of floxetine in major depression: Serial changes and the relationship to clinical response. *Biol.Psychiatry, 48*(8), 830–843.

Mayberg, H.S., Lozano, A.M., Voon, V., McNeely, H.E., Seminowicz, D., Hamani, C., Schwalb, J.M. & Kennedy, S.H. (2005). Deep brain stimulation for treatment-resistant depression. *Neuron, 45*, 651–660.

Mayer, E., Martory, M.D., Pegna, A.J., Landis, T., Delavelle, J. & Annoni, J.M. (1999). A pure case of Gerstmann syndrome with a subangular lesion. *Brain, 122*(6), 1107–1120.

McCormick, D.A. & Huguenard, J.R. (1992). A model of the electrophysiological properties of thalamocortical relay neurons. *J Neurophysiol, 68*, 1384–1400.

Mcrone, J. (2002). The first word. *Lancet Neurol, 1*(1), p72.

Menon, V., Adleman, N.E., White, C.D., Glover, G.H. &Reiss, A.L. (2001). Error-related brain activation during a Go/NoGo response inhibition task. *Human Brain Mapping, 12*,131–143.

Mesulam, M. & Guela, C. (1988). Nucleus basalis (Ch4) and cortical cholinergic innervation in the human brain: Observations based on the distribution of acetylcholinesterase and choline acetyltransferase. *Journal of Comparative Neurology, 275*(2), 216–240.

Minamimoto, T., Hori, Y. & Kimura, M. (2009). Roles of the thalamic CM-PF complex-basal ganglia circuit in externally driven rebias of action. *Brain Research Bulletin, 78*(2–3), 75–79.

Moran, J.M., Wigg, G.S., Adams, R.B., Janata, P. & Kelly, W.M. (2004). Neural correlates of humour detection and appreciation. *Neuroimage, 21*(3), 1055–1060.

Nagai, M., Hoshide, S. & Kario, K. (2010). The insular cortex and cardiovascular system: a new insight into the brain-heart axis. *Journal of the American Society of Hypertension, 4*(4), 174–182.

Nee, D.E., Kastner, S. & Brown, J.W. (2011). Functional heterogeneity of conflict, error, task-switching, and unexpectedness effects within medial prefrontal cortex. *NeuroImage, 54*(1), 528–40.

Netter, F.H. (1997). *Atlas of Human Anatomy.* 2nd Edition. Havas Medi Media. Canada: Friesens Corporation.

Northoff, G., Heinzel, A., de Greck, M., Bermpohl, F., Dobrowolny, H. & Panksepp, J. (2006). Self-referential processing in our brain—A meta-analysis of imaging studies on the self. *NeuroImage 31*, 440 – 457.

Nusslock, R., Almeida, J.R.C., Forbes, E.E., Versace, A., Frank, E., LaBarbara, E.J., Klein, C.R. & Phillips, M.L. (2012). Waiting to win: elevated striatal and orbitofrontal cortical activity during reward anticipation in euthymic bipolar disorder adults. *Bipolar Disord*er, *14,* 249–260.

Ochsner, K. N. & Gross, J. J. (2005). The cognitive control of emotion. *Trends in Cognitive Sciences*, *9*(5), 242–249.

Ongur, D. (2000). The Organization of Networks within the Orbital and Medial Prefrontal Cortex of Rats, Monkeys and Humans. *Cerebral Cortex, 10*(3), 206–219.

Oppenheimer, S. (2001). Forebrain lateralization and the cardiovascular correlates of epilepsy. *Oxford Journals, Medicine, Brain, 124*(12), 2345–2346.

Oppenheimer, S.M., Gelb, A., Girvin, J.P. & Hachinski, V.C. (1992). Cardiovascular effects of human insular cortex stimulation, *Neurology, 42*, 1727–1732.

Paquette, V., Beauregard, M. & Beaulieu-Prévoste, D. (2009). Effect of a psychoneurotherapy on brain electromagnetic tomography in individuals with major depressive disorder. *Psychiatry Research*: *Neuroimaging, 174*(3), 231–239.

Pascual-Marqui, R.D. (2002). The sLORETA method: Standardized low-resolution brain electromagnetic tomography (sLORETA): technical details. *Methods and Findings in Experimental and Clinical Pharmacology, 24*(Supplement D), 5–12.

Pascual-Marqui, R.D., Esslen, M., Kochi, K. & Lehmann, D. (2002). Functional imaging with low-resolution electromagnetic tomography (LORETA): A review. *Methods and Findings in Experimental and Clinical Pharmacology, 24C*, 91–95.

Pasqual-Marqui, R.D., Michel, C.M. & Lehmann, D. (1994). Low resolution eletromagnetic tomography : a new method for localizing electrical activity in the brain. *International Journal of Psychophysiology, 18*(1), 49–65.

Penfield, W. & Jasper, H. (1954). *Epilepsy and the Functional Anatomy of the Human Brain.* Boston: Little Brown & Co.

Penfield, W. & Perot, P. (1963). The brain's record of auditory and visual experience. A final summary and discussion, *Brain, 86,* 595–696. (also *Brain, 128*(3), 449–450).

Persinger, M.A. & Saroka, K.S. (2012). Protracted parahippocampal activity associated with Sean Harribance, *Int J Yoga, 5*, 140–150.

Petersen, S.E., Fox, P.T., Snyder, A.Z. & Raichle, M.E. (1990). Activation of extrastriate and frontal cortical areas by visual words and word-like stimuli. *Science*, *249*(4972), 1041–1044.

Pfeifer, H., Iacoboni, M., Mazziotta, C. & Dapretto, M. (2005). Mirror neuron system activity in children and its relation to empathy and interpersonal competence. In Abstract Viewer/Itinerary Planner, *Soc Neurosci Abstr, 660*(24).

Pizzagalli, D.A., Iosifescu, D., Hallett, L.A., Ratner, K.G. & Fava, M. (2008). Reduced hedonic capacity in major depressive disorder: Evidence from a probabilistic reward task. *Journal of Psychiatric Research, 43*(1), 76–87.

Pizzagalli, D.A., Nitschke, J.B., Oakes, T.R., Hendrick, A.M., Horras, K.A., Larson, C.L., Abercrombie, H.C., Schaefer, S.M., Koger, J.V., Benca, R.M., Pascual-Marqui, R.D. & Davidson, R.J. (2002). Brain electrical tomography in depression: The importance of symptom severity, anxiety, and melancholic features. *Biological Psychiatry*, *52(*2), 73–85.

Porges, S.W. (2003). Social engagement and attachment: A phylogenetic perspective. *Annals of the New York Academy of Sciences, 1008,* 31–47.

Porges, S.W. (2004). The Vagus: A mediator of behavioral and physiologic features associated with autism. In M. L. Bauman and T. L. Kemper (Eds.), *The Neurobiology of Autism.* (pp. 65 – 78). Baltimore: Johns Hopkins University Press.

Porges, S.W. (2007). The Polyvagal Perspective . *Biological Psychiatry*, *74*, 116 – 143.

Posner, M.I. & Petersen, S.E. (1990). The attention system of the human brain. *Annual Review of Neuroscience, 13,* 25–42.

Prather, A.A., Marsland, A.L., Hall, M., Neumann, S.A., Muldoon, M.F. & Manuck, S.B. (2009). Normative variation in self-reported sleep quality and sleep debt is associated with stimulated pro-inflammatory cytokine production. *Biological Psychology, 82,* 12–17.

Prather, A.A., Rabinovitz, M., Pollock, B.G. & Lotrich, F.E. (2009). Cytokine-induced depression following IFN-α treatment: the role of IL-6 and sleep quality. *Brain, Behavior, and Immunity, 23,* 1109–1116.

Raichle, M.E. (2010). Two views of brain function. *Trends in Cognitive Sciences, 14*(4), 180–90.

Raichle, M.E., MacLeod, A.M., Snyder, A.Z., Powers,W.J., Gusnard, D.A. & Shulman, G.L. (2003). A default mode of brain function, National Academy of Sciences, *Proc Natl Acad Sci USA, 98* (2), 676–682.

Ramachandran, V.S., & Oberman, L.M. (2006). Broken mirrors. *Scientific American, 295*(5), 62–69.

Read, D. (1981). Solving deductive-reasoning problems after unilateral temporal lobectomy. *Brain and Language, 12*:116–127.

Robbins, T.W., & Everitt, B.J. 2009. Limbic-striatal memory systems and drug addiction. *Neurobiol Learn Mem, 78*(3), 625–636

Rosenfeld, J.P. (1997). EEG Biofeedback of frontal alpha asymmetry in affective disorders. *Biofeedback, 25*(1), 8–25.

Rosenfeld, J.P., Baehr, E., Baehr, R., Gotlib, I. & Ranganath, C. (1996). Preliminary evidence that daily changes in frontal alpha asymmetry correlate with changes in affect in therapy sessions. *International Journal of Psychophysiology, 23,* 241–258.

Ross, E.D. (1981). The aprosodias: Functional-anatomic organization of the affective components of language in the right hemisphere. *Archives of Neurology, 38,* 561–569.

Sacks, O. (1985). *The Man Who Mistook His Wife for a Hat.* New York: Summit Books.

Sapolsky, R. (2010). This is your brain on metaphors, *Opinionator, The Stone, The New York Times,* Nov. 14, 2010 (http://opinionator.blogs.nytimes.com/2).

Sara, S.J. & Bouret, S. (2012). Orienting and reorienting: The locus coeruleus mediates cognition through arousal. *Neuron, 76*(1), 130–141.

Sarter, M., Givens, B. & Bruno, J.P. (2001). The cognitive neuroscience of sustained attention: Where top-down meets bottom-up. *Brain Research Reviews, 35,* 146–160.

Seeley, W., Menon, V., Schatzberg, A., Keller, J., Glover, G., Kenna, H., Reiss, A. & Greicius, M. (2007). Dissociable intrinsic connectivity networks for salience processing and executive control. *The Journal of Neuroscience, (27)*9, 2349–2356.

Seger, C.A., Stone, M. & Keenan, J.P. (2004). Cortical activations during judgments about the self and another person. *Neuropsychologia, 42,* 1168–1177.

Shah, S.G., Klumpp, H., Angstadt, M., Nathan, P.J. & Phan, K.L. (2009). Amygdala and insula response to emotional images in patients with generalized anxiety disorder. *J Psychiary Neurosci, 34*(4), 296–302.

Sheline, Y.I., Barch, D.M., Price, J.L., Rundle, M.M., Vaishnavi, S.N., Snyder, A.Z., Mintun, M.A., Wang, S., Coalson, R.S. & Raichlem M.E. (2009). The default mode network and self-referential processes in depression. *Proc Natl Acad Sci USA, 106*(6), 1942–1947.

Smith, C.G. (1962). *Basic Neuroanatomy.* Toronto, Canada: University of Toronto Press.

Smith, Y., Surmeier, D.J., Redgrave, P. & Kimura, M. (2011). Thalamic contributions to basal ganglia-related behavioral switching and reinforcement. *The Journal of Neuroscience : The Official Journal of the Society for Neuroscience, 31*(45), 16102–6.

Sridharan, D., Levitin, J. & Menon, V. (2008). A causal role for the right fronto-insular cortex in switching between executive-control and default-mode networks, *Proceedings of the National Academy of Sciences, 105*(34):12569–12574.

Sterman, M.B. & Wyrwicka, W. (1967). EEG correlates of sleep: Evidence for separate forebrain substrates. *Brain Res. 6,* 143–163.

Sterman M.B. & Thompson, L.M. (2014). Neurofeedback for seizure disorders: Origins, mechanisms, and best practice, Chapter 12 in D. Cantor & J. Evans (Eds.), *Clinical Neurotherapy: Application of Techniques for Treatment.* Kidlington, Oxford, U.K.: Elsevier Ltd.

Supekar, K., Uddin, L.Q., Prater, K., Amin, H,.,Greicius, M.D. & Menon,V. (2010). Development of functional and structural connectivity within the default mode network in young children, *J. Neuroimage 52,* 290–301

Suthana, N., Haneef, Z., Stern, J., Mukamel, R., Behnke, E., Knowlton, B. & Fried, I. (2012). Memory enhancement and deep-brain stimulation of the entorhinal area. *New England Journal of Medicine, 366*(6), 502–510.

Talairach, J. & Tournoux, P. (1988). *Co-Planar Stereotactic Atlas of the Human Brain: 3-Dimensional Proportional System: An Approach to Cerebral Imaging.* Trans. by M. Rayport. New York: Thieme Classics.

Tan, C.O. & Bullock, D. (2008). A dopamine-acetylcholine cascade: Simulating learned and lesion-induced behavior of striatal cholinergic interneurons. *Journal of Neurophysiology, 100*(4), 2409–21.

Tekin, S. & Cummings, J.L. (2002). Frontal-subcortical neuronal circuits and clinical neuropsychiatry: An update. *Journal of Psychosomatic Research, 53*(2), 647–54.

Thatcher, R. (2007). Neuroguide Delux, 2.3.7, Applied Neuroscience Inc. (www.appliedneuroscience.com)

Thatcher, R.W. (2012). *Handbook of Quantitative Electroencephalography and EEG Biofeedback: Scientific Foundations and Practical Applications*. www.appliedneuroscience.com, Self Published, Page 35, 305, In Prepublication Adobe Format supplied by Author.

Thatcher, R.W. (2012). *Handbook of Quantitative Electroencephalography and EEG Biofeedback: Scientific Foundations and Practical Applications*. www.appliedneuroscience.com.

Thayer, J.F., Åhs, F., Fredrikson, M., Sollers III, J.J. & Wager, T.D. (2012). A meta-analysis of heart rate variability and neuroimaging studies: Implications for heart rate variability as a marker of stress and health. *Neuroscience & Biobehavioral Reviews, 36*(2), 747–756.

Thayer, J.F. & Lane, R.D. (2009). Claude Bernard and the heart–brain connection: Further elaboration of a model of neurovisceral integration. *Neurosci Biobehav Rev 33*, 81–88.

Thompson, J. & Hagedorn, D. (2012). Multimodal analysis: New approaches to the concussion conundrum. *Journal of Clinical Sport Psychology, 6*, 22–46.

Thompson, L. & Thompson M. (1998). Neurofeedback combined with training in metacognitive strategies: Effectiveness in students with ADD. *Applied Psychophysiology and Biofeedback, 23*(4), 243–263.

Thompson, L., Thompson, M. & Reid, A. (2010) Neurofeedback outcomes in clients with Asperger's syndrome. *Journal of Applied Psychophysiology and Biofeedback, 35(*1), 63–81.

Thompson, M., Thompson, J. & Wu, W. (2008). *Brodmann Areas (BA) Correlated with 10-20 Sites and their Primary Functions.* San Rafael, Calif.: International Society for Neurofeedback and Research.

Thompson, M. & Thompson, L. (2002). Biofeedback for movement disorders (Dystonia with Parkinson's Disease): Theory and preliminary results. *Journal of Neurotherapy, 6*(4), 51–70.

Thompson, M. & Thompson, L. (2003). *The Neurofeedback Book: An Introduction to Basic Concepts in Applied Psychophysiology*, Wheat Ridge, CO: Association for Applied Psychophysiology. Polish translation 2012.

Thompson, M. & Thompson, L. (2006). Improving attention in adults and children: Differing electroencephalograhy profiles and implications for training. *Biofeedback*, Fall.

Thompson, M. & Thompson, L. (2007). Neurofeedback for stress management. In P. Lehrer, R. Woolfolk & W. Sime (Eds.) *Principles and Practice of Stress Management, 3rd Edition*, 249–287. New York: Guilford Publications.

Thompson, M. & Thompson, L. (2010). Functional neuroanatomy and the rationale for using EEG biofeedback for clients with Asperger's syndrome. *Journal of Applied Psychophysiology and Biofeedback, (35)*1, 39–61.

Thompson, M., Thompson, L., Reid-Chung, A. & Thompson, J. (2013). Managing TBI: Appropriate assessment and a rationale for using neurofeedback and biofeedback to enhance recovery in postconcussion syndrome. *Biofeedback, 41*(4).

Thompson, M., Thompson, L., Thompson, J. & Hagedorn, D. (2011). Networks: A compelling rationale for combining neurofeedback, biofeedback and strategies. *NeuroConnections*, Summer.

Thompson, M.G.G. & Havelkova, M. (1983). Childhood psychosis. In P. Steinhauer & Q. Rae-Grant (Eds.) *Psychological Problems of the Child in the Family*. New York: Basic Books, Inc.

Thompson, M.G.G. & Patterson, P.G.R. (1986). The Thompson- Patterson Scale of Psychosocial Development I: Theoretical Basis. *Canadian Journal of Psychiatry,* 31(5).

Tower of London Test (1982). Colorado Assessment Tests. www.catstests.com/prod03.htm

Tranel, D., Rudrauf, D., Vianna, E.P.M. & Damasio, H. (2008). Does the clock drawing test have focal neuroanatomical correlates? *Neuropsychology, 22*(5), 553–562.

Uecker, A., Barnes, C.A., McNaughton, B.L. & Reiman, E.M. (1997). Hippocampal glycogen metabolism, EEG, and behavior. *Behav Neurosci 111*, 283–291.

Ungerleider, L.G. & Mishkin, M. (1982). Reported in Kim M.S, Robertson L.C. (2001). Implicit representations of space after bilateral parietal lobe damage. *J Cogn Neurosci, 13* (8), 1080–1087.

Vertes, R.P., Hoover, W.B., Szigeti-Buck, K. & Leranth, C. (2007). Nucleus reuniens of the midline thalamus: Link between the medial prefrontal cortex and the hippocampus. *Brain Research Bulletin 71*(6), 601–609.

Wang, J., Rao, H., Wetmore, G.S., Furlan, P.M., Korcyowski, M., Dinges, D.F. & Detre, J.A. (2005). Perfusion functional MRI reveals cerebral blood flow pattern under psychological stress. B.S. McEwen, Ed., *Proc Natl Acad Sci USA, 102*(49), 17804–17809.

Whalen, P.J. (2003). Remembering people: Neuroimaging takes on the real world. *Learning & Memory*, *10*(4), 240–241.

Yang, T.T., Simmons, A.N., Matthews, S.C., Tapert, S.F., Bishoff-Grethe, A., Frank, G.K., Arce, E. & Paulus, M.P. (2007). Increased amygdala activation is related to heart rate during emotion processing in adolescent subjects. *Neurosci Lett, 428*(2–3), 109–114.

Zhou, Y., Dougherty, Jr., J.H., Hubner, K.F., Bai, B., Cannon, R.L. & Hutson, R.K. (2008). Abnormal connectivity in the posterior cingulate and hippocamus in early Alzheimer's disease and mild cognitive impairment. *Alzheimer Dement.*, *4*(4), 265–270.

Zoeller, Jr., R.F. (2007). Physical activity: Depression, anxiety, physical activity, and cardiovascular disease: What is the connection? *American Journal Lifestyle Med, 1*, 175–180.